Molecular Innovations in Cancer

This book offers a comprehensive overview of the latest breakthroughs transforming cancer research and treatment. Integrating insights from molecular biology, pharmacology, microbiomics, and artificial intelligence (AI), this volume highlights how cross-disciplinary innovations are redefining oncology.

The book explores the applications of multi-omics and computational tools, the potential of heterocyclic and bioactive compounds, and the promise of probiotic-based nanomedicine in advancing personalized cancer therapy. It further examines the emerging roles of the gut microbiome, pharmacomicrobiomics, and AI-driven diagnostics in enhancing therapeutic precision and enabling early cancer detection. Addressing a wide spectrum of cancer types from colorectal and breast cancers to gliomas, the book also discusses contemporary challenges such as microplastic exposure, mitochondrial dysfunction, and the importance of evidence-based clinical practices in oncology. Beyond therapeutics, it highlights cutting-edge diagnostic innovations, including AI-assisted screening tools and microbiome-based biomarkers for early colorectal cancer detection. The volume concludes with evidence-based insights into clinical practices, such as blood transfusion protocols in oncology, effectively bridging laboratory research with real-world clinical applications.

With contributions from leading experts across disciplines, this book serves as a valuable reference for oncologists, biomedical researchers, clinicians, and students, offering a forward-looking perspective on how integrated scientific approaches are shaping the future of cancer care.

Molecular Innovations in Cancer

Genomics, Microbiomics Approaches

Edited by
Surajit Pathak and Antara Banerjee

CRC Press
Taylor & Francis Group
Boca Raton London New York

CRC Press is an imprint of the
Taylor & Francis Group, an **informa** business

Designed cover image: Shutterstock

First edition published 2026
by CRC Press
2385 NW Executive Center Drive, Suite 320, Boca Raton FL 33431

and by CRC Press
4 Park Square, Milton Park, Abingdon, Oxon, OX14 4RN

CRC Press is an imprint of Taylor & Francis Group, LLC

ISBN: 9781041082118 (hbk)
ISBN: 9781041082125 (pbk)
ISBN: 9781003644309 (ebk)

DOI: 10.1201/9781003644309

Typeset in Times
by KnowledgeWorks Global Ltd.

Contents

Preface vii
About the Editors ix

Chapter 1 Multi-Omics, Computational Approaches, and AI Tools in Oncotherapeutics: Recent Advances and Perspectives 1

Rohit Yadav, Saumya Shukla, Bhawna Rathi, and Shivani Sharda

Chapter 2 Exploring Small Heterocyclic Compounds as Promising Agents in Cancer Therapy 19

Sandip Paul, Pinki Saha Sardar, and Anjoy Majhi

Chapter 3 Probiotic-Based Nanomedicine: A Next-Generation Strategy for Personalized Cancer Therapy 31

Lakshmi Shanmugam, Prathiba Varadhan, Sree Kathyayani Sundara Raman, Sahana R. K., and Megala Jayaraman

Chapter 4 Pharmacomicrobiomics and AI Designs in GI Tract Cancers 49

Naman Kapoor, Harsh Kashyap, Bhawna Rathi, Shivani Sharda, Pallavi Somvanshi, and Swarna Kanchan Kesheri

Chapter 5 Gut Microbiome: A Novel Screening Tool for Colorectal Cancer 79

Rayvathy Balasubramanian and Sudhasri Ganeshan

Chapter 6 The Intersection of Oncology and Infectious Diseases in Human Health: The Battle between Pathogens 92

Anu Shibi Anilkumar, Sheena Mariam Thomas, and Ramakrishnan Veerabathiran

Chapter 7 Artificial Intelligence-Integrated Precision Oncology of Colorectal Cancer 115

Maduravani Ramasundaram and Thirumurthy Madhavan

Chapter 8 Precision Medicine in Breast Cancer: An Immuno-Oncology Approach 125

Juvin Ann Thomas and Suboj Babykutty

Chapter 9 Harnessing Probiotics for Personalized Cancer Therapy: A Holistic Approach 147

Adheena M, Reshma K V, and Jayamurthy Purushothaman

Chapter 10 Mitochondrial Dysfunction in Gliomas: Pathophysiological Insights and Therapeutic Targets 165

Charles Emmanuel Jebaraj Walter, Tina Sara Biju, Zioni Sangeetha Shankaran, Lawrence D. Cruze, Thanka Johnson, Jezra Emmanuel Walter, and Christhunesa Soundararajan Christudass

Chapter 11 Plastic Pollution and Cancer: The Emerging Role of Microplastics in Oncology 194

Niketha Manoj and Shabina Ashraf

Chapter 12 Bioactive Compounds in Colorectal Cancer Therapy: Emerging Challenges and Future Directions 214

Ashiq Shibili P, Sneha Pallatt, Antara Banerjee, and Surajit Pathak

Chapter 13 Evidence-Based Blood Transfusion Practices 235

R. Raj Bharath

Index 247

Preface

Cancer remains one of the most formidable challenges in modern medicine, demanding not only advances in diagnosis and therapy but also a holistic, multidisciplinary approach to treatment and prevention. Over the past decades, rapid progress in molecular biology, computational sciences, pharmacology, and biotechnology has transformed the oncology landscape, opening new frontiers of hope for patients worldwide. Yet, the complexity of cancer requires continued collaboration across diverse fields to translate innovation into meaningful clinical outcomes. This book, *Molecular Innovations in Cancer: Genomics, Microbiomics Approaches*, brings together contributions from researchers to showcase emerging strategies, technologies, and paradigms in cancer research and therapy. The chapters span a wide spectrum of themes, ranging from the role of multiomics and artificial intelligence in drug discovery and diagnostics, to the potential of probiotics and microbiome-based interventions, precision medicine, and the impact of environmental factors such as microplastics on cancer risk.

The volume highlights the revolutionary convergence of diverse scientific disciplines in modern cancer research and management. It explores topics such as bioactive compounds in personalized therapies, next-generation small heterocyclic agents, and probiotic nanoparticles for targeted treatment. Additionally, it delves into novel fields such as pharmacomicrobiomics and computational oncology, emphasizing how these advancements are shaping therapeutic designs. The gut microbiome is discussed not only as a powerful diagnostic tool but also as a critical element in developing personalized therapies and identifying biomarkers for cancer. Other chapters address important intersections of oncology, such as the relationship between pathogens and cancer, computational approaches to diagnostics, and precision medicine strategies, including immuno-oncology and breast cancer treatment. Complex challenges such as mitochondrial dysfunction in gliomas and the emerging role of microplastics in cancer progression are also examined, with practical examples provided to illustrate their clinical and research relevance.

By integrating perspectives from pharmacology, computational sciences, microbiology, immunology, and clinical oncology, this book underscores the interconnected nature of modern cancer research. Collectively, these multidisciplinary insights present a forward-looking vision of oncology, where the integration of molecular biology, computational technologies, microbiome research, and environmental health paves the way for innovative and personalized cancer care. We envision this volume as a valuable resource for students, researchers, and healthcare professionals seeking to keep pace with the latest advancements in oncology. We hope that the insights presented here will not only inspire innovation but also encourage collaboration and help bridge the gap between laboratory research and clinical practice in the ongoing fight against cancer.

We extend our sincere gratitude to the contributing authors for their scholarly efforts and to the scientific community for its unwavering commitment to advancing the field of oncology.

Prof. Surajit Pathak
Prof. Antara Banerjee
Editors
Chennai, Tamil Nadu, India

About the Editors

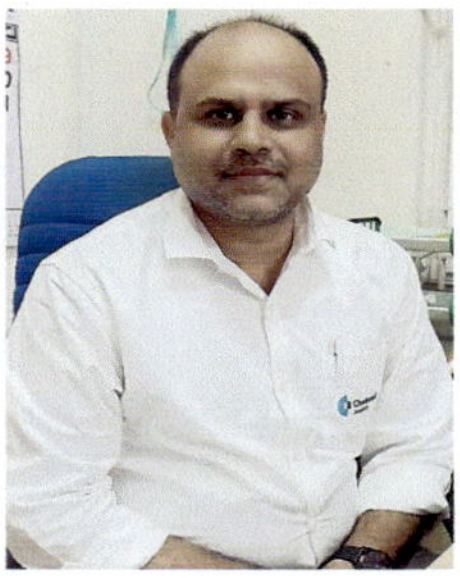

Surajit Pathak, Ph.D., is a leading researcher and academic, currently Professor at Chettinad Academy of Research and Education in Chennai. He has previously held esteemed positions as Principal Research Scientist at Linkoping University, Sweden, with a Ph.D. from India (2007) and an extensive post-doctoral journey at renowned institutions such as the University of Alabama (USA), University of Padova (Italy), and University of Linkoping (Sweden), his research focuses on microRNAs for early colorectal cancer detection. Prof. Pathak has published over 150 research and review articles, earning more than 5000 citations (Google Scholar) and an h-index of 39. Prof. Pathak is a member of national research societies.

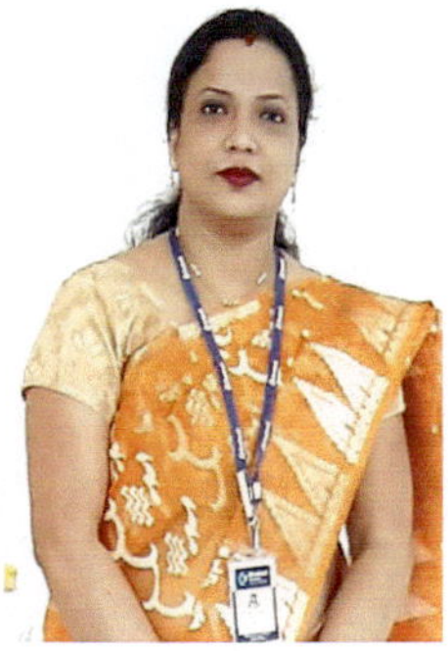

Antara Banerjee, Ph.D., is currently working as Professor at Chettinad Academy of Research and Education (CARE), Chennai. Dr. Banerjee pursued her post-doctoral research on Cancer Biology and Regenerative Medicine at the University of Padova, Italy, and Linkoping University. She has published over 120 articles with an h-index of 34 and 3804 citations (Google Scholar) with two patents awarded and five filed and secured national and international grants. Dr. Banerjee has edited several books on stem cells and cancer. She is affiliated with professional research bodies and is a member of several national research societies.

1 Multi-Omics, Computational Approaches, and AI Tools in Oncotherapeutics

Recent Advances and Perspectives

Rohit Yadav, Saumya Shukla, Bhawna Rathi, and Shivani Sharda
Amity Institute of Biotechnology, Amity University Noida, India

1.1 INTRODUCTION

Oncotherapeutics are medical treatments designed to fight against cancer and to provide effective treatment to patients globally. These medical treatments aim at the target specific sites to destroy or control the growth of cancerous cells and minimize the damage caused to healthy tissue. Oncotherapy is applied according to the types and stage of cancer and condition of patient's immune level and overall health. To diagnose the disease at early stages, various tools and techniques have been introduced. Molecular profiling identifies specific genetic alterations, biomarkers, and expression of protein, which lead to tumor growth—by using tools such as next-generation sequencing (NGS) (Satam et al., 2023).

Bioinformatics and computational approaches have changed the field of oncology, allowing for deep understanding of cancer biology and development of targeted therapeutic agents. They allow researchers to evaluate and interpret large-scale genomic, transcriptomic, proteomic, and other biological information to better understand disease initiation, advancement, and metastasis. Bioinformatics has made an enormous contribution to the field of precision medicine. Researchers are designing personalized therapeutic strategies by identifying the specific genetic mutations responsible for tumorigenesis, thereby enabling targeted interventions that address the underlying molecular drivers of an individual patient's tumor. By tailoring treatments to the individual's specific cancer biology, this approach has the potential to result in more effective therapies with reduced side effects. Bioinformatics tools can also be used to identify potential drug targets and to screen large libraries of molecules for novel therapeutic agents (Adeniji, Dulal, & Martin, 2021). The intricate networks of cancer-relevant genes and proteins can be studied using computational methods as well. Researchers can then characterize these networks and identify pathways that are involved in tumorigenesis and devise ways to stop them. In addition, bioinformatics can also be used to predict cancer progression and discover biomarkers for monitoring disease status and treatment response (Masucci, Karlsson, Blomqvist, & Ernberg, 2024). Additionally, advances in bioinformatics have also led to the rise of liquid biopsies, which provide a less intrusive way to detect and monitor cancer. Researchers can detect genetic changes associated with cancer and monitor the disease's progression by analyzing DNA shed from blood or other bodily fluids. This method has important implications for early detection, treatment-monitoring, and, ultimately, personalized therapies (Jeon et al., 2014).

DOI: 10.1201/9781003644309-1

The integrated approach of bioinformatics, artificial intelligence (AI), multi-omics, computational tools, precision medicines, and NGS techniques has led to improved diagnostics and treatments. The omics-based technology is a compact tool used to identify potential therapeutic targets, such as genes, proteins, or metabolic pathways that are involved in cancer. Omics technologies can also help identify clinical phenotypes, such as tumor types and subtypes, drug responses, and survival outcomes. These omics techniques when used in precision medicine help to predict the patient response to a particular treatment regime (Chakraborty et al., 2024).

Conventional methods often fail in early detection, treatment design, and drug discovery. As one of the most innovative technologies of recent years, AI is revolutionizing cancer treatment. AI is transforming oncology procedures, with its ability to process large amounts of data and find patterns that human specialists might miss. Recent advancements in machine learning and deep neural networks have enabled the development of AI systems and algorithms that can assist in processes from imaging diagnoses to tailoring individualized treatment protocols (Yu, Beam, & Kohane, 2018; Topol, 2019). The goal of this chapter is to summarize the current landscape of AI-related solutions in oncology, describe real-world case studies, limitations, and ethical dilemmas of AI in the clinical space, and finally highlight potential directions in research and application in oncotherapy. By analyzing genetic data and other biomarkers, AI can predict patient-specific responses to treatments, helping doctors choose the most effective treatment with the fewest side effects.

1.2 OMICS-BASED TECHNOLOGIES

Omics-based techniques refer to the large-scale experimental techniques used to study biological systems. It encompasses various disciplines such as genomics, transcriptomics, proteomics, and metabolomics. Bioinformatics plays a crucial role in analyzing the vast datasets generated by these techniques. Omics technologies simultaneously measure biomolecules in a biological sample. These technologies can be used to study complex molecular mechanisms and generate large amounts of data about molecules. An omics-based test that is more accurate can be obtained using standard clinical approaches via classical methods. Omics technologies have revolutionized our understanding of cancer biology by allowing comprehensive analyses at the genomic, epigenomic, transcriptomic, proteomic, and metabolomic levels. Each of these domains contributes unique insights into the molecular underpinnings of cancer (Yang et al., 2020) (**Figure 1.1**).

1.2.1 Genomics

Genomic analyses focus on the DNA sequence and its variations, including single nucleotide variations (SNVs) and copy number variations (CNVs). Microarrays have traditionally been used for genotyping, but NGS has become the standard. NGS involves aligning sequence data to a reference genome and employs various tools for variant discovery and annotation. Regulatory guidelines, such as those from the FDA, outline best practices for the development and validation of NGS-based diagnostics (Kosugi & Terao, 2024).

1.2.2 Epigenomics

Epigenomics studies chemical modifications to DNA and histone proteins, which can regulate gene expression and are critical in cancer. Techniques such as ChIP-Seq analyze protein–DNA interactions, while tools for assessing DNA methylation and chromatin accessibility are essential for understanding gene regulation in cancer. The dynamic nature of the epigenome provides a complementary perspective to genomic data, revealing potential biomarkers and therapeutic targets (Sharma, Sharma, Bansal, & Kumar, 2020).

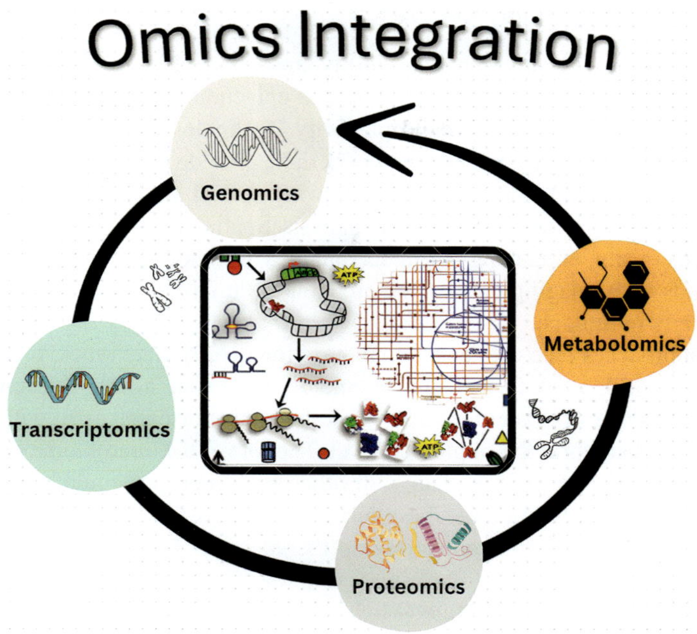

FIGURE 1.1 Integration of omics-based technologies through which genetic potential, gene function, and activity of target sequence can be performed by using genomics, transcriptomics, metabolomics, and proteomics.

1.2.3 Transcriptomics

Transcriptomics measures RNA abundance and gene expression, serving as a biological "barcode" for cellular states. Technologies such as RNA-sequencing and microarrays are employed to analyze gene expression profiles, which can highlight differences in cancer phenotypes. The analysis involves several steps: Data acquisition, quality control, normalization, and differential expression analysis. Tools including DESeq2 and edgeR facilitate the exploration of transcriptomic data, while alignment-free methods such as Kallisto and Salmon are tailored for cancer research to detect fusion transcripts (Sager et al., 2015).

1.2.4 Proteomics

Proteomics identifies and quantifies proteins within biological samples, with mass spectrometry being the predominant technology. Although proteomics has historically lagged behind genomics, it holds promise for discovering cancer biomarkers and therapeutic targets. Analysis workflows involve data acquisition and peptide identification, often utilizing tools available in the Bioconductor ecosystem and the MaxQuant platform (Urbiola-Salvador, Miroszewska, Jabłońska, Qureshi, & Chen, 2022).

1.2.5 Metabolomics and Lipidomics

Metabolomics focuses on metabolic changes in cancer, while lipidomics examines lipid profiles. Both fields rely on mass spectrometry for analysis. Tools such as the metab and lipidr packages assist in data processing and functional analysis, aiming to uncover insights into cancer metabolism and potential therapeutic strategies (Creative Proteomics, 2021; Suri, Kaur, Carbone, & Shinde, 2023).

1.2.6 Single-Cell and Imaging Approaches

Cancer is heterogeneous, with significant variability among individual cells. Single-cell sequencing techniques allow researchers to explore genomic and epigenomic features at the single-cell level, revealing insights into tumor evolution and plasticity. Technologies such as scRNA-seq generate data that, while sparser and more variable than bulk data, provide a detailed view of cellular behavior. Imaging techniques complement omics by allowing spatial analysis of tissues, with tools like CellProfiler facilitating high-throughput image analysis. Spatial transcriptomics (ST) captures gene expression patterns in situ, enhancing our understanding of tumor microenvironments. Combining single-cell methods with imaging enables the creation of "tumor atlases," which map cellular and spatial heterogeneity in tumors.

Multi-omics approaches face challenges in integrating diverse data types, often requiring innovative experimental designs, such as using organoids that better mimic the tumor environment. The immune system's role in cancer response is another active research area, with methods such as CITE-Seq providing insights at the single-cell level. The role of the microbiome in cancer is gaining recognition. Integrating metagenomic data with other omic analyses could unveil critical aspects of cancer pathogenesis and treatment. These technologies provide a multifaceted view of cancer biology, driving advancements in diagnostics and therapeutics. The continuous evolution of these technologies and their integration into holistic frameworks holds the promise of improved patient outcomes through personalized medicine (Micheel, Nass, & Omenn, 2012; de Anda-Jáuregui & Hernández-Lemus, 2020).

1.3 ROLE OF MULTI-OMICS IN ONCOTHERAPEUTICS

Advanced multi-omics techniques in genome screening are whole genome sequencing (WGS) and whole exome sequencing (WES), which have given detailed insights into DNA methylation patterns and gene expression data, which was not possible earlier with classical methods. Single-cell omics technology provides new information about the gene activity and cellular properties at the microscopic level. These advancements in mass spectrometry give accurate detection results of vast numbers of proteins and metabolites by using various proteomics and metabolomics approaches. This new technology has led to a growing efficacy and accuracy in developing data-driven high-throughput computational and mathematical methods for analyzing high-dimensional datasets from various analytical tools. Multi-omics techniques were discovered to integrate diverse omics datasets obtained from cancer patients to develop personalized medicines using precision oncology, which helped in identifying consistent molecular or clinical traits across multiple datasets.

Multi-omics approaches target biological features and patient groups based on various symptoms and biomarkers contributing to the development of cancer therapies and drugs. Multi-omics research creates new avenues for personalized cancer treatment, offering opportunities to determine the correlation between molecular markers and responses to targeted therapies through integrative techniques and extensive multi-omics datasets, enhanced understanding of the molecular traits of tumors, which may facilitate more accurate therapy predictions, potentially improving therapeutic efficacy or overcoming drug resistance (Chakraborty, Sharma, Sricheta Karmakar, & Banerjee, 2024).

1.4 ROLE OF COMPUTATIONAL TOOLS IN ONCOTHERAPEUTICS

In the realm of drug discovery, bioinformatics tools can accelerate the process by simulating the interactions between drug molecules and their targets. Various treatment methods and medications have been developed, including chemotherapy, radiotherapy, and various anti-cancer drugs. Anti-cancer drug discovery started in 1940 and is still emerging and paving the way in the field of oncotherapeutics.

From 1940 to 1950 development of the early cancer drugs took place; in the next decade till 1960, combinatorial chemotherapy was introduced. More recently the technology evolved very drastically. In 1980, NONMEM, a population PK technology, was introduced and was applied to the cancer drug approach in 1990. Till 2010 various developments occurred in computational drug discovery (CDD) methods, and in present times the advancements in technology have risen. Computational discovery of drugs in the field of oncotherapeutics includes various steps such as target identification, use of structure- or ligand-based methods for drug designing, and drug targeting (Hung & Chen, 2014). Some of the drugs introduced using computational biology are Gefitinib, Crizotinib, and Abiraterone (approved by the FDA). This computational modeling can help researchers identify potential drug candidates and optimize their properties, reducing the time and cost associated with traditional drug development (Park, 2019). The various computational techniques included in the field of oncotherapeutics are target identification, visualizing, characterizing, and predicting the interactions between ligand and target. Some of the techniques are discussed in the following sections.

1.4.1 Structure-Based Drug Discovery

This technique depends on the already-specified structural data of the template and target. This method focuses on the interaction between the compound and receptor. This structural information of biological compounds was obtained using various spectroscopic methods such as NMR and X-ray crystallography. The structure-aided approach in drug discovery facilitates strong interactions between ligands and their molecular targets, thereby improving target-specific therapeutic activity and after this technique structure-based pharmacophore (SBP) mapping is also a helpful method. It improves pharmacophore modeling and in lead optimization process. Drugs such as Axitinib and β-lapachone are made using these techniques (Tian, Basu, & Capriotti, 2015).

1.4.1.1 Molecular Docking

This technique is the most acceptable form of computational tools in the CDD techniques. It predicts 3D structures of complexes and ligand-binding interaction. Determination of 3D structure of target and ligand protein is done by cryo-electron microscopy, NMR, X-ray crystallography, etc. Some of the databases such as protein databases (PDB) are used for the analysis of structure, active sites, and characteristics of the biological molecules. Examples of this software are AutoDock Vina Extended (2021), Medusa Dock 2.0 (2019), and CABS-Dock (2019).

1.4.2 Ligand-Based Drug Discovery

This ensures the supramolecular interactions with specific biological targets and triggers or blocks their biological reaction. This is considered the most appropriate method of CDD. If any molecule under observation shows higher compatibility with predicted pharmacophore, the drug is considered effective against the targeted disease. This technique was further used in novel anti-cancer compounds.

1.4.2.1 QSAR Modeling

QSAR stands for quantitative structure–activity relationship modeling. This technique was built to perform virtual screening methods of ligand-based approach to drug discovery. This method is very fast and has a reasonable hit rate with high-throughput efficiency. Some oncotherapeutic drugs made through QSAR modeling target and inhibit isopropyl benzoylhydrazone, withanolide analogs, etc. (Iwaloye et al., 2023) (**Figure 1.2**).

1.5 ROLE OF ARTIFICIAL INTELLIGENCE IN ONCOTHERAPEUTICS

AI refers to the intelligence demonstrated by machines, developed by humans. It is an interdisciplinary field that encompasses computer science, cybernetics, neurophysiology, psychology, and

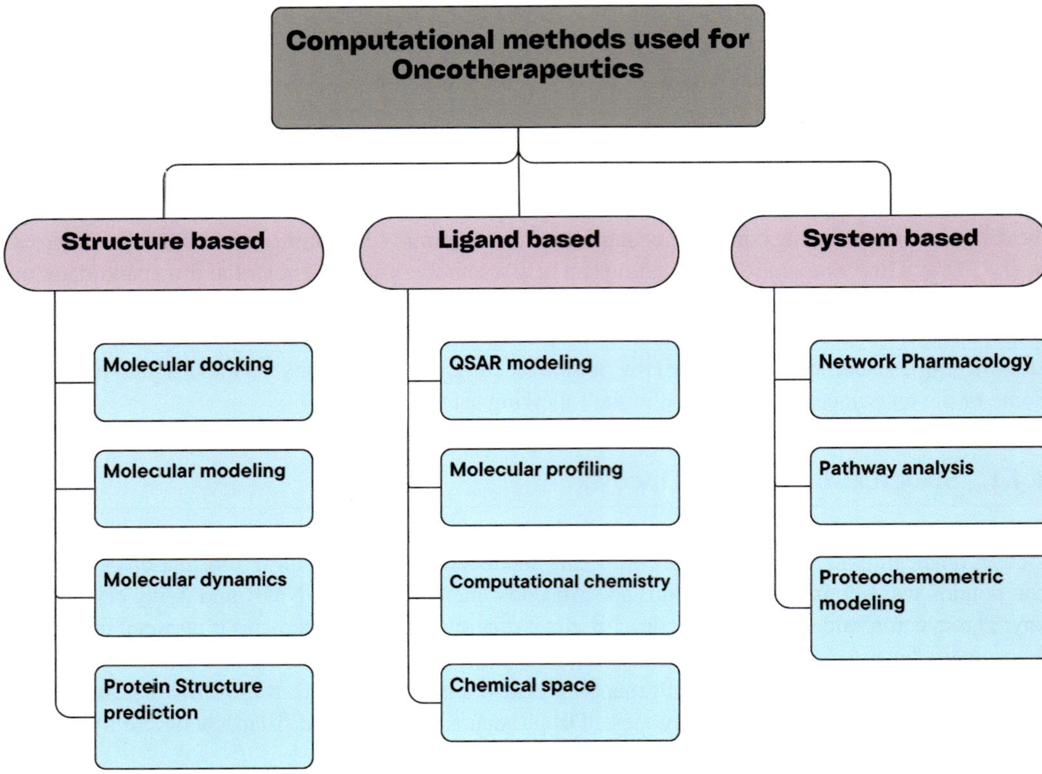

FIGURE 1.2 Different approaches of computational methods used in oncotherapeutics, including structure, ligand, and system-based approaches.

linguistics. AI as a concept is widely considered to have originated at the Dartmouth Conference in 1956. Over the decades, its definition has broadened to include various technologies, such as artificial neural networks, machine learning, and deep learning. Deep learning, a crucial subset of AI, enables machines to analyze vast amounts of data and autonomously extract meaningful patterns. Notably, it can identify details in images that may be imperceptible to the human eye, making it especially valuable in the early detection of tumors from medical imaging. Beyond diagnosis, AI plays an increasingly important role in cancer treatment by leveraging its multi-layered neural network structures. These systems possess advanced reasoning and learning capabilities, allowing AI to mimic human thought processes. Much like the human brain, AI can rapidly assess situations and provide precise, data-driven insights to solve complex problems. Given these strengths, AI has the potential to transform and enhance existing cancer research methodologies (Liang, Fan, Luo, & Zhu, 2020).

AI is playing a significant role in predicting the effectiveness of anti-cancer drugs and supporting drug development. Since different types of cancer—and even the same cancer treated with identical drugs—can respond in varying ways, high-throughput screening data are essential in uncovering links between cancer cell genetics and drug activity. The researchers created a predictive model using random forest algorithms, integrating screening data with machine learning techniques. Their model assesses how anti-cancer drugs interact with cancer cells based on their genetic mutations and developed a drug sensitivity prediction model using elastic net regression, a machine learning approach. These models have successfully predicted drug responses in patients with ovarian, gastric, and endometrial cancers. After this approach the patients were identified as drug-resistant by the AI models—such as ovarian cancer patients treated with tamoxifen, gastric cancer patients receiving 5-FU, and endometrial cancer patients on paclitaxel—and were later confirmed to have

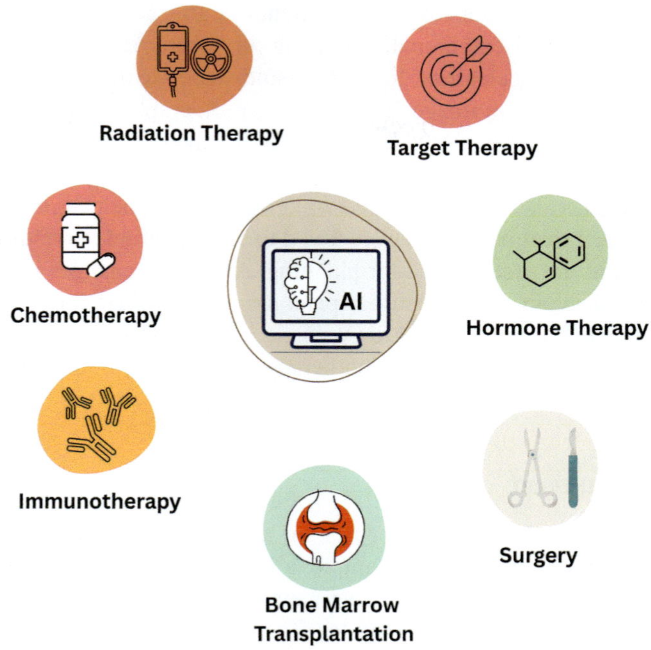

FIGURE 1.3 Various fields of oncotherapeutics where AI has been implemented for the treatment.

poor prognoses (Wang et al., 2023). This ability to rapidly process and interpret complex biological data underscores AI's transformative potential in oncology (**Figure 1.3**).

1.5.1 AI in Chemotherapy

One central focus of AI in this field is to decipher drug–patient interactions specifically in the context of cancer chemotherapy. Its primary utilization has been in controlling chemotherapy drug utilization, predicting the tolerance of patients to these drugs, and optimizing chemotherapy treatment plans. AI is instrumental in optimizing combination therapies, streamlining, and expediting the process. For instance, researchers have turned to "CURATE. AI," the AI platform powered by the National University of Singapore, which employs deep learning and other technologies to determine the best dose of ZEN-3694 and enzalutamide. This method improved the effectiveness and tolerance of the combined therapy. PARP inhibitors are used for treating HRD breast cancer. Researchers designed a deep learning-based HR defect screening system that can detect HR defects in cancer cells with an accuracy rate of 74%, potentially identifying which patients would benefit the most from taking PARP inhibitors. A sympatric machine learning algorithm was developed to predict breast cancer patients' sensitivity to chemotherapy. That study, which examined how chemotherapy and patients' genes interact, was able to distinguish the effects of two chemotherapy drugs, taxol and gemcitabine. Drug sensitivity prediction, drug resistance analysis, optimizing drug combinations and dosages, image-based tumor monitoring, virtual clinical trials, and drug discovery are the steps followed in the study of chemotherapy by using AI tools (Liang, Fan, Luo, & Zhu, 2020; Rasool, Mohammed, Hallit, Malaeb, & Hosseini, 2025).

1.5.2 AI in Radiotherapy

In the field of cancer radiotherapy, AI technology has more specific applications, helping radiologists in tasks such as mapping target areas or automatically planning radiation treatment regimens.

Scientists used a three-dimensional (3D) convolutional neural network (3D CNN) to automatically delineate nasopharyngeal carcinoma, achieving an accuracy of 79%, which is comparable to the results of radiotherapy specialists. In another study, deep learning has been combined with radiomics (a method that extracts image features from radiographic scans) to create a predictive model for evaluating the response of bladder cancer to treatment. A deep learning–based automation software that drastically reduced the time required to plan radiation therapy, completing the task in just a few hours, has also been developed which has majorly helped in the field of oncotherapeutics. The AI-generated treatment plans were found to be comparable to traditional ones, but with a significant reduction in the time needed for planning. AI detects changes in daily imaging scans and recommends modifications to the treatment plan. RayStation (RaySearch), Eclipse AI (Varian), MIM Maestro, Ethos AI (Varian), HyperArc (Varian), AlignRT (Vision RT), and Calypso System (Varian) are some of the AI tools used in radiotherapy (Liang, Fan, Luo, & Zhu, 2020); (Siddique & Chow, 2020).

1.5.3 AI in Immunotherapy

In cancer immunotherapy, AI primarily focuses on assessing treatment outcomes and assisting doctors in adjusting treatment plans. For example, a team of scientists developed an AI platform powered by machine learning to predict the therapeutic effects of programmed cell death protein 1 (PD-1) inhibitors (Tempus AI, IBM Watson for Oncology, BioXcel AI). This platform provides accurate evaluations of immunotherapy effectiveness for patients with advanced solid tumors who respond to PD-1 inhibitors (Atomwise, Insilico Medicine, and BenevolentAI). Additionally, work has also been conducted on a machine learning approach that utilizes a human leukocyte antigen (HLA) mass spectrometry database, improving the identification of cancer neoantigens and enhancing the overall effectiveness of cancer immunotherapy (QinLab Radiomics, ImmunoMap, ArteraA) (Liang, Fan, Luo, & Zhu, 2020; Xu et al., 2021).

1.6 ONCOTHERAPEUTIC DRUG DISCOVERY USING OMICS, COMPUTATIONAL BIOLOGY, AND AI-BASED TOOLS

1.6.1 Omics Tools-Based Drugs

1.6.1.1 Imatinib (Gleevec)

It is a drug used in targeted, personalized cancer therapy, and its development involves genomics and proteomics tools and techniques. Imatinib targets the BCR-ABL tyrosine kinase protein for chronic myeloid leukemia (CML) progression and it helps in targeted chemotherapy. It is a revolutionized therapy that can be applied in the treatment of CML and gastrointestinal stromal tumors (GISTs). It specifically inhibits the BCR-ABL tyrosine kinase enzyme, which is a product of a genetic mutation in CML. This targeted approach in the field of oncotherapeutics has significantly improved outcomes and survival rates for patients with these conditions.

In a case study reported where patients were diagnosed with CML, the Philadelphia chromosome, a genetic abnormality associated with CML, was first identified through karyotyping, a technique that visualizes chromosomes under a microscope as well as a technique called cytogenetic analysis. This chromosome is the result of a translocation between chromosomes 9 and 22. The researchers performed gene expression profiling by using quantitative PCR (qPCR) to determine the expression levels of BCR-ABL fusion gene in CML patients. Functional genomics approaches, including RNA interference (RNAi), were used to confirm the involvement of the BCR-ABL fusion protein in CML. As BCR-ABL has been shown to contribute to the development and proliferation of cancer cells, the ability to silence that gene allows the researcher to focus on the impact of cancer cell proliferation itself, allowing for very precise therapeutic target identification.

Techniques (e.g., mass spectrometry) from proteomics were applied in the characterization and identification of the BCR-ABL fusion protein. This in turn enabled researchers to understand its structure and function and how it interacts with other proteins in the cell. Several techniques including the Western blotting were used to detect and quantify the BCR-ABL protein in CML patient samples, confirming its overexpression and role in the disease. To validate BCR-ABL as a target, protein kinase assays were conducted to evaluate BCR-ABL tyrosine kinase activity. Using the BCR-ABL protein in the biochemical assays, they showed that BCR-ABL protein was constitutively active, and the oncogenic protein had potential as a drug target. The BCR-ABL protein was screened for activity using small molecules, in vitro binding studies drug-screening, and using proteomics techniques. This involved developing high-throughput screening assays to discover Imatinib as a highly effective BCR-ABL tyrosine kinase inhibitor.

Oncotherapeutic drug observations, in vitro testing, and theoretical-based considerations have led to the conclusions that have allowed Imatinib to thrive. Based on the BCR-ABL protein structure presented from proteomics studies, chemists implemented structure-based drug design to generate Imatinib. The drug–Gleevec–specifically binds to the ATP-binding site of the BCR-ABL tyrosine kinase and inhibits its activity. Imatinib had been evaluated in both preclinical models and clinical trial settings. Understanding the genomics and proteomics of CML meant that we had a decent chance of knowing the right molecular pathways to hit with drugs (a standard that, fortunately, worked, and Imatinib passed through the approvals hurdles and is now used to treat CML). The foundation for CML therapy was genomics, which revealed the genetic abnormalities in the causative driver of CML, while proteomics identified and confirmed the fusion protein as a drug target. These techniques were integral together in the development of Imatinib as a targeted treatment for CML. Imatinib is a small molecule kinase inhibitor which was the first targeted therapy approved for cancer treatment and has been a major advancement in the treatment of chronic myeloid leukemia, with increased effectiveness and decreased toxicity compared with traditional chemotherapy. Its success is reflected in the dramatically improved prognosis for CML patients, a generation of whom now achieve long-term remission (National Cancer Institute, 2018).

1.6.1.2 Trastuzumab

The development of Trastuzumab (Herceptin), a targeted therapy for HER2-positive breast cancer, involves various omics techniques. Trastuzumab is a monoclonal antibody that targets the HER2 protein, which is overexpressed in breast cancers and other tumors. By binding to HER2, Trastuzumab helps inhibit tumor growth and promotes immune system attack on cancer cells.

Many tools and techniques have been involved in making this medication a successful anticancer drug, including the identification of HER2 gene (also known as *ERBB2*); amplifications were done by using karyotyping to detect chromosomal abnormalities associated with breast cancer. Researchers discovered that the breast cancer patient had an abnormality on chromosome 17, which led to the amplification of the HER2 gene. So, the techniques such as fluorescence in situ hybridization (FISH) were carried out to visualize and quantify HER2 gene amplification directly in tumor tissue samples. Sequencing helps in understanding the genetic context of HER2 overexpression and any associated mutations; this helps in early stage diagnosis of breast cancer. Functional genomics approaches, such as RNA interference (RNAi), have been used to study the effects of HER2 knockdown on cancer cell proliferation and survival.

Proteomics techniques, such as mass spectrometry, were used to identify the characteristics of HER2 protein, including its structure and function. This helped confirm that HER2 is a receptor for tyrosine kinase involved in cell signaling pathways that promote tumor growth. Western blotting was employed to detect and quantify HER2 protein levels in breast cancer tissue samples. This technique validated the overexpression of HER2 in certain tumors and helped establish its role in the disease. Immunohistochemistry (IHC) was used to visualize HER2 protein expression in tissue samples. Proteomics techniques like in vitro binding assays helped in screening and identifying monoclonal antibodies that could specifically bind to HER2. These assays were crucial for developing Trastuzumab, which was designed to target the extracellular domain of the HER2 protein (Bradley et al., 2021).

Genetic engineering forms the basis of the design and testing process, which in this case involved the creation of monoclonal antibodies, as well as preclinical trials. Drawing on findings from proteomics studies, scientists were able to develop Trastuzumab, a monoclonal antibody with specificity for the HER2 receptor. It is a humanized monoclonal antibody that targets the HER2 extracellular domain, preventing HER2 activation and subsequent signaling cascades that underlie tumor proliferation. It was evaluated in preclinical models and clinical trials to assess the potential activity of Trastuzumab on HER2-positive breast cancer. Genomic and proteomic data ensured the therapy was targeting the right molecular pathway. The genomics enabled the understanding of the HER2 gene amplification and its role in breast cancer, while proteomics characterized the HER2 protein and validated it as a therapeutic target. These approaches combined enabled the discovery of Herceptin, targeted therapy that has dramatically changed the outcome for patients with the HER2-positive subtype of breast cancer. Trastuzumab has greatly improved prognosis in patients with HER2-positive breast cancer. This has resulted in increased rates of remission and survival, and its success has also spurred the development of other HER2-targeted treatments.

1.6.1.3 Olaparib (Lynparza)

It is a groundbreaking drug used in mutated breast cancer therapy, particularly for tumors with BRCA1 or BRCA2 mutations. Its development involved omics-based techniques that helped identify its mechanism of action and optimize its therapeutic potential. The concept of synthetic lethality was central to Olaparib's development. In BRCA1/2-deficient cancer cells, which already have compromised DNA repair pathways, inhibiting PARP (Poly ADP-Ribose Polymerase) further exacerbates DNA damage, leading to cell death.

Mutations in both genes were identified by genetic sequencing tools such as whole-genome sequencing (WGS) and whole-exome sequencing (WES). These genes are essential for homologous recombination-based DNA repair. Note that mutations in these genes result in defective DNA repair mechanisms, a feature associated with certain forms of cancer—including breast and ovarian cancers. Functional genomics approaches such as RNAi are used to study the effects of BRCA1 and BRCA2 gene silencing in cancer cells. This model showed that loss of BRCA function resulted in PARP sensitivity, providing a rationale for the use of PARP inhibitors in cancers with these mutations. Genomic Testing: Comprehensive genomic profiling (CGP) of tumors can identify BRCA mutations and other genomic alterations that may affect sensitivity to Olaparib. Tumor genomic profiling is pivotal to customize treatment and ensure appropriate use of the drug (Tutt, 2021).

Mass spectrometry and other proteomics approaches led to the identification and characterization of the PARP (poly ADP-ribose polymerase) family of proteins. PARP enzymes are involved in repairing single-strand DNA breaks. Knowledge of their structure and function was important for the design of drugs that target these proteins, and Western blotting was used to identify and quantify PARP proteins and their post-translational modifications. It provided the understanding of mechanism of action between PARP and DNA—specifically how PARP binds and which repair processes are involved—, and it suggested overall detailed characterization of cells known as PARP proteins. Olaparib's specific inhibition of PARP enzymes was validated by binding assays using proteomics techniques. These studies showed that Olaparib binds to the PARP enzyme and inhibits it from repairing DNA, resulting in the accumulation of DNA damage in cancer cells carrying BRCA mutations (Orsini, Diquigiovanni, & Bonora, 2023).

It used genomic profiling of patient's tumors to select individuals whose tumors had BRCA mutations and were most likely to benefit from treatment with Olaparib. Efficacy data from clinical trials in these patients resulted in its approval. The genetic basis of cancer-associated BRCA mutations was elucidated by genomics, and by proteomics the action of PARP proteins was explored, leading to their validation as drug targets. These methods combined allowed for the development of Olaparib as a potent treatment option for BRCA-deficient cancers. Despite this, Olaparib has proved

TABLE 1.1
Omics-Based Tools Used in the Discovery of Imatinib, Trastuzumab, and Olaparib

S. No.	Medicine	Omics-Based Tools Used	Function
1	Imatinib (Gleevec)	*Genomics*: Karyotyping, qPCR, RNA interference (RNAi) for BCR-ABL gene expression and validation. *Proteomics*: Mass spectrometry, Western blotting, protein kinase assays, in vitro binding studies for drug screening.	Targets BCR-ABL tyrosine kinase, inhibiting its activity in chronic myeloid leukemia (CML) and gastrointestinal stromal tumors (GISTs).
2	Trastuzumab (Herceptin)	*Genomics*: Karyotyping, fluorescence in situ hybridization (FISH), RNA interference (RNAi) for HER2 gene analysis. *Proteomics*: Mass spectrometry, Western blotting, immunohistochemistry (IHC), in vitro binding assays for monoclonal antibody screening.	A monoclonal antibody that binds to the HER2 receptor, inhibiting tumor growth in HER2-positive breast cancer.
3	Olaparib (Lynparza)	*Genomics*: Whole-genome sequencing (WGS), whole-exome sequencing (WES), RNA interference (RNAi) for BRCA gene mutations. *Proteomics*: Mass spectrometry, Western blotting, protein binding assays for PARP protein analysis.	A PARP inhibitor that induces synthetic lethality in BRCA1/2-mutated cancers (e.g., breast and ovarian cancer).

particularly successful in treating ovarian cancer and has demonstrated efficacy in additional malignancies with the presence of BRCA mutations. It has offered longer progression-free survival for these patients, and it is a major advance in personalized medicine. These factors have led to the successful development of Olaparib (Orsini, Diquigiovanni, & Bonora, 2023) (**Table 1.1**).

1.6.2 Computational Tools-Based Drugs

1.6.2.1 Crizotinib

This drug is a successful example of applying structure-based design techniques. Crizotinib has been acknowledged as a selective and potent cMet/ALK dual inhibitor, which was approved by the FDA in 2011. c-Met is also known as HGFR (hepatocyte growth factor receptor), and its corresponding natural ligand HGF (hepatocyte growth factor) plays a critical role in different cell activities. An abnormal overexpression of c-Met protein has been often detected in human cancers (including SCLC and non-small cell lung cancer (NSCLC)), and abnormal function of c-Met signaling was observed in various solid and blood tumor cancers. Thus, c-MET is an effective and promising oncology target to treat cancer. Molecular docking was used to predict how Crizotinib binds to the ALK protein where molecular docking simulations involve placing Crizotinib into the 3D model of the ALK protein's binding site (Boulos et al., 2021). Algorithms calculate the best orientation and position of the drug within the active site of the protein, predicting the strength and nature of the interaction. Computational biology software such as AutoDock, Glide, and DOCK are commonly used for this purpose. The outcomes of these techniques allowed us to identify the possible binding modes and provide estimates of the binding affinity which are critical for selecting promising drug candidates.

Crizotinib was designed using structure-based drug design methods based on the 3D structure of ALK. Using structural data collected from techniques such as X-ray crystallography or cryo-electron microscopy, scientists model the way that different chemical compounds interact with the ALK protein. Based on structure, we can even modify the antibody to increase the relative affinity or specificity. Automatic structure generation and correction were performed using programs such as Schrödinger's Maestro, MOE (Molecular Operating Environment), and Coot for these tasks. It yields optimized drug candidates that dock tightly in the protein's active site.

The potential drug-like compounds were identified by virtual screening from large libraries. It showed that thousands of compounds can be run through a computer-based screening process to predict which are more likely to bind successfully to ALK. It employs scoring functions to assess the potential for each compound. Types of ligands docking screenings, which are performed through tools such as PyRx, LigandFit, and AutoDock Vina, narrow your search to the most promising candidates and streamline the drug discovery process by narrowing the varieties of candidates that laboratory experiments are performed on. Dynamic stability of Crizotinib–ALK complex was observed through molecular dynamics (MD) simulations. MD simulations include the running of computer simulations to see how Crizotinib and the ALK protein interact following a span of time. These simulations help model the movement of atoms and molecules to gain insight into the stability and conformational changes seen in the drug–protein complex. MD simulations use software packages such as GROMACS, AMBER, and NAMD to describe the plasticity of the binding site and how Crizotinib binding could be influenced by protein conformational changes.

QSAR Modeling Data Set: This technique is used to fully understand and predict the relationship between chemical structure and biological activity. QSAR model: It correlates data obtained from previous experiments pertaining to chemical features of drug candidates and their biological activity. QSAR analysis is typically performed using software such as Dragon, QSAR Plus, and ChemOffice. It gives clues to the chemical modifications that would enhance the efficacy and selectivity for Crizotinib. HLP: Binding Affinity Prediction: The HLP predicts the strength of Crizotinib binding to ALK. Computational methods measure the binding affinity of Crizotinib through the free energy of binding; these techniques include scoring functions and free energy perturbation methods. This meaningful interaction between receptors induces immense pressure that helps to determine the evolution of small molecules docking in the receptors as the primary database of many programs such as GOLD, Smina, and PMV (Python Molecular View) which helps to predict binding affinity. It provides an estimate of how well Crizotinib binds to its target, aiding in the evaluation of its potential effectiveness (Cui et al., 2020; Iwaloye et al., 2023).

1.6.2.2 Axitinib

This orally active compound is derived from a lead agent that was found through computational biology methods that focused on the renal cell carcinoma (RCC) disease area and has been used to treat patients with advanced RCC. These techniques played a critical role in identifying and optimizing the drug's efficacy, selectivity, and safety profile. Based on the detailed 3D structure of the vascular endothelial growth factor receptors (EGFRs) (VEGFRs), structure-based drug design optimizes Axitinib. It enables the fine-tuning of the chemical structures to promote binding and selectivity. Instructions on the use of programs, such as Maestro from Schrödinger and Molecular Operating Environment, are common. This ultimately resulted in the creation of Axitinib, a more tailored compound with enhanced interactions and better selectivity for VEGFRs. The method of virtual screening happens to computationally check a large array of compounds to discover those able to bind to VEGFRs effectively. PyRx, LigandFit, and AutoDock Vina are some examples of software for virtual screening. It reduces the list of compounds to those that are most likely to work, expediting the drug discovery process. QSAR modeling was performed to understand the connection between the chemical structure of Axitinib and its biological activity. SAR or QSAR modeling defines a relationship between the biological activity of drug candidates and their chemical properties or structures. Statistical and computational methods predict how changes to the chemical structure could influence the drug's efficacy and safety. Most common software are Dragon, QSAR Plus, and ChemOffice for the QSAR analysis (Leelananda & Lindert, 2016; Cui et al., 2020).

The binding of Axitinib to its target proteins, specifically VEGFRs, was predicted by molecular docking. This includes inserting Axitinib inside the 3D structure of VEGFRs and calculating how tightly this drug can attach to the active site of the receptor. Just to note, docking scores are used to refine binding affinity and potential interaction of Axitinib and VEGFR. This has been done by simulating binding between compounds and targets using computational biology software such as AutoDock, Glide, and DOCK. It offers the binding mode and affinity of the drug, which are important for both the respective mechanism of action and to tailor the drug. MD simulations accurately model atom and molecule motion in the Axitinib–VEGFR complex. These simulations show how the drug binds to the receptor in physiological conditions, including conformational changes that might influence binding. MD simulations are run using GROMACS, AMBER, NAMD, and so on. Enlightening the stability/rigidity of drug–receptor complex required for thin therapeutic action, aiding in drug engineering. Binding affinity prediction model estimates the strength of binding of Axitinib to each of the VEGFRs. Axitinib is a small molecule, and computational methods are used to predict the affinity on the basis of the free energy of binding. One such evaluation is how well the drug binds to the target receptor. Binding affinity estimation is done by programs such as GOLD, Smina, and PMV (Python Molecular View). It helps assess the potential effectiveness of Axitinib and guide the optimization of its chemical structure (Cui et al., 2020).

1.6.2.3 Gefitinib

Genetic algorithms were utilized in the development of the oral-targeted therapy Gefitinib for NSCLC. These include the specific computational methods employed in the development of Gefitinib.

Molecular docking predicts the binding pattern of drug to EGFR. The attachment of Gefitinib within the 3D model of the EGFR tyrosine kinase domain occurs through molecular docking simulations (56). We aim to analyze how tightly Gefitinib binds onto the active site of EGFR and to predict their affinity and bond. Some of the frequently used software of this type are AutoDock, Glide, and DOCK. Details binding interactions, necessary to interpret the inhibition of EGFR activity by Gefitinib.

Structure-based drug design helps in designing of Gefitinib on the basis of 3D structure of EGFR protein. Researchers model how different chemical structures interact with EGFR using detailed structural information obtained by techniques such as X-ray crystallography. Drug designs are optimized and refined by software such as Schrödinger's Maestro and Molecular Operating Environment. So, you end up with a drug that is selected for EGFR specifically, which improves the therapeutic efficacy. It uses large chemical libraries to find potential drug candidates or drug-like compounds against a specific target through virtual screening. This process employs programs such as PyRx, LigandFit, and AutoDock Vina. It aide in choosing the most promising candidates for continued experimental validation. The relationship between chemical structure of Gefitinib and its biological activity is studied using QSAR modeling. CQSAR (Chem Quant Struct Act Rel): This relates chemical characteristics of Gefitinib and related drugs to their biological activities. This analysis allows for predictions of how modifications to chemical structure may influence activity and selectivity. This analysis is done using QSAR tools such as Dragon, QSAR Plus, and ChemOffice. It shares updates on data leading to the designer of a chemically optimized Gefitinib, with a focus on improving its efficacy and reducing side effects.

MD simulations aid in studying the dynamic interactions of Gefitinib with EGFR over time. MD simulations allow you to simulate the interaction of Gefitinib with EGFR at physiological conditions. The simulation show how the drug and receptor move, and how binding might change over time. MD simulations software such as GROMACS, AMBER, and NAMD provide insights into the stability and flexibility of the Gefitinib–EGFR complex, which may help in optimizing the drug. The prediction power is binding affinity prediction, which predicts how well Gefitinib binds and interacts with EGFR. The free energy of binding is calculated to predict binding affinity of Gefitinib to EGFR using these methods. This means looking at how strongly the drug binds to the receptor. Affinity prediction by GOLD, Smina, and PMV (Python Molecular View) methods aids in assessing the potential efficacy of Gefitinib and leads to further fine-tuning. These computational biology techniques were crucial in the development of Gefitinib, allowing for the design and optimization of

TABLE 1.2
Computational Tools Used in the Discovery of Crizotinib, Axitinib, and Gefitinib

S. No.	Medicine	Computational Tools Used	Function
1	Crizotinib	Molecular docking (AutoDock, Glide, DOCK)	Predicts binding to ALK protein
		Virtual screening (PyRx, LigandFit, AutoDock Vina)	Identifies potential drug-like compounds
		Molecular dynamics (GROMACS, AMBER, NAMD)	Analyzes stability of drug–protein interaction
		QSAR modeling (Dragon, QSAR Plus, ChemOffice)	Predicts structure–activity relationship
2	Axitinib	Structure-based drug design (Schrödinger's Maestro, MOE)	Optimizes interaction with VEGFRs
		Virtual screening (PyRx, LigandFit, AutoDock Vina)	Screens potential VEGFR inhibitors
		QSAR modeling (Dragon, QSAR Plus, ChemOffice)	Correlates chemical structure with activity
		Molecular docking (AutoDock, Glide, DOCK)	Predicts Axitinib binding to VEGFRs
3	Gefitinib	Molecular docking (AutoDock, Glide, DOCK)	Predicts binding to EGFR
		Structure-based drug design (Schrödinger's Maestro, MOE)	Designs drug based on EGFR structure
		QSAR modeling (Dragon, QSAR Plus, ChemOffice)	Analyzes structure–activity relationships
		Binding affinity prediction (GOLD, Smina, PMV)	Estimates drug binding strength to EGFR

a targeted therapy that specifically inhibits EGFR, thus improving treatment outcomes for patients with NSCLC (Cui et al., 2020; Mao, Lin, Zhang, & Zhou, 2021) (**Table 1.2**).

1.6.3 AI Tools-Based Drugs

1.6.3.1 AI-Designed Cancer Drug: "DSP-1181"

DSP-1181 is a novel drug developed for the treatment of psychotic disorders, but it has shown potential for oncological applications as well. Atomwise, an AI platform that uses deep learning algorithms, was used to predict and discover potential drug candidates by analyzing the interaction of small molecules with target proteins in cancer cells.

AI tool used to design this drug was Atomwise (AI platform) which uses deep learning models to predict how molecules will behave in the body and whether they will interact with certain cancer-related proteins. The AI identified DSP-1181 as a promising candidate for various cancers due to its ability to bind effectively with the target receptors involved in tumor progression. DSP-1181 is currently in clinical trials for various indications, including cancer. The drug was among the first to be discovered using AI and is an example of how AI can accelerate drug development in oncology (Farghali, Kutinová Canová, & Arora, 2021).

1.6.3.2 AI-Driven Drug Repurposing: "Ibrutinib"

It is a drug originally developed for chronic lymphocytic leukemia (CLL); it is now used in the treatment of several cancers, including mantle cell lymphoma and Waldenström's macroglobulinemia. Although the discovery of Ibrutinib predates many AI tools, the concept of drug repurposing using AI was instrumental in identifying Ibrutinib (Imbruvica) as an effective therapy for CLL and other cancers.

AI tool used for making Ibrutinib was BenevolentAI which utilized its platform to analyze various datasets of cancer genomics and biological pathways. The AI system identified that Ibrutinib

TABLE 1.3
AI Tools Used in the Discovery of DSP-1181, Ibrutinib, and BMS-986205

S. No.	Medicine	AI Tool Used	Function
1	DSP-1181	Atomwise (AI platform)	Uses deep learning to predict molecular interactions and identify drug candidates for cancer.
2	Ibrutinib	BenevolentAI	AI-driven drug repurposing identified Ibrutinib as an effective therapy for multiple cancers by targeting BTK enzyme.
3	BMS-986205	Insilico Medicine	AI-driven drug discovery optimized molecular design for targeting the CCR2 receptor in immune cells for cancer treatment.

could block a key enzyme called Bruton's tyrosine kinase (BTK), which plays a role in tumor growth and immune cell signaling. This repurposing led to the FDA approval of Ibrutinib for several cancers. Ibrutinib is approved and widely used for several types of blood cancers, and AI techniques continue to identify similar repurposing opportunities for other existing drugs (Brown et al., 2023).

1.6.3.3 AI for Targeted Therapy: "BMS-986205"

It is an immune checkpoint inhibitor drug. Insilico Medicine is using AI-driven drug discovery tools to create novel targeted therapies, one of which is BMS-986205, a drug that targets the CCR2 receptor in immune cells. The drug is part of a class of immune checkpoint inhibitors and has been shown to modulate immune responses in tumors. AI tools used in Insilico Medicine's deep learning tools were used to identify potential druggable targets and predict how small molecules would interact with the CCR2 receptor. The AI system also optimized the chemical structure of candidate molecules to enhance their potency and selectivity. BMS-986205 is currently undergoing clinical trials for various cancers, including solid tumors (Atene et al., 2023) (**Table 1.3**).

1.7 FUTURE RESEARCH DIRECTIONS AND OPPORTUNITIES

The fight against cancer is being transformed by the integration of omics-based approaches, computational tools, and AI, offering new hope for precision medicine, early detection, and innovative treatments. By combining genomics, transcriptomics, proteomics, and metabolomics, scientists are gaining a more detailed understanding of tumor behavior and are uncovering new biomarkers that can help predict how a patient will respond to treatment. AI plays a crucial role in drug discovery by rapidly identifying potential therapeutic targets and repurposing existing drugs, significantly reducing the time and cost involved in developing new treatments. Personalized oncology is advancing with AI-powered digital twins—virtual models of a patient's tumor that allow doctors to simulate treatment responses and create customized therapies. In immuno-oncology, AI helps to identify unique cancer-specific antigens, improving the development of personalized cancer vaccines and engineered immune cells such as CAR-T therapy, which enhances the body's natural ability to fight cancer.

AI transforms the landscape of early cancer detection and prognosis by processing information acquired from non-invasive liquid biopsies, radiomics studies, and histopathological slides, allowing for real-time monitoring and earlier treatment. Computational modeling reveals how tumors grow, spread, and resist treatment—insights that are power the development of more effective and targeted therapies. AI also has applications in making clinical trials more effective, and using real-world data analytics for patient recruitment, anticipating side effects, and enabling better treatment choices using a large amount of electronic health record (EHR) data. But in order for these technologies to be adopted at scale, some hurdles need to be cleared—such as ensuring data quality, creating more transparent AI models, working through ethical concerns, and getting through regulatory approvals.

The future of cancer therapy is harnessing AI and computational tools to make the treatment more precise, personalized, and accessible. Their applications include AI-enabled decision-support systems for oncologists, blockchain for secure data-sharing, and federated AI models that allow research institutions to collaborate globally while maintaining patient-level privacy. The progress being made is significant, despite challenges such as bias in AI models and the complexities of incorporating these tools into healthcare. AI technology, when paired with omics-based research, will continue to advance the prediction, prevention, and personalized treatment of cancer, resulting in improved quality of life and increases in survival for patients.

1.8 CONCLUSION

AI and computational biology and omics technologies are revolutionizing cancer treatment in truly profound ways; this is evident from better early detection to development of targeted therapies. Together, these novel AI-driven predictive models with detailed omics data provide a greater capability to target cancer pathways that give rise to the disease state and offer opportunities for therapeutics that generate better cancer therapies with less toxicity. These technologies are still evolving, but they have the potential to transform oncotherapeutics and increase the personalized, efficient, and successful treatment of cancer. Thus, the convergence of AI, computational biology, and omics technologies is fundamentally changing the paradigm of cancer treatment. These cutting-edge technologies facilitate more accurate diagnoses, tailor-made treatments, and faster drug development. AI and computational models can examine large volumes of biological, genetic, and clinical data to identify patterns and predict treatment outcomes, enabling more effective and targeted therapies. Omics technologies, including genomics, proteomics, and metabolomics, enable more in-depth investigation of the molecular basis of cancer, paving the way for the discovery of novel biomarkers and drug targets. Encouragingly, ongoing technological advancements of this nature offer the potential not only to greatly enhance patient outcomes through targeted therapies but also to reduce side effects associated with treatment, revolutionizing cancer care and enabling a future in which such treatments can be more personalized, efficient, and successful. The integration of all the methods, including computational, AI, and omics-based tools helped in the evolvement of treatment of cancer and benefited the patients of cancer.

REFERENCES

Adeniji, A. A., Dulal, S., & Martin, M. G. (2021). Personalized Medicine in Oncology in the Developing World: Barriers and Concepts to Improve Status Quo. *World Journal of Oncology*, *12*(2–3), 50–60. https://doi.org/10.14740/wjon1345

Atene, C. G., Fiorcari, S., Mesini, N., Maffei, R., Martinelli, S., Pilato, F., …, & Marasca, R. (2023). The Unique BCR Inhibiting Properties of BMS-986205 in Chronic Lymphocytic Cells. *Blood*, *142*(1), 6516. https://doi.org/10.1182/blood-2023-189127

Boulos, J. C., Saeed, M. E. M., Chatterjee, M., Bülbül, Y., Crudo, F., Marko, D., …, & Efferth, T. (2021). Repurposing of the ALK Inhibitor Crizotinib for Acute Leukemia and Multiple Myeloma Cells. *Pharmaceuticals*, *14*(11), 1126. https://doi.org/10.3390/ph14111126

Bradley, R., Braybrooke, J., Gray, R., Hills, R., Liu, Z., Peto, R., …, & Romond, E. (2021). Trastuzumab for Early-Stage, HER2-Positive Breast Cancer: A Meta-Analysis of 13 864 Women in Seven Randomised Trials. *The Lancet Oncology*, *22*(8), 1139–1150. https://doi.org/10.1016/S1470-2045(21)00288-6

Brown, J. R., Eichhorst, B., Hillmen, P., Jurczak, W., Kaźmierczak, M., Lamanna, N., …, & Osterborg, A. (2023). Zanubrutinib or Ibrutinib in Relapsed or Refractory Chronic Lymphocytic Leukemia. *New England Journal of Medicine*, *388*(4), 319–332. https://doi.org/10.1056/nejmoa2211582

Chakraborty, S., Sharma, G., Karmakar, S., Chatterjee, P., Sinha, S., Ghosh, P., & Banerjee, S. (2024). Abstract 4490: Targeting NQO1 with Episesaminol: A New Therapeutic Option Identified for Colorectal Cancer Using Integrated Systems Biology and Structural Biology-Based Approach. *Cancer Research, 84*(6_Supplement), 4490–4490. https://doi.org/10.1158/1538-7445.am2024-4490

Chakraborty, S., Sharma, G., Karmakar, S., & Banerjee, S. (2024). Multi-OMICS Approaches in Cancer Biology: New Era in Cancer Therapy. *Biochimica et Biophysica Acta (BBA) - Molecular Basis of Disease, 1870*(5), 167120–167120. https://doi.org/10.1016/j.bbadis.2024.167120

Creative Proteomics. (2021). Lipidomics in Cancer Research and Disease Understanding. Retrieved from Creative Proteomics Website: https://www.creative-proteomics.com/resource/lipidomics-cancer-research-disease-understanding.htm

Cui, W., Aouidate, A., Wang, S., Yu, Q., Li, Y., & Yuan, S. (2020). Discovering Anti-Cancer Drugs via Computational Methods. *Frontiers in Pharmacology, 11*(733). https://doi.org/10.3389/fphar.2020.00733

de Anda-Jáuregui, G., & Hernández-Lemus, E. (2020) Computational Oncology in the Multi-Omics Era: State of the Art. *Frontiers in Oncology*, 10:423. https://doi.org/10.3389/fonc.2020.00423

Farghali, H., Kutinová Canová, N., & Arora, M. (2021). The Potential Applications of Artificial Intelligence in Drug Discovery and Development. *Physiological Research, 70*(30), S715–S722. https://doi.org/10.33549/physiolres.934765

Hung, C.-L., & Chen, C.-C. (2014). Computational Approaches for Drug Discovery. *Drug Development Research, 75*(6), 412–418. https://doi.org/10.1002/ddr.21222

Iwaloye, O., Paul, O., Olawale, F., Babalola, O., Elekofehinti, O. O., Kikiowo, B, …, & Shityakov, S. (2023). Computer-Aided Drug Design in Anti-Cancer Drug Discovery: What Have We Learnt and What Is the Way Forward? *Informatics in Medicine Unlocked, 41*(101332), 101332–101332. https://doi.org/10.1016/j.imu.2023.101332

Jeon, J., Nim, S., Teyra, J., Datti, A., Wrana, J. L., Sidhu, S. S., …, & Kim, P. M. (2014). A Systematic Approach to Identify Novel Cancer Drug Targets Using Machine Learning, Inhibitor Design and High-Throughput Screening. *Genome Medicine, 6*(7). https://doi.org/10.1186/s13073-014-0057-7

Kosugi, S., & Terao, C. (2024). Comparative Evaluation of SNVs, Indels, and Structural Variations Detected With Short- and Long-Read Sequencing Data. *Human Genome Variation, 11*(1). https://doi.org/10.1038/s41439-024-00276-x

Leelananda, S. P., & Lindert, S. (2016). Computational Methods in Drug Discovery. *Beilstein Journal of Organic Chemistry, 12*(1), 2694–2718. https://doi.org/10.3762/bjoc.12.267

Liang, G., Fan, W., Luo, H., & Zhu, X. (2020). The Emerging Roles of Artificial Intelligence in Cancer Drug Development and Precision Therapy. *Biomedicine & Pharmacotherapy, 128*, 110255. https://doi.org/10.1016/j.biopha.2020.110255

Mao, K., Lin, F., Zhang, Y., & Zhou, H. (2021). Identification of Key Genes and Pathways in Gefitinib-Resistant Lung Adenocarcinoma Using Bioinformatics Analysis. *Evolutionary Bioinformatics, 17*(1), 117693432110237–117693432110237. https://doi.org/10.1177/11769343211023767

Masucci, M., Karlsson, C., Blomqvist, L., & Ernberg, I. (2024). Bridging the Divide: A Review on the Implementation of Personalized Cancer Medicine. *Journal of Personalized Medicine, 14*(6), 561. https://doi.org/10.3390/jpm14060561

Micheel, C. M., Nass, S. J., & Omenn, G. S. (2012). Omics-Based Clinical Discovery: Science, Technology, and Applications. *Evolution of translational omics: Lessons learned and the path forward (pp. 33–66).* In *www.ncbi.nlm.nih.gov*. National Academies Press (US). Retrieved from https://www.ncbi.nlm.nih.gov/books/NBK202165/

National Cancer Institute. (2018, April 11). How Gleevec Transformed Leukemia Treatment. Retrieved from National Cancer Institute website: https://www.cancer.gov/research/progress/discovery/gleevec

Orsini, A., Diquigiovanni, C., & Bonora, E. (2023). Omics Technologies Improving Breast Cancer Research and Diagnostics. *International Journal of Molecular Sciences, 24*(16), 12690. https://doi.org/10.3390/ijms241612690

Park, K. (2019). A Review of Computational Drug Repurposing. *Translational and Clinical Pharmacology, 27*(2), 59. https://doi.org/10.12793/tcp.2019.27.2.59

Rasool, A., Mohammed, A. H., Hallit, S., Malaeb, D., & Hosseini, H. (2025). Exploring the Role of Artificial Intelligence in Chemotherapy Development, Cancer Diagnosis, and Treatment: Present Achievements and Future Outlook. *Frontiers in Oncology, 15*(1475893). https://doi.org/10.3389/fonc.2025.1475893

Sager, M., Yeat, N. C., Pajaro-Van der Stadt, S., Lin, C., Ren, Q., & Lin, J. (2015). Transcriptomics in Cancer Diagnostics: Developments in Technology, Clinical Research and Commercialization. *Expert Review of Molecular Diagnostics, 15*(12), 1589–1603. https://doi.org/10.1586/14737159.2015.1105133

Satam, H., Joshi, K., Mangrolia, U., Waghoo, S., Zaidi, G., Rawool, S., …, & Malonia, S. K. (2023). Next-Generation Sequencing Technology: Current Trends and Advancements. *Biology*, *12*(7), 997. https://doi.org/10.3390/biology12070997

Sharma, A., Sharma, K. L., Bansal, C., & Kumar, A. (2020). Updates on "Cancer Genomics and Epigenomics." *World Journal of Clinical Oncology*, *11*(11), 890–897. https://doi.org/10.5306/wjco.v11.i11.890

Siddique, S., & Chow, J. C. L. (2020). Artificial Intelligence in Radiotherapy. *Reports of Practical Oncology & Radiotherapy*, *25*(4), 656–666. https://doi.org/10.1016/j.rpor.2020.03.015

Suri, G. S., Kaur, G., Carbone, G. M., & Shinde, D. (2023). Metabolomics in Oncology. *Cancer Reports*, *6*(3). https://doi.org/10.1002/cnr2.1795

Tian, R., Basu, M. K., & Capriotti, E. (2015). Computational Methods and Resources for the Interpretation of Genomic Variants in Cancer. *BMC Genomics*, *16*(S8). https://doi.org/10.1186/1471-2164-16-s8-s7

Tutt, A. N. J. (2021). Adjuvant Olaparib for Patients with BRCA1- or BRCA2-Mutated Breast Cancer. *New England Journal of Medicine*, *384*(25), 2394–2405. https://doi.org/10.1056/nejmoa2105215

Urbiola-Salvador, V., Miroszewska, D., Jabłońska, A., Qureshi, T., & Chen, Z. (2022). Proteomics Approaches to Characterize the Immune Responses in Cancer. *Proteomics Approaches to Characterize the Immune Responses in Cancer. Biochimica et Biophysica Acta (BBA) – Molecular Cell Research*, *1869*(8), 119266–119266. https://doi.org/10.1016/j.bbamcr.2022.119266

Wang, L., Song, Y., Wang, H., Zhang, X., Wang, M., He, J., …, & Cao, L. (2023). Advances of Artificial Intelligence in Anti-Cancer Drug Design: A Review of the Past Decade. *Pharmaceuticals*, *16*(2), 253. https://doi.org/10.3390/ph16020253

Xu, Z., Wang, X., Zeng, S., Ren, X., Yan, Y., & Gong, Z. (2021). Applying Artificial Intelligence for Cancer Immunotherapy. *Acta Pharmaceutica Sinica B*, *11*(11), 3393–3405. https://doi.org/10.1016/j.apsb.2021.02.007

Yang, W., Zhang, R., Xu, J., Wang, L., Li, Z., Zou, F., …, & Wang, Y.. (2020). The Electrophysiology Correlation of the Cognitive Bias in Anxiety Under Uncertainty. *Scientific Reports*, *10*(1). https://doi.org/10.1038/s41598-020-68427-y

Yu, K.-H., Beam, A. L., & Kohane, I. S. (2018). Artificial Intelligence in Healthcare. *Nature Biomedical Engineering*, *2*(10), 719–731. https://doi.org/10.1038/s41551-018-0305-z

2 Exploring Small Heterocyclic Compounds as Promising Agents in Cancer Therapy

Sandip Paul and Pinki Saha Sardar
The Bhawanipur Education Society College, Kolkata, India

Anjoy Majhi
Presidency University, Kolkata, India

2.1 INTRODUCTION

Cancer is the second leading cause of mortality worldwide [1–3], and consequently, a major focus of research efforts has been directed toward its prediction, early detection, and effective treatment. Protein kinases play a critical role in regulating cell growth and signal transduction. Among them, the vascular endothelial growth factor receptor (VEGFR) has been reported to govern cellular differentiation and signaling pathways, highlighting its importance in the pathophysiology of cancer [4]. Tumor suppressor glutathione S-transferase (GSTP) is implicated in multiple types of cancer, such as lung, breast, and nephrological tissue cancer [5]. VGFR2 and GSTP1 have a strong correlation with cancer phenotypes that are multidrug resistant (MDR). Therefore, it is imperative to expand the development of innovative small chemical entities like VEGFR2 and GSTP1 inhibitors. Bufuralol is a well-known non-selective β-adrenoceptor blocking agent. Recent studies have demonstrated that β-blockers possess therapeutic potential in the management of several cancers, including pancreatic, prostate, lung, melanoma, and breast malignancies [6]. This has prompted researchers to design and identify novel compounds structurally related to bufuralol with potential anticancer activity. In the post-genomic era, drug discovery has been significantly advanced by *in silico* approaches, which enable efficient prediction of chemical leads while reducing both cost and time [7]. Hundreds of drugs have been taken off the market in the last ten years due to clinical trial failures. Druglikeness, absorption, distribution, metabolism, excretion, and toxicity (ADMET) can all be filtered or predicted using computational methods [8]. Using a variety of algorithms, the toxicity prediction primarily looks at the potential irritating, carcinogenic, mutagenic, tumorigenic, and reproductive toxicity of the suggested substances. Clinical research on these qualities is costly and time-consuming. Consequently, computational methods could show to be highly beneficial prior to the costly in vitro, in vivo, and clinical trial stages. The druglikeness of a molecule can be determined using empirical methods such as the Ghose filter, the Viber rule, and Lipinski's rules of five. Other rules that may be utilized include lead likelihood and PAINS.

A considerable proportion of currently utilized anticancer pharmaceuticals are derived from natural sources [9, 10]. These natural products possess distinct chemical structures and exhibit diverse mechanisms of action, enabling them to interact with a wide range of therapeutic targets

DOI: 10.1201/9781003644309-2

implicated in complex pathological conditions. While plants constitute a major source of naturally occurring anticancer compounds, both microorganisms and marine organisms have also yielded several clinically important chemotherapeutic agents [9]. Notable examples of anticancer agents of natural origin include bleomycin, dactinomycin, and doxorubicin from microbial sources; bryostatins, sarcodictyin, and cytarabine from marine organisms; and vincristine, vinblastine, paclitaxel, camptothecin, and topotecan from plants. The remarkable structural diversity and broad spectrum of biological activities exhibited by natural compounds derived from the vast array of plant, marine, and microbial species have ushered in a new era of potential therapeutic anticancer agents. Chemotherapy remains a standard approach for cancer treatment. However, despite extensive research advancements, improvements in survival rates have been limited, and cancer persists as a significant global public health challenge [11]. For over five decades, natural products have served as a vital source of therapeutic agents in cancer chemotherapy, providing both established drugs and novel lead compounds for synthetic modification, with relevant cellular and molecular mechanisms of action [9]. More than 60% of anticancer medications on the market today have some sort of natural origin. One study found that around 49% of the 175 small-molecule anticancer medications utilized in affluent nations were derived from natural materials or directly sourced from organisms [9]. Although only a limited fraction of isolated natural products advance to clinically approved therapeutics, nature remains an abundant reservoir of biologically active and structurally diverse chemotypes. These molecules frequently work as models for more effective counterparts. Note that effective chemotherapy for cancer frequently requires the use of combination regimens (also known as combination chemotherapy), which can include medicines from both synthetic and natural sources. There has been much written on the critical role that natural products play in the identification and development of new anticancer drugs, as well as the value of interdisciplinary cooperation in the optimization of new molecular leads derived from natural product sources [12].

Since pathological angiogenesis is a defining feature of cancer, several FDA-approved anticancer medications work by blocking angiogenesis through various mechanisms. Redundancy, multiplicity, and the formation of compensatory mechanisms that remodel blood vessels have all presented challenges in the development of the most effective anti-angiogenics. To further improve the effectiveness of anti-angiogenesis medications, it has been demonstrated that the identification of broad-spectrum anti-angiogenesis targets is necessary. According to this viewpoint, a thorough comprehension of the structure–activity relationship (SAR) of the most current anti-angiogenic drugs is necessary [13]. Over the years, many anti-angiogenic classes have been discovered; the most promising are the heterocyclic organic compounds, with multiple FDA-approved medications belonging to this family. Heterocyclic compounds are considered to be an essential branch of organic chemistry. Their innate adaptability and distinctive physicochemical features, together with the presence of most heterocycle molecules and often common heterocycle fragments in the bulk of currently available medications, have established them as genuine pillars of medicinal chemistry [14, 15]. Besides the medications currently available on the market, many other compounds are under investigation for their potential in treating various cancers. Research in anticancer therapy has particularly benefited from the intrinsic versatility and dynamic core structure of these molecules. The synthesis of a wide range of biologically active compounds has led to the development of numerous agents exhibiting antibacterial, analgesic, anti-inflammatory, antioxidant, anticancer, local anesthetic, anticoagulant, and antithrombotic activities. In oncology and other conditions where treatment responses can vary significantly among individuals, heterocyclic compounds play a crucial role in advancing personalized therapy. Personalized medicine aims to tailor treatment based on a patient's unique genetic makeup, environmental factors, and lifestyle. Often, this approach involves combining multiple drugs to address different pathways involved in disease progression, with heterocyclic compounds frequently forming part of these therapies. By analyzing the molecular characteristics of a patient's disease, clinicians can design drug regimens that specifically target the underlying mechanisms driving that individual's cancer.

2.2 FINDING OF ANTICANCER AGENTS WITH VARIOUS NATURAL ORIGIN

A current collaborative, multidisciplinary research initiative is focused on isolating, structurally characterizing, chemically modifying, and biologically evaluating novel natural product-based anticancer agents derived from diverse organisms, including filamentous fungi, aquatic and terrestrial cyanobacteria, and tropical plants. Recent progress in this project is highlighted, along with detailed descriptions of the methods used to collect and process these organisms. The isolated pure compounds, chromatographic fractions, and initial extracts are assessed using appropriate bioassays. The identification of several promising bioactive lead compounds from each major organism type underscores the extensive chemical diversity present in these natural sources.

Years of anticancer research have led to notable improvements in cancer management, largely through the discovery and development of natural substances and their derivatives. Many of these compounds target conventional cytotoxic pathways expressed by cancer cells and some normal proliferative cells, often interacting with nonspecific macromolecules. Most natural products are heterocyclic organic compounds exhibiting potent medicinal properties. Examples include plant- and microbe-derived drugs such as actinomycin D, mitoxantrone HCl, bleomycin, and anthracycline derivatives (daunorubicin, idarubicin, doxorubicin, epirubicin, and valrubicin) [16]. In developed countries, four primary groups of plant-derived anticancer agents are widely used in clinical practice: taxanes (paclitaxel, docetaxel, and cabazitaxel), semi-synthetic epipodophyllotoxins (etoposide, teniposide, and etoposide phosphate), and camptothecin derivatives (irinotecanand topotecan) [17].

Marine-derived compounds have also expanded the anticancer arsenal. Trabectedin (ET-743), approved in the past decade, acts as a DNA-intercalating agent to disrupt transcription [18]. Similarly, the synthetic derivative of the marine macrolide Halichondrin B, eribulin mesylate, functions as a microtubule inhibitor [19]. Romidepsin, obtained from a soil bacterium, is an FDA-approved histone deacetylase inhibitor effective against T-cell lymphoma. Ixabepilone, a semisynthetic microbial derivative, shows efficacy against metastatic breast cancer by inhibiting microtubules, while omacetaxine mepesuccinate, an alkaloid from plants, inhibits protein translation [20]. Topically applied ingenol mebutate, another plant-derived agent, has been approved for treating actinic keratosis. Numerous natural product-based compounds continue to be evaluated in clinical trials as potential new anticancer agents [21].

Flavonoids, particularly flavone derivatives, have emerged as a significant class of natural product-based anticancer agents, acting as selective dual inhibitors of Raf1 and JNK1 kinases [22]. Several flavonoids, including apigenin, kaempferol, myricetin, luteolin, and quercetin, have been reported to reduce the risk of developing cancers of the respiratory tract [23]. Multiple studies have investigated the protective role of flavonoids against various malignancies, showing that apigenin, for example, can lower both the incidence and recurrence of several cancers, including those of the skin, gastrointestinal tract, prostate, breast, and hematologic system [24]. Alkaloids have become extremely popular in the age of herbal remedies because of their wide range of biological actions [9]. Many plants have employed the alkaloids as a defense against herbivorous animals [25]. Alkaloids were studied extensively to determine their pharmacological profile from the start of the 19th century, and as a result, they became a key ingredient in many anticancer medications. Alkaloids are the largest group of low molecular weight organic nitrogenous chemicals originating from terrestrial and marine sources among the various naturally occurring secondary metabolites [26, 27]. About 17,000 compounds have demonstrated noteworthy biological and pharmacological actions, including anti-inflammatory, antibacterial, and anticancer properties, out of the many identified alkaloids [9].

Merely 5% of all accessible marine sources have been investigated for their potential pharmacological effects [24]. In vitro, in vivo, and human investigations revealed substantial anticancer efficacy for several substances obtained from marine sources. Few of these have received FDA approval for use in humans, despite the fact that several of them have reached clinical trials [28]. A handful of these FDA-approved substances, such as cytarabine, trabectedin, eribulin, and a synthetic derivative based on the structure of halichondrin B, have been covered in this chapter.

2.3 PREDICTION OF THE SELECTED INHIBITORS BASED ON DRUG LIKENESS AND ABSORPTION DISTRIBUTION METABOLISM EXCRETION (ADME)

Computational methods have become indispensable in multidisciplinary drug discovery, offering valuable support at different stages of the development pipeline. Harnessing the full potential of these tools is essential for generating meaningful outcomes, as they significantly improve the identification and evaluation of prospective therapeutic compounds [29]. However, strong inhibitory interactions with receptor proteins or enzymes alone are not sufficient to establish a compound's druglikeness. Therefore, absorption, distribution, metabolism, and excretion (ADME) studies play a pivotal role in drug development [30]. Guided by Lipinski's rule of five, ADME profiling helps determine the suitability of inhibitors within biological systems. Indeed, poor ADME properties and unfavorable toxicity profiles are among the leading causes of drug candidate failures during clinical trials [31]. In addition to safety and efficacy concerns, inadequate pharmacokinetics and low bioavailability contribute substantially to drug development setbacks [32]. Two critical pharmacokinetic parameters that must be evaluated throughout the process are gastrointestinal absorption and brain penetration [33].

2.4 HETEROCYCLIC COMPOUNDS CONTAINING NITROGEN ATOM

Nitrogen-containing heterocycles are a distinct and critically important group of compounds in organic chemistry, garnering considerable research interest for the creation of new molecules and their derivatives. Many naturally occurring N-heterocyclic compounds exhibit important physiological and pharmacological activities and serve as fundamental scaffolds in biologically essential molecules, including vitamins, nucleic acids, pharmaceuticals, antibiotics, dyes, and agrochemicals. Notably, purines and pyrimidines, key classes of N-heterocycles, form the bases of DNA and RNA, such as guanine, cytosine, adenine, and thymine. The ability of the nitrogen atom to readily form hydrogen bonds with biological targets makes N-heterocyclic frameworks valuable building blocks for novel drug candidates with broad therapeutic potential. Indeed, numerous nitrogen-containing heterocyclic compounds have been reported to possess diverse pharmacological activities, including anti-tubercular, anti-HIV, anticancer, antimalarial, antimicrobial, and antidiabetic effects [34].

An indication of the structural importance of nitrogen-based heterocycles in the fight against cancer is the number of anticancer prospects that contain a nitrogen heterocycle [34]. Heterocyclic moieties containing nitrogen make up more than 75% of medications that have been approved by the FDA and are currently on the market [35]. Over the past two decades, medicinal chemistry research has increasingly shifted toward the exploration of more complex nitrogen-based heterocyclic scaffolds. Among these, triazolothiadiazoles and triazolothiadiazines represent polycyclic frameworks ingeniously constructed through the fusion of triazoles with thiadiazoles or thiadiazines. These hybrid scaffolds have emerged as biologically significant structural motifs with notable relevance in oncology [14]. The anticancer potential of newly synthesized 1,2,4-triazoles, triazolothiadiazoles, and triazolothiadiazines has been systematically investigated, highlighting their promise as therapeutic candidates [14].

VEGFRs are critical signaling molecules that play a central role in the development of the circulatory system and in angiogenesis, the process by which new blood vessels form from existing vasculature [36, 37]. The expression of VEGF is upregulated by activated oncogenes, hypoxic conditions, and various cytokines [38]. Beyond stimulating endothelial cell proliferation and promoting cell

TABLE 2.1
Several Clinically Approved or Well-Studied Heterocyclic Compounds Used as Anticancer Drugs

Drug Name	Heterocyclic Core(s)	Clinical Use/Cancer Type
Imatinib	Pyrimidine, piperazine	Chronic myeloid leukemia (CML)
Gefitinib	Quinazoline	Non-small cell lung cancer (NSCLC)
Sunitinib	Indole, pyrrole	Renal cell carcinoma, GIST
Sorafenib	Pyridine, urea	Liver, kidney, and thyroid cancers

migration, VEGF also functions to inhibit apoptosis [39]. Moreover, VEGF contributes to increased vascular permeability and serves as a key regulator of vasculogenesis [40]. Several nitrogen-based heterocyclic drugs have been developed to inhibit VEGF activity. For example, FDA-approved sunitinib, a pyrrolidinone-derived VEGFR tyrosine kinase inhibitor (TKI), is used for the treatment of renal cell carcinoma (RCC) and gastrointestinal stromal tumors (GISTs) resistant to imatinib [41]. Similarly, vatalanib, a phthalazine-based compound, is under clinical investigation for its potential in treating non-small cell lung cancer (NSCLC) and metastatic colorectal cancer (**Table 2.1**) [42]. The indole scaffold also plays a significant role in VEGF inhibition [43]. Notably, panobinostat, an indole-derived agent approved in 2015 for the treatment of multiple myeloma, has demonstrated strong efficacy in suppressing cancer cell proliferation, growth, and invasion [44].

2.5 HETEROCYCLIC SULFONAMIDES

Sulfonamides constitute a broad class of compounds with diverse pharmacological activities, including diuretic, anticancer, and carbonic anhydrase inhibitory effects [45]. A wide range of structurally unique heterocyclic sulfonamide derivatives have been shown to have strong anticancer activity [13]. Most anticancer sulfonamides operate on angiogenesis through many mechanisms, while their exact mode of action varies.

Although there are a number of intriguing possibilities being investigated, there are currently no FDA-approved heterocyclic sulfonamide anti-angiogenics available on the market. One such lead is E7820, which is currently undergoing a phase II clinical study to treat colorectal cancer by inhibiting integrin α2 [13]. Integrins are transmembrane receptors that play a pivotal role in the pathophysiology of various human diseases. They facilitate interactions between cells and the extracellular matrix [13], thereby influencing a wide range of cellular responses such as adhesion, spreading, migration, growth and survival signaling, protease secretion, and invasion through the transmission of extracellular cues [46]. Numerous studies have reported that increased expression of integrin α2 is closely associated with enhanced cancer metastasis [13]. Hypoxia-inducible factors (HIFs) also serve as potent anti-angiogenic targets [47], as the progression of macroscopic tumors is heavily dependent on an adequate oxygen supply [13]. Tumor angiogenesis arises from an imbalance characterized by increased production of pro-angiogenic factors and reduced synthesis of anti-angiogenic factors, thereby fulfilling this oxygen demand [48]. Under hypoxic conditions, tumor cells undergo metabolic adaptations that alter the balance between pro- and anti-apoptotic factors, enhancing survival by increasing glucose uptake and glycolysis while reducing oxygen dependence [13]. Among these, HIF-1 plays a central role in regulating tumor angiogenesis, being activated by multiple stimuli.

2.6 HETEROCYCLIC COMPOUNDS CONTAINING OXYGEN ATOM

An estimated 15% of all FDA-approved medications are heterocycles based on oxygen [49]. As of right now, the FDA has approved a number of oxygen-based anti-angiogenic cancer medications. Certain medications, such cabazitaxel (Jevtana) and paclitaxel (PTX, Taxol), function by targeting microtubules and are based on the oxetane ring [50]. Cytoskeletal components called microtubules are essential for a variety of processes, such as cell division, morphogenesis, intracellular transport, and motility [13]. The protofilament of the tube is formed by the sequential assembly of α–β tubulin heterodimers, which constitute the microtubules [13]. The two ends of the microtubule become characteristically heterogeneous as a result of this microtubule polymerization, which results in distinct kinetics for the addition and subtraction of heterodimers at the two ends [51]. The kinetics of polymerization and depolymerization are faster at the "plus" end than they are at the opposite, slower, so-called minus end. The microtubule-organizing center is where microtubules inside the cell are connected by their minus ends, with their plus ends toward the cell border [13]. The plus ends are continuously growing and getting shorter, which is an essential characteristic for cell division and other cellular functions [52]. Normal cells may stop during mitosis due to disruptions in the dynamic characteristics of microtubules, which act as a "pulling device" for the duplicate chromosomes by rapidly polymerizing and depolymerizing [53]. Microtubule-targeting agents, or MTAs, work by keeping microtubules stable against depolymerization [13]. Paclitaxel is one of the most promising microtubule-targeting drugs.

Heterocycles that have both nitrogen and oxygen in their ring structure are also quite promising. Felipe Rodrigues and colleagues investigate the antiproliferative properties of 23 distinct mefloquine-oxazolidine derivatives, which are cyclic molecules with nitrogen and oxygen atoms. IC50 values varied from 0.59 to 4.79 μg/mL after cell viability tests in HCT8 (colorectal), OVCAR8 (ovarian), HL60 (peripheral blood), and SF295 (nervous system). This was the first investigation to assess the derivatives of mefloquine and oxazolidine's anticancer potential [54]. Saulo Andrade et al. have examined oxazolidine complexes as possible anticancer agents in another study [55]. Furthermore, additional research evaluating the anticancer qualities of oxazolidine compounds was conducted, consistently demonstrating strong toxicities with low IC50 values. This suggests that these families of oxygen- and nitrogen-based heterocycles represent a novel and developing field of study [14].

The occurrence of drastically varied toxicities for several of the heterocycles currently undergoing pre-clinical study, depending on the type of oxygen-based heterocycle, its overall structure, ligands, ring size, and aromaticity. Given the examples of eribulin and cabazitaxel, the pharmaceutical industry is likely to continue to take advantage of the findings that oxygen-based heterocycle scaffolds have been showing potential anticancer effects in order to build better chemotherapeutic cancer treatments. However, the precise method by which many of these novel heterocycle medications or scaffolds achieve their therapeutic effects is yet unknown.

2.7 BIOACTIVE COMPOUNDS DERIVED FROM PLANTS AS POTENTIAL ANTICANCER AGENTS

Pharmaceutical research has primarily concentrated on discovering novel and effective anticancer agents from natural sources, owing to the immense chemical diversity found in animals, plants, and microorganisms, which makes them valuable reservoirs of therapeutic compounds. Natural products, either directly or in modified forms, have contributed to the development of over 60% of currently available anticancer drugs. Over the past decade, extensive studies have examined the ethnopharmacological and ethnomedicinal properties of numerous plant-derived bioactive compounds, with recent investigations also highlighting their antibacterial and antibiofilm activities [56]. The most widely used anticancer medicines originating from plants are terpenes, podophyllotoxin and its semi-synthetic analogs, camptothecin and its derivatives, and vinca alkaloids and their derivatives. Vincristine and vinblastine, two alkaloids that were isolated from plants utilizing *Catharanthus roseus* and Madagascar periwinkle, established the use of plants as anticancer medicines [57]. Over the course of around 50 years, these medications have been utilized in oncology. In order to accomplish their goal, they prevent tubulin molecules from polymerizing, which prevents the development of mitotic spindles and causes apoptosis or metaphase arrest [58]. Natural alkaloids originating from plants are used as anticancer medications. Examples of these include vincristine, vinblastine, vinorelbine, vinflunine, veratridine, and berbamine.

2.8 SMALL-MOLECULE TRIAZOLE AS HETEROCYCLIC COMPONENT

Triazoles are highly versatile heterocyclic compounds with a broad range of applications, particularly in medicinal chemistry, materials science, and catalysis. Their ability to interact with biological targets through the nitrogen atoms of the ring makes them valuable pharmacophores in drug design. The rich chemistry of triazoles, combined with efficient synthetic routes like click chemistry, allows for the creation of diverse derivatives with tailored properties for various applications. 1,2,4-Triazole derivatives have been explored in the design of anticancer agents due to their ability to inhibit enzymes like aromatase (involved in estrogen biosynthesis), which plays a role in the development of breast cancer [59, 60]. Triazole derivatives have shown potential as anticancer agents by targeting specific enzymes involved in cell cycle regulation or apoptosis [61]. Voriconazole, a 1,2,3-triazole derivative, originally an antifungal drug [62], has now been investigated for its potential anticancer effects. Studies have shown that voriconazole can inhibit tumor growth in various cancer models, possibly through angiogenesis inhibition [63, 64]. Several triazole molecules have been reported for potential fluorescent probe that might useful in cancer therapy [65, 66]. Triazole-containing metal complexes: Some triazole derivatives can coordinate with metal ions *viz.* Cu and Pt, forming metal–drug complexes [67]. These complexes may enhance the anticancer activity of the triazole scaffold by targeting metal-dependent enzymes or increasing DNA binding affinity [68]. Several small molecules that feature triazole units linked to other pharmacophores, e.g. quinolines, have shown promise in clinical trials. These molecules often target multiple cancer-related pathways simultaneously, improving their efficacy as anticancer agents [69, 70].

2.9 SPECIFIC HETEROCYCLIC COMPOUNDS USED FOR ANTICANCER DRUG

Cyclophosphamide, a chemotherapeutic agent belonging to the class of alkylating agents, exerts its effect by disrupting DNA, thereby preventing cancer cells from proliferating and dividing. It is widely used in the treatment of various malignancies, including leukemia, lymphoma, and breast cancer. Beyond oncology, cyclophosphamide is also prescribed as an immunosuppressant for autoimmune disorders such as lupus [71]. However, its use is associated with several adverse effects, including immunosuppression, hair loss, nausea, and vomiting. In some patients, bladder irritation may occur, making it essential to maintain adequate hydration during therapy.

Another substance that is classified as a disease-modifying antirheumatic drug (DMARD) that has dual uses as a chemotherapeutic agent is methotrexate. It functions by blocking the dihydrofolate reductase enzyme, which is required for the production of DNA. This reduces the growth of cells that divide quickly, such cancer cells or those involved in autoimmune diseases [72].

Personalized medicine is greatly advanced by heterocyclic compounds, which allow for the creation of highly selective treatments based on a patient's genetic and molecular cancer profile. Their ability to precisely target important oncogenic pathways, including VEGFR, PD-1/PD-L1, and Wnt/β-catenin, reduces off-target effects and enhances treatment results. Through the use of certain biomarkers, these tiny molecules facilitate the transition from generic chemotherapy to

TABLE 2.2
Comparison of Natural and Synthetic Heterocyclic Compounds in Anticancer Drug Development

S/N	Features	Natural Heterocyclic Compounds	Synthetic Heterocyclic Compounds
1	Source	Derived from plants, microbes, or marine organisms (e.g., alkaloids, flavonoids, and anthracyclines)	Designed and synthesized in laboratories using chemical approaches
2	Examples	Vincristine, Vinblastine, Doxorubicin, Camptothecin, Trabectedin	Imatinib, Gefitinib, Sorafenib, Sunitinib, Panobinostat
3	Structural Diversity	High diversity due to natural biosynthetic pathways	Controlled diversity Structures can be optimized by medicinal chemists
4	Mechanism of Action	Often broad, sometimes nonspecific (DNA intercalation, microtubule inhibition, and enzyme inhibition)	Highly specific Designed to target particular pathways (e.g., VEGFR, PD-1/PD-L1, and Wnt/β-catenin)
5	Advantages	Rich source of novel scaffolds; evolutionary "pre-tested" for biological activity	Greater control over structure–activity relationship (SAR) Improved pharmacokinetics and selectivity
6	Limitations	Low yield, complex isolation, possible toxicity, and limited availability	Development may be costly Risk of off-target effects if design is not optimal
7	Role in Drug Discovery	Provide lead compounds and templates for semisynthetic derivatives	Enable rational drug design, high-throughput screening, and precision medicine applications

tailored regimens that improve effectiveness and lower toxicity. Therefore, heterocyclic compounds are essential to the development of precision oncology, providing patients with more tailored, safer, and better cancer treatments.

The targeted therapy medication imatinib (Gleevec) is mainly used to treat GISTs and chronic myeloid leukemia (CML). It is a member of the class of medications known as TKIs, which function by preventing the action of particular proteins (tyrosine kinases) that promote the proliferation of cancer cells [73].

Targeting topoisomerase I, an enzyme essential to DNA replication, topotecan and irinotecan are both topoisomerase inhibitors. By blocking this enzyme, they stop DNA from correctly unwinding, which damages DNA and eventually kills cancer cells. The main purpose of these medications is to treat specific types of cancer [74].

The development of contemporary targeted cancer medicines relies heavily on heterocyclic compounds because of their structural variety, bioavailability, and capacity to alter particular molecular targets linked to carcinogenesis. In contrast to traditional chemotherapeutic drugs, which frequently kill rapidly dividing cells without showing any specificity, targeted therapies aim to disrupt particular signaling pathways or biological mechanisms that are abnormally active in cancer cells. While reducing systemic toxicity and side effects, this focused strategy can improve treatment efficacy.

The invention of TKIs that target VEGFR, a crucial factor in tumor angiogenesis, has made substantial use of heterocyclic molecules. Through the inhibition of the VEGFR signaling pathway, these medicines prevent the development of new blood vessels that provide oxygen and nutrition to tumors. The comparison of natural and synthetic heterocyclic compounds in anticancer drug development is mentioned in **Table 2.2**.

2.10 CONCLUSION

Heterocyclic compounds represent a cornerstone of modern anticancer drug discovery owing to their structural diversity, biological versatility, and wide-ranging therapeutic potential. Both naturally derived and synthetically designed heterocycles have contributed significantly to the current repertoire of chemotherapeutic and targeted therapies, with several clinically approved agents demonstrating efficacy against diverse malignancies. Natural products, particularly those obtained from plants, microorganisms, and marine organisms, continue to provide invaluable lead structures that inspire synthetic modification and optimization, thereby expanding the pool of potential anticancer agents. Despite substantial progress, major challenges remain, including issues of toxicity, drug resistance, limited selectivity, and suboptimal pharmacokinetic profiles. Advances in computational modeling, SAR studies, and ADME/T optimization are now helping to address these limitations, while the integration of heterocyclic scaffolds into precision medicine offers new opportunities for patient-specific therapeutic strategies.

Looking forward, the synergy between natural product chemistry, synthetic heterocyclic design, and emerging technologies such as nanomedicine and molecular docking is expected to accelerate the development of safer, more effective anticancer agents. Ultimately, the continued exploration and rational modification of heterocyclic compounds will remain pivotal to overcoming current therapeutic barriers and achieving meaningful improvements in cancer treatment outcomes.

ACKNOWLEDGMENTS

Authors acknowledge the SERB for research grant (ref: EEQ/2019/000194) for financial support. The authors are also extremely thankful to the Presidency University, Kolkata, and The Bhawanipur Education Society College, Kolkata, for research grant and providing facilities.

Author's contribution Include all authors.

REFERENCES

1. Tarver, T. (2012). American cancer society. Cancer facts and figures 2014. *Journal of Consumer Health on the Internet*, *16*, 366–367.
2. Paul, S., & Majhi, A. (2024). Chemical approaches to stem cell and signaling pathways for therapeutics. In *Cancer Stem Cells and Signaling Pathways* (pp. 309–321). Academic Press.
3. Majhi, A., Paul, S., & Sardar, P. S. (2024). Addressing the diagnosis and therapeutics of malignant tumor cells. In *Biomarkers in Cancer Detection and Monitoring of Therapeutics* (pp. 99–116). Academic Press.
4. Takahashi, Y., Kitadai, Y., Bucana, C. D., Cleary, K. R., & Ellis, L. M. (1995). Expression of vascular endothelial growth factor and its receptor, KDR, correlates with vascularity, metastasis, and proliferation of human colon cancer. *Cancer Research*, *55*(18), 3964–3968.
5. Kumar, U., Sharma, U., & Rathi, G. (2017). Reversal of hypermethylation and reactivation of glutathione S-transferase pi 1 gene by curcumin in breast cancer cell line. *Tumor Biology*, *39*(2), 1010428317692258.
6. Akbar, S., & Alsharidah, M. S. (2014). Are beta blockers new potential anticancer agents? *Asian Pacific Journal of Cancer Prevention*, *15*(22), 9567–9574.
7. Xu, C., Cheng, F., Chen, L., Du, Z., Li, W., Liu, G., …, & Tang, Y. (2012). In silico prediction of chemical Ames mutagenicity. *Journal of Chemical Information and Modeling*, *52*(11), 2840–2847.
8. Cheng, F., Li, W., Zhou, Y., Shen, J., Wu, Z., Liu, G., …, & Tang, Y. (2012). admetSAR: A comprehensive source and free tool for assessment of chemical ADMET properties, *Journal of Chemical Information and Modeling*, *52*(11), 3099–3105.
9. Singh, M., Sharma, P., Singh, P. K., Singh, T. G., & Saini, B. (2020). Medicinal potential of heterocyclic compounds from diverse natural sources for the management of cancer. *Mini Reviews in Medicinal Chemistry*, *20*(11), 942–957.
10. Paul, S., Majhi, A., & Sardar, P. S. (2024). Recent advancement in the use of medicinal plants in brain aging. In *Neuroprotective Effects of Phytochemicals in Brain Ageing* (pp. 317–331). Springer Nature Singapore.

11. Singh, R. K., Kumar, S., Prasad, D. N., & Bhardwaj, T. R. (2018). Therapeutic journery of nitrogen mustard as alkylating anticancer agents: Historic to future perspectives. *European Journal of Medicinal Chemistry*, *151*, 401–433.
12. Cragg, G. M., & Newman, D. J. (2009). Nature: A vital source of leads for anticancer drug development. *Phytochemistry Reviews*, *8*, 313–331.
13. Nada, H., Elkamhawy, A., & Lee, K. (2021). Structure activity relationship of key heterocyclic anti-angiogenic leads of promising potential in the fight against cancer. *Molecules*, *26*(3), 553.
14. Martins, P., Jesus, J., Santos, S., Raposo, L. R., Roma-Rodrigues, C., Baptista, P. V., & Fernandes, A. R. (2015). Heterocyclic anticancer compounds: Recent advances and the paradigm shift towards the use of nanomedicine's tool box. *Molecules*, *20*(9), 16852–16891.
15. Paul, S., Ghanti, R., Sardar, P. S., & Majhi, A. (2019). Synthesis of a novel coumarin derivative and its binding interaction with serum albumins. *Chemistry of Heterocyclic Compounds*, *55*, 607–611.
16. Saklani, A., & Kutty, S. K. (2008). Plant-derived compounds in clinical trials. *Drug Discovery Today*, *13*(3–4), 161–171.
17. De Sanctis, R., Marrari, A., & Santoro, A. (2016). Trabectedin for the treatment of soft tissue sarcomas. *Expert Opinion on Pharmacotherapy*, *17*(11), 1569–1577.
18. Huyck, T. K., Gradishar, W., Manuguid, F., & Kirkpatrick, P. (2011). Eribulinmesylate. *Nature Reviews Drug Discovery*, *10*(3), 173.
19. Allan, E. K., Holyoake, T. L., Craig, A. R., & Jørgensen, H. G. (2011). Omacetaxine may have a role in chronic myeloid leukaemia eradication through downregulation of Mcl-1 and induction of apoptosis in stem/progenitor cells. *Leukemia*, *25*(6), 985–994.
20. Lebwohl, M., Swanson, N., Anderson, L. L., Melgaard, A., Xu, Z., & Berman, B. (2012). Ingenolmebutate gel for actinic keratosis. *New England Journal of Medicine*, *366*(11), 1010–1019.
21. Leal, M., Sapra, P., Hurvitz, S. A., Senter, P., Wahl, A., Schutten, M., …, & Kabbarah, O. (2014). Antibody–drug conjugates: An emerging modality for the treatment of cancer. *Annals of the New York Academy of Sciences*, *1321*(1), 41–54.
22. Knekt, P., Järvinen, R., Seppänen, R., Heliövaara, M., Teppo, L., Pukkala, E., & Aromaa, A. (1997). Dietary flavonoids and the risk of lung cancer and other malignant neoplasms. *American Journal of Epidemiology*, *146*(3), 223–230.
23. Clere, N., Faure, S., Carmen Martinez, M., & Andriantsitohaina, R. (2011). Anticancer properties of flavonoids: Roles in various stages of carcinogenesis. *Cardiovascular & Hematological Agents in Medicinal Chemistry (Formerly Current Medicinal Chemistry-Cardiovascular & Hematological Agents)*, *9*(2), 62–77.
24. Shukla, S., & Gupta, S. (2010). Apigenin: A promising molecule for cancer prevention. *Pharmaceutical Research*, *27*, 962–978.
25. Mithöfer, A., & Boland, W. (2012). Plant defense against herbivores: Chemical aspects. *Annual Review of Plant Biology*, *63*(1), 431–450.
26. Zenk, M. H., & Juenger, M. (2007). Evolution and current status of the phytochemistry of nitrogenous compounds. *Phytochemistry*, *68*(22–24), 2757–2772.
27. Ramirez-Llodra, E., Brandt, A., Danovaro, R., De Mol, B., Escobar, E., German, C. R., …, & Vecchione, M. (2010). Deep, diverse and definitely different: Unique attributes of the world's largest ecosystem. *Biogeosciences*, *7*(9), 2851–2899.
28. Newman, D. J., & Cragg, G. M. (2016). Drugs and drug candidates from marine sources: An assessment of the current "state of play". *Plantamedica*, *82*(09/10), 775–789.
29. Bajorath, J. (2015). Computer-aided drug discovery. *F1000Research*, *4*.
30. Zhang, P., Xu, S., Zhu, Z., & Xu, J. (2019). Multi-target design strategies for the improved treatment of Alzheimer's disease. *European Journal of Medicinal Chemistry*, *176*, 228–247.
31. Di, L., & Kerns, E. H. (2015). *Drug-Like Properties: Concepts, Structure Design and Methods from ADME to Toxicity Optimization*. Academic press.
32. Daina, A., & Zoete, V. (2016). A boiled-egg to predict gastrointestinal absorption and brain penetration of small molecules. *Chem Med Chem*, *11*(11), 1117–1121.
33. Alavijeh, M. S., Chishty, M., Qaiser, M. Z., & Palmer, A. M. (2005). Drug metabolism and pharmacokinetics, the blood-brain barrier, and central nervous system drug discovery. *NeuroRx*, *2*, 554–571.
34. Akhtar, J., Khan, A. A., Ali, Z., Haider, R., & Yar, M. S. (2017). Structure-activity relationship (SAR) study and design strategies of nitrogen-containing heterocyclic moieties for their anticancer activities. *European Journal of Medicinal Chemistry*, *125*, 143–189.

35. Kerru, N., Gummidi, L., Maddila, S., Gangu, K. K., & Jonnalagadda, S. B. (2020). A review on recent advances in nitrogen-containing molecules and their biological applications. *Molecules*, *25*(8), 1909.
36. Peng, F. W., Liu, D. K., Zhang, Q. W., Xu, Y. G., & Shi, L. (2017). VEGFR-2 inhibitors and the therapeutic applications thereof: A patent review (2012-2016). *Expert Opinion on Therapeutic Patents*, *27*(9), 987–1004.
37. Pandey, A. K., Singhi, E. K., Arroyo, J. P., Ikizler, T. A., Gould, E. R., Brown, J., …, & Moslehi, J. (2018). Mechanisms of VEGF (vascular endothelial growth factor) inhibitor–associated hypertension and vascular disease. *Hypertension*, *71*(2), e1–e8.
38. Farina, A. R., Cappabianca, L., Sebastiano, M., Zelli, V., Guadagni, S., & Mackay, A. R. (2020). Hypoxia-induced alternative splicing: The 11th Hallmark of Cancer. *Journal of Experimental & Clinical Cancer Research*, *39*(1), 30.
39. Yan, X., Hui, Y., Hua, Y., Huang, L., Wang, L., Peng, F., & Wang, F. (2019). EG-VEGF silencing inhibits cell proliferation and promotes cell apoptosis in pancreatic carcinoma via PI3K/AKT/mTOR signaling pathway. *Biomedicine & Pharmacotherapy*, *109*, 762–769.
40. Schafer, C. M., Gurley, J. M., Kurylowicz, K., Lin, P. K., Chen, W., Elliott, M. H., & Griffin, C. T. (2020). An inhibitor of endothelial ETS transcription factors promotes physiologic and therapeutic vessel regression. *Proceedings of the National Academy of Sciences*, *117*(42), 26494–26502.
41. Motzer, R. J., Hutson, T. E., Cella, D., Reeves, J., Hawkins, R., Guo, J., & Choueiri, T. K. (2013). Pazopanib versus sunitinib in metastatic renal-cell carcinoma. *New England Journal of Medicine*, *369*(8), 722–731.
42. Scagliotti, G., & Govindan, R. (2010). Targeting angiogenesis with multitargeted tyrosine kinase inhibitors in the treatment of non-small cell lung cancer. *The Oncologist*, *15*(5), 436–446.
43. Liu, J. C., Narva, S., Zhou, K., & Zhang, W. (2019). A review on the antitumor activity of various nitrogenous-based heterocyclic compounds as NSCLC inhibitors. *Mini Reviews in Medicinal Chemistry*, *19*(18), 1517–1530.
44. Garnock-Jones, K. P. (2015). Panobinostat: First global approval. *Drugs*, *75*, 695–704.
45. Gulçin, İ., & Taslimi, P. (2018). Sulfonamide inhibitors: A patent review 2013-present. *Expert Opinion on Therapeutic Patents*, *28*(7), 541–549.
46. Hytönen, V. P., & Wehrle-Haller, B. (2016). Mechanosensing in cell–matrix adhesions–Converting tension into chemical signals. *Experimental Cell Research*, *343*(1), 35–41.
47. Tan, C., de Noronha, R. G., Devi, N. S., Jabbar, A. A., Kaluz, S., Liu, Y., & Van Meir, E. G. (2011). Sulfonamides as a new scaffold for hypoxia inducible factor pathway inhibitors. *Bioorganic & Medicinal Chemistry Letters*, *21*(18), 5528–5532.
48. Baeriswyl, V., & Christofori, G. (2009, October). The angiogenic switch in carcinogenesis. In *Seminars in cancer biology* (Vol. 19, No. 5, pp. 329–337). Academic Press.
49. Delost, M. D., Smith, D. T., Anderson, B. J., & Njardarson, J. T. (2018). From oxiranes to oligomers: Architectures of US FDA approved pharmaceuticals containing oxygen heterocycles. *Journal of Medicinal Chemistry*, *61*(24), 10996–11020.
50. Han, X., Chen, J., Jiang, M., Zhang, N., Na, K., Luo, C., …, & Wang, Y. (2016). Paclitaxel–paclitaxel prodrugnanoassembly as a versatile nanoplatform for combinational cancer therapy. *ACS Applied Materials & Interfaces*, *8*(49), 33506–33513.
51. Vemu, A., Atherton, J., Spector, J. O., Moores, C. A., & Roll-Mecak, A. (2017). Tubulin isoform composition tunes microtubule dynamics. *Molecular Biology of the Cell*, *28*(25), 3564–3572.
52. Janke, C., & Magiera, M. M. (2020). The tubulin code and its role in controlling microtubule properties and functions. *Nature Reviews Molecular Cell Biology*, *21*(6), 307–326.
53. Checchi, P. M., Nettles, J. H., Zhou, J., Snyder, J. P., & Joshi, H. C. (2003). Microtubule-interacting drugs for cancer treatment. *Trends in Pharmacological Sciences*, *24*(7), 361–365.
54. Rodrigues, F. A., Bomfim, I. D. S., Cavalcanti, B. C., Pessoa, C., Goncalves, R. S., Wardell, J. L., & de Souza, M. V. (2014). Mefloquine–oxazolidine derivatives: A new class of anticancer agents. *Chemical Biology & Drug Design*, *83*(1), 126–131.
55. Saulo F. Andrade, Bárbara G. Oliveira, Larissa C. Pereira, Jonas P. Ramos, Angélica R. Joaquim, Martin Steppe, Elaine M. Souza-Fagundes, Ricardo J. Alves, (2017). Design, synthesis and structure-activity relationship studies of a novel focused library of 2,3,4-substituted oxazolidines with antiproliferative activity against cancer cell lines, *European Journal of Medicinal Chemistry*, *138*, 13–25.
56. ErtasOnmaz, N., Demirezen Yilmaz, D., Imre, K., Morar, A., Gungor, C., Yilmaz, S., & Gungor, G. (2022). Green synthesis of gold nanoflowers using *Rosmarinus officinalis* and *Helichrysum italicum* extracts: Comparative studies of their antimicrobial and antibiofilm activities. *Antibiotics*, *11*(11), 1466.

57. Verma, A. K., & Singh, R. R. (2010). Induced dwarf mutant in *Catharanthus roseus* with enhanced antibacterial activity. *Indian Journal of Pharmaceutical Sciences*, *72*(5), 655–657.
58. Jordan, M. A., Thrower, D., & Wilson, L. (1991). Mechanism of inhibition of cell proliferation by *Vinca* alkaloids. *Cancer Research*, *51*(8), 2212–2222.
59. Pathak, C., Matore, B. W., Singh, J., Roy, P. P., & Kabra, U. D. (2024). Discovery of potential 1,2,4-triazole derivatives as aromatase inhibitors for breast cancer: Pharmacophore modelling, virtual screening, docking, ADMET and MD simulation. *Molecular Simulation*, *50*(15), 1206–1219.
60. Mohamed, T.-E. M., Almutairi, T. M., Bräse, S., Salem, O. I. A., Bahaa, G. M. Y., & Mahmoud, M. S. (2023). New 1,2,3-triazole/1,2,4-triazole hybrids as aromatase inhibitors: Design, synthesis, and apoptotic antiproliferative activity. *Molecules*, *28*(20), 7092.
61. El-Sherief, H. A. M., Youssif, B. G. M., Bukhari, S. N. A., Abdel-Aziz, M., & Abdel-Rahman, H. M. (2018). Novel 1,2,4-triazole derivatives as potential anticancer agents: Design, synthesis, molecular docking and mechanistic studies. *Bioorganic Chemistry*, *76*, 314–325.
62. Greer, N. D. (2003). Voriconazole: The newest triazole antifungal agent. *Baylor University Medical Center Proceedings*, *16*(2), 241–248.
63. Ikeya,S., Sakabe,J. I., Yamada,T., Naito,T., & Tokura,Y. (2018). Voriconazole-induced photocarcinogenesis is promoted by aryl hydrocarbon receptor-dependent COX-2 upregulation. *Scientific Reports* *8*(1), 5050.
64. Xia,M., Song,X., Lu,Z., Wang,Y., Zhou,Q., Geng,P., Wang,S., Zhou,Y., Wu,Q., & Han,A. (2023). Evaluation of the inhibitory effect of azoles on pharmacokinetics of lenvatinib in rats both in vivo and in vitro by UPLC-MS/MS. *Thoracic Cancer*, *14*(33), 3331–3341.
65. Misra, S., Pakrashy, S., Paul, S., Maurya, P. K., SahaSardar, P., Bose, A., & Majhi, A. (2024). Interaction of a new triazole compound with Serum albumins and Proteolytic enzyme Bromelain by Steady state fluorescence and Molecular docking techniques. *Indian Journal of Biochemistry and Biophysics*, *61*, 305–313.
66. Paul, S., Roy, P., Das, S., Ghosh, S., SahaSardar, P., & Majhi, A. (2021). Addressing the exigent role of a coumarinfluorophore toward finding the suitable microenvironment of biomimicking and biomolecular systems: Steering to project the drug designing and drug delivery study. *ACS Omega*, *6*(18), 11878–11896.
67. Czylkowska, A., Pitucha, M., Lanka, S., Raducka, A., Rogalewicz, B., Szczesio, M., Świątkowski, M., Żarczyński, A., Klepacz-Smółka, A., Szczytko, J., Camargo, B., Drabińska, A., & Szymański, P. (2024). Triazole-based Mn(II), Fe(II), Ni(II), Cu(II) and Zn(II) complexes as potential anticancer agents – Physicochemical properties, in silico predictions and in vitro activity. *Polyhedron*, *261*, 117106.
68. Andrés, C. M. C., Pérez de la Lastra, J. M., Bustamante Munguira, E., Andrés Juan, C., & Pérez-Lebeña, E. (2024 Jul 3). Anticancer activity of metallodrugs and metallizing host defense peptides-current developments in structure-activity relationship. *International Journal of Molecular Sciences*, *25*(13), 7314.
69. Al Sheikh Ali, A., Khan, D., Naqvi, A., Al-blewi, F. F., Rezki, N., Reda Aouad, M., & Hagar, M. (2021). Design, synthesis, molecular modeling, anticancer studies, and density functional theory calculations of 4-(1,2,4-triazol-3-ylsulfanylmethyl)-1,2,3-triazole derivatives. *ACS Omega*, *6*(1), 301–316.
70. Mohan Ilakiyalakshmi, M., & Napoleon, A. A. (2022). Review on recent development of quinoline for anticancer activities. *Arabian Journal of Chemistry*, *15*(11), 104168.
71. Baumann, F., & Preiss, R. (2001). Cyclophosphamide and related anticancer drugs. *Journal of Chromatography B: Biomedical Sciences and Applications*, *764*, 173–192.
72. Rafique, B., Khalid, A. M., Akhtar, K., & Jabbar, A. (2013). Interaction of anticancer drug methotrexate with DNA analyzed by electrochemical and spectroscopic methods. *Biosensors and Bioelectronics*, *44*, 21–26.
73. Capdeville, R., Buchdunger, E., Zimmermann, J., & Matter, A. (2002). Glivec (STI571, imatinib), a rationally developed, targeted anticancer drug. *Nature Reviews Drug Discovery*, *1*(7), 493–502.
74. Mathijssen, R. H., Loos, W. J., Verweij, J., & Sparreboom, A. (2002). Pharmacology of topoisomerase I inhibitors irinotecan (CPT-11) and topotecan. *Current Cancer Drug Targets*, *2*(2), 103–123.

3 Probiotic-Based Nanomedicine

A Next-Generation Strategy for Personalized Cancer Therapy

Lakshmi Shanmugam, Prathiba Varadhan, Sree Kathyayani Sundara Raman, Sahana R. K., and Megala Jayaraman
SRM Institute of Science and Technology, SRM Nagar, Kattankulathur, Chennai, Tamil Nadu, India

3.1 INTRODUCTION

Gastrointestinal (GI) cancer, one of the most dreadful cancers in humans, is estimated to cause one-third of cancer-related deaths worldwide (Globocon, 2024). Despite advancements in detection and conventional treatments, the prognosis remains unfavorable, especially for advanced-stage malignancies. Although advanced treatment strategies such as immunotherapy have exhibited proven efficacy and sustained clinical responses in certain patients, their overall effectiveness in gastrointestinal cancers is often limited by intrinsic or acquired drug resistance mechanisms (Yao et al., 2024). Hence, probiotic-based therapy assists in recognizing the individual patient's microbiota and facilitates the provision of personalized treatment.

Personalized medicine is transforming modern healthcare by transitioning from uniform treatment procedures to tailored strategies that incorporate genetic, molecular, and environmental factors. This shift was particularly crucial in oncology, as variations in tumor biology, immune responses, and metabolism influence individual therapeutic responses. Personalized oncology aims to develop highly precise and effective treatment protocols by integrating various disciplines, including genetics, analytics, and targeted therapies (Singh & Natraj, 2021). Probiotic-based personalized cancer treatment offers numerous advantages, as represented in **Figure 3.1**. The term "probiotics" was introduced by Stillwell and Lilley in 1965 to designate these beneficial bacteria (Gupta & Garg, 2009). In the 1980s, key attributes of probiotics were outlined, encompassing the ability of strains to exert a positive influence by exhibiting substantial quantities of non-pathogenic, non-toxic, non-allergenic substances, compatibility with the gut environment, and possessing storage stability (Amara & Shibl, 2015). From the outset, probiotics have been recognized for their positive impact on gut health, with studies confirming their associations with various chronic diseases.

3.1.1 GI CANCER – AN OVERVIEW

GI cancer includes esophageal cancer, gastric cancer (GC), colorectal cancer (CRC), and cancer of the accessory organs of digestion, such as the liver and pancreas (Arnold et al., 2020). Esophageal cancer generally arises from chronic inflammation in the esophagus, disrupting regular cellular communication and growth mechanisms. The condition was categorized into two subtypes: esophageal adenocarcinoma and esophageal squamous cell carcinoma. The risk factors for this type of

DOI: 10.1201/9781003644309-3

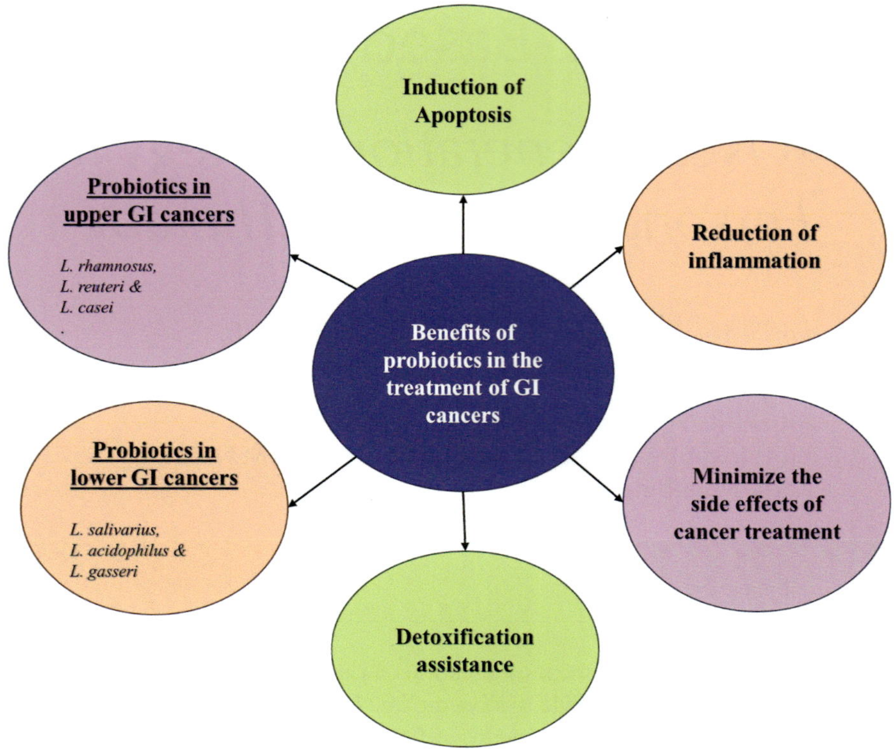

FIGURE 3.1 Applications of probiotics for personalized cancer therapy.

cancer include gastroesophageal reflux disease (GERD), smoking, dietary factors, alcohol consumption, and Barrett's esophagus (Yang et al., 2020). GC is classified into two primary subsites: cardia and non-cardia. Non-cardia GC refers to tumors that develop in the primary portion of the stomach. A significant risk factor associated with this type of cancer is *Helicobacter pylori* infection, which disrupts the plasticity and homeostasis of gastric epithelial cells, contributing to their tumorigenesis (Kumar et al., 2020). Cardia GC, on the other hand, is a type of cancer that occurs in the cardia region, which is situated at the junction of the stomach and esophagus. The risk factors associated with this type of cancer are obesity and GERD (Plummer et al., 2016).

CRC is characterized by the abnormal growth of glandular epithelial cells in the colon or rectum, resulting in its emergence. CRC was classified into three primary types: sporadic, hereditary, and colitis-associated. Factors such as environmental, genetic, and nutritional elements contribute to the development of CRC. While the precise microbial community associated with CRC remains unclear, studies have revealed that *Fusobacterium nucleatum*, *Escherichia coli*, and *Bacteroides fragilis* contribute to tumor progression by causing DNA damage and activating other signaling pathways (Pandey et al., 2023). Hepatocellular carcinoma (HCC), the most predominant form of primary liver cancer, is commonly linked to chronic hepatitis C virus (HCV) and hepatitis B virus (HBV) infection, non-alcoholic liver disease, alcoholic liver disease, and exposure to dietary toxins, such as aflatoxin B1. These risk factors contribute to liver damage and fibrinogenesis, which can lead to cirrhosis and HCC (Thilakarathna et al., 2021).

There are two main types of tumors associated with pancreatic cancer: pancreatic ductal adenocarcinoma (PDAC) and pancreatic neuroendocrine tumors (PanNET). PDAC tumors are the most common type and originate from exocrine epithelial cells within the pancreatic ducts. On the other hand, PanNETs arise from islet cells and can be functional endocrine tumors that secrete hormones such as insulin and glucagon (Sexton et al., 2022). While infectious factors are known to cause approximately 10–20% of all cancers worldwide, there is no specific microbe that has been identified as the causative agent for pancreatic cancer. However, several studies suggest that changes in the composition and proportions of the microbiome, including *Bacteroides/Bifidobacteria*, *Fusobacterium*, *Porphyromonas*, *Actinomycetes*, *Streptococcus*, and *Neisseria* species, may be associated with the development and occurrence of pancreatic cancer (Wang et al., 2019).

3.1.2 Microbes and Cancer

Although cancer was regarded as a disease brought on by genetic characteristics and environmental factors, research suggests that microorganisms may play a role in approximately 20% of the cancers that affect humans. In recent years, there has been a growing interest in the relationship between the microbiome and cancer. The compositions of these microbes are influenced by various factors, such as the host's genetics, dietary habits, lifestyle, and exposure to microbes at birth (Zitvogel et al., 2017). Numerous studies indicate variations in oxygen levels and intestinal pH among bacterial populations inhabiting various parts of the GI tract. Furthermore, the concentration of these bacteria is high in the stomach and rectum (Lozupone et al., 2012). Over the past three decades, researchers have explored many gene-based and culture-based methods for analyzing microbiome profiling. Currently, it is widely documented that *Actinobacteria*, *Firmicutes*, *Bacteroidetes*, and *Proteobacteria* phyla are the primary components of the human gut microbiota (Ağagündüz et al., 2023). These microbiomes induce GI carcinogenesis by targeting various signaling pathways, as given in **Table 3.1**.

3.1.3 Global Burden of GI Cancer

In 2020, more than 4.8 million fresh cases of GI cancer were documented. According to GLOBOCON 2020 data, CRC ranked third in terms of incidence with 1.9 million cases, and second in mortality. Globally, 1 million new cases of stomach cancer have been reported, ranking fifth in incidence and fourth in mortality. Liver cancer was the sixth most prevalent type of cancer, with 90,600 new cases diagnosed, and it is the third leading cause of cancer-related deaths. Esophageal cancer ranked seventh in incidence, with 60,400 new cases, and sixth in mortality. Due to its poor prognosis, pancreatic cancer was ranked as the seventh leading cause of cancer-related deaths (Sung et al., 2021).

Owing to the high mortality rate and the susceptibility of the microbiota in the GI tract, this chapter seeks to investigate the correlation between GI cancer and the gut microbiome, as well as the prospective therapeutic function of probiotic nano-formulation (PNF) in treating GI cancers, with an emphasis on personalized cancer therapy.

3.2 THE IMPACT OF PROBIOTICS ON GUT MICROBES

In the 20th century, it was observed that infants receiving their mothers' milk were found to be healthy, displaying the presence of *Bifidobacteria* in their gut microbiota, establishing a positive connection between health and gut microbiota. This discovery prompted extensive research to unravel the underlying mechanisms, revealing certain bacteria's positive correlation with overall health. While *Lactobacillus* is the most employed probiotic, numerous other beneficial microbes exist, and their usage was contingent upon their origin and health-friendly attributes. Each bacterial strain possesses specific properties; some are effective in addressing obesity, others in treating diabetes mellitus (DM), some contribute to chronic kidney disease (CKD) management, and some are involved in osteoporosis care (Abraham & Quigley, 2017). Beyond these, numerous studies have affirmed the beneficial role of probiotics in irritable bowel syndrome (IBS) and wound healing (Abraham & Quigley, 2017; Mu et al., 2018). Furthermore, probiotics have been explored for their potential in promoting oral health and enhancing the

TABLE 3.1
List of Microbiomes and Their Mechanistic Role in GI Carcinogenesis

GI Cancers	Carcinogenic Microbiome	Mechanism of Action	Reference
Esophageal cancer	*Fusobacterium nucleatum*	Increased expression of chemokines, activation of TLR4 triggering NFκB pathway	Zhou et al. (2021)
	Helicobacter pylori	Production of genotoxins and upregulating ROS	
Gastric cancer	*H. pylori*	Activation of β-catenin and Ras/MEK/ERK pathway, overexpression of cyclin D1	Nasr et al. (2020)
	Non-H. pylori gastric bacteria *(Porphyromonas gingivalis* and *F. nucleatum)*	Increased reactive oxygen species activity	
Colorectal cancer	*F. nucleatum, Streptococcus bovis/gallolyticus, H. pylori*, enterotoxigenic *Bacteroides fragilis*	Increased expression of β-catenin, NFκB pathways, impairs the anti-tumor immune response	Vogtmann and Goedert (2016)
	Escherichia coli	Causes DNA double-stranded breaks	
	Enterococcus faecalis and *Peptostreptococcus anaerobius*	DNA damage by reactive oxygen species and extra superoxide	
	F. nucleatum	Activates NF-κB in intestinal epithelial cells via the ALPK1/TIFA/TRAF6 pathway	Martin-Gallausiaux et al. (2024)
Liver cancer	*Ruminococcus, Enterococcus*	Activation of TLR-2 and mTOR pathway by deoxycholic acid (DCA)	Yu and Schwabe (2017)
	Enterobacteriaceae, Veillonellaceae	TLR-4 upregulates expression of epiregulin	
Pancreatic cancer	*P. gingivalis, Actinobacillus actinomycetemcomitans*	LPS-TLR4 interaction activates NFκB and activator-protein 1	Wang et al. (2019a)

immune system (Iqbal Khan, 2019). According to the latest survey, a high percentage of gastroenterologists (97%) and nutritionists (98%) have endorsed the efficacy of probiotics in GI tract management and have affirmed their safety (Valdovinos-García et al., 2019). Further, recent advancements in sequencing technology have shown that the gut microbiota plays a significant role in the onset and sequence of different tumors. Particularly, alterations in gut microbial biochemicals, such as short-chain fatty acids (SCFAs) and tryptophan metabolites, resulted in a significant impact on the development of different types of tumors (Jaye et al., 2022). Thus, focusing on the gut microbiota could represent a novel curative approach for personalized cancer therapy.

3.3 THE SIGNIFICANCE OF PROBIOTICS AGAINST GI CANCERS

The scientific community has shown a growing interest in utilizing probiotic therapy for preventing and treating various GI disorders (**Figure 3.1**). Additionally, epidemiological evidence supports the protective role of probiotics against cancer. Extensive research has demonstrated that probiotics have antiproliferative or pro-apoptotic effects in GI cancers (**Table 3.2**), with a particular focus on colon and GC cells (De Preter et al., 2011; Kumar et al., 2010).

TABLE 3.2
Mechanism of Probiotics and PNFs in Inducing Anticancer Activity in Relation to GI Cancers

Probiotics/PNFs	Types of GI Cancer	Mechanisms Involved in Prevention of GI Cancers	References
Bifidobacterium longum and *Lactobacillus acidophilus*	Esophageal cancer	Reduction in the expression of CDX1 (caudal type homeobox 1), COX-2, TNF-α, and p53. Conversely, there was an upregulation in the expression level of IL-18	Spechler (2013)
Lactobacillus casei, *Bifidobacterium* spp., and *Lacticaseibacillus rhamnosus*	Esophageal cancer	Inhibition of tumor growth by influencing genes associated with signal transduction pathways	Abbaszadegan et al. (2018)
Lactobacillus casei	Pancreatic cancer	Inhibition of cancer growth triggering the expression of DNA damage-inducible transcript-3 (DDIT3)	Iwama et al. (2021)
Lactobacillus plantarum and *L. rhamnosus*	Gastric cancer	Increased expression of MUC2 and MUC3 genes suggests their ability to restore gastric mucosal integrity and prevent pathogenic bacterial adhesion	Borruel et al. (2003)
Lactobacilli	Gastric cancer	Inhibit *Helicobacter pylori* through various immunological and non-immunological mechanisms	
Lactobacillus reuteri	Gastric cancer	Inhibit cancer metastasis by decreasing the expression of uPA and uPAR genes	Borruel et al. (2003)
L. gasseri	Gastric cancer	Reducing TNF and IL-6 secretion in macrophages by enhancing IgA levels and strengthening mucosal barriers	Zhang et al. (2020)
F. nucleatum	Colon cancer	Hinder human T-cell responses, disturb the cell cycle, prompt apoptotic cell death in specific immune cells, and regulate the tumor microenvironment, thus slowing down tumor progression	Lee et al. (2018)
L. acidophilus, *B. longum*, and *L. gasseri*	Colon cancer	Reducing tumor size and burden and inhibiting the expression of COX-2 and β-catenin in colon cancer	Gong et al. (2017)
Ligilactobacillus salivarius	Colon cancer	Suppresses DMH-induced colon cancer	Zhang et al. (2020)
Lacticaseibacillus paracasei SD1 and *L. rhamnosus* SD11	Colon cancer	Inhibits the growth of Caco-2 cells, although their effect on HIEC-6 cells	Dikeocha et al. (2021)
L. rhamnosus and *Pediococcus pentosaceus*	Colon cancer	Effectively impedes the proliferation of DLD-1 cells, inducing G2 cell cycle arrest by downregulating CDK1/Cyclin B1 expression	Khaleel et al. (2023)
L. casei	Pancreatic cancer	Immune checkpoint inhibitors	Chaib et al. (2022a)
Bifidobacterium pseudolongum	Pancreatic cancer	Inhibit the cancer cell growth in both mouse model and pancreatic cancer cell lines	Iwama et al. (2021)
AuNP-bacteria–EPS–MNP	Gastric cancer	Magnetic hyperthermia and photothermal therapy	Garcés et al. (2022)

(*Continued*)

TABLE 3.2 (*Continued*)
Mechanism of Probiotics and PNFs in Inducing Anticancer Activity in Relation to GI Cancers

Probiotics/PNFs	Types of GI Cancer	Mechanisms Involved in Prevention of GI Cancers	References
Curto-Cumin AuNP	Gastric cancer	Upregulation of p53, Bcl-associated X protein (Bax), and caspase-9/caspase-3 and activation of autophagy flux-related biomarkers, such as LC3b/a, Beclin-1, p62, and caspase-8	Dhandapani et al. (2021)
L. paracasei GMNL-133	Gastric cancer	Upregulation of cleaved PARP, caspase-8, caspase-9, and caspase-3	Huang et al. (2024)
Escherichia coli/BPQDs	Colon cancer	By simulating high level of ROS inside cancer cells	Ding et al. (2021)
E. coli nanobodies	Colon cancer	Targeting PD-L1 and CTLA-4	Gurbatri et al. (2020)
Selenium nanoparticle–enriched *L. casei*	Colon cancer	Upregulation of TRAILR1/DR4, TRAILR2/DR5, XIAP, PON2, and catalase and downregulation of survivin, cIAP-1, HIF-1a, and cytochrome-c	Spyridopoulou et al. (2021)
DOX/SOR/Spore-DA and DOX/SOR/Spore-HA	Colon cancer	Upregulation of caspase-3, caspase-9, and Bax and downregulation of Bcl-2	Song et al. (2019)
EcN@TTVP	Colon cancer	Cherenkov radiation-induced photodynamic therapy	Zhu et al. (2023)
SPORE-MGEM	Pancreatic cancer	Intratumoral drug accumulation in the pancreatic tumor site	Han et al. (2022)

3.3.1 Role of Probiotics against Esophageal Cancer

Barrett's esophagus is a medical condition characterized by damage to the lining of the lower esophagus, typically resulting from exposure to stomach acid. This condition is associated with the development of esophageal cancer. Conversely, the intervention with both probiotic strains caused an increased expression level of IL-18 (Spechler, 2013). Research investigations indicate a notable change in the microbial community in the esophagus during esophagitis episodes or esophageal cancer. Notably, in cases of esophageal cancer, there was a drop in *Streptococcal* species and an increase in gram-negative anaerobic bacteria or microaerophiles, including *Peptostreptococcus*, *Prevotella*, *Fusobacterium*, and *Neisseria* (Mozaffari Namin et al., 2015). When esophageal cancer patients were compared to healthy persons, Deng et al. (2021) identified a reduction in energy metabolism pathways (Deng et al., 2021).

GI bacteria regularly produce the SCFAs butyrate, propionate, and acetate as metabolites. SCFAs play a critical role in controlling apoptosis, cellular differentiation, and inflammation in host cells, essential for the metabolism of bacterial energy and general health. SCFAs also have anticancer qualities and serve as molecular signals. Additionally, Deng's research showed that individuals with esophageal cancer had higher levels of *Firmicutes* and *Actinobacteria* but lower levels of *Bacteroides*, which led to an increased *Firmicutes*-to-*Bacteroides* ratio. These changes in the gut microbiota may be related to inflammation and dysbiosis in patients with esophageal cancer (Ge et al., 2021). Probiotic microbes such as *Lactobacilli* are widely known for having significant anti-tumor effects. Also, the cell wall peptidoglycans, heat-killed cells, and cytoplasmic extracts can induce apoptosis in several cancer cell types. Moreover, research has shown that *Bifidobacterium* and *Lactobacillus casei* cytoplasmic extracts can affect cancer cell growth and multiplication. Furthermore, *Lacticaseibacillus rhamnosus* has demonstrated the prevention of tumor growth through its influence on genes related to signal transduction pathways (Abbaszadegan et al., 2018). In a study by Namin et al. (2015), it was found that treatment with *Bifidobacterium longum* and *Lactobacillus acidophilus* in cell lines associated with Barrett's esophagus led to a decrease in the interaction of COX-2, TNF-α, CDX1 (caudal type homeobox 1), and p53, thereby inhibiting cancer cell proliferation. These pathways offer intriguing targets for cancer treatment and are important players in the initiation and progression of cancer (Mozaffari Namin et al., 2015).

3.3.2 Role of Probiotics in Combating Pancreatic Cancer

Ferrichromes are tiny, high-affinity molecules that bacteria produce for iron chelation and have shown anti-tumor potential by promoting the expression of DNA damage-inducible transcript-3 (DDIT3) in colon, pancreatic, and stomach cancer cells (Iwama et al., 2021). In a recent study, Chaib et al. (2022) emphasized the possibility of treating pancreatic cancer with immune checkpoint inhibitors, including PD-L1 inhibitors, in combination with ferrichrome (Chaib et al., 2022).

3.3.3 Role of Probiotics in Treating Gastric Cancer

GC stands as a prominent worldwide threat of mortality, with *H. pylori* infection frequently implicated in its onset by colonizing the stomach lining. Probiotics exhibit promise in ameliorating *H. pylori*-linked ailments by provoking inflammatory reactions against *H. pylori*. It elevates pro-inflammatory cytokine levels like IL-2, IL-8, IL-6, IL-1β, and TNF-α in the stomach lining (Borruel et al., 2003; Maleki-Kakelar et al., 2019), thereby inhibiting bacterial adhesion to epithelial cells which hinders the *H. pylori* replication. In addition, probiotics attack *H. pylori* by emitting antimicrobial substances like hydrogen peroxide, lactic acid, bacteriocins, SCFA, and molecules that resemble reuterin and reutericyclin.

Lactobacillus and *Bifidobacterium* rank among the most prevalent probiotic strains, with *Lactobacilli* particularly exhibiting inhibitory effects on *H. pylori* via diverse immunological and non-immunological mechanisms (Borruel et al., 2003). Studies investigating the effect of probiotics on GC have revealed that Lactobacillus *plantarum* might have a role in modulating PTEN/AKT signaling pathways associated with *H. pylori*-induced gastric carcinogenesis. The potential of *L. plantarum* and *L. rhamnosus* to restore gastric mucosal integrity and prevent pathogenic bacterial adhesion has been proven by the elevated expression of MUC2 and MUC3 genes in research (Keikha & Karbalaei, 2021). Additionally, *Lactobacillus reuteri* exhibits the potential to curtail cancer metastasis by reducing uPA and uPAR gene expression. Also, various *Lactobacillus* strains demonstrate efficacy in diminishing *H. pylori* attachment and invasion of gastric epithelial cells, along with IL-8 reduction. Furthermore, *Lactobacillus gasseri* has shown promise in dampening IL-6 and TNF secretion in macrophages, suggesting the role of probiotics in pathogenic inhibition through heightened IgA levels and fortified mucosal barriers (Ballesteros-Álvarez et al., 2023; Zhang et al., 2020).

UroA, a metabolite produced by the gut microbiota from ellagitannins and their derivatives, demonstrated anti-GC application by inducing cell apoptosis *in vitro* and *in vivo* (Ballesteros-Álvarez et al., 2023). Furthermore, UroA was found to stimulate autophagy, subsequently activating the downstream Hippo pathway. This activation led to the suppression of the Warburg effect, a metabolic phenomenon associated with cancer cells, and facilitated cell apoptosis, suggesting the potential of UroA in the treatment of GC (Qiao et al., 2024).

3.3.4 Role of Probiotics in Suppressing Colorectal Cancer

CRC, being the most prevalent GI malignancy, represents a significant health concern. Recent research underscores a unique connection between probiotics and CRC, highlighting their ability to regulate the gut microbiota and deter cancer progression (Thirabunyanon et al., 2009). The composition of the gut microbiome profoundly influences the immune system, with specific attention drawn to *F. nucleatum*'s role in CRC. Research suggests that *F. nucleatum* can hinder human T-cell responses, interrupt the cell cycle, trigger apoptotic cell death in specific immune cells, and alter the tumor microenvironment, thereby impeding tumor progression. These immunosuppressive effects may impact the mortality rates of CRC patients (Nosho, 2016).

Moreover, a study conducted by Compare and Nardone (2014) demonstrated that probiotics, such as VSL#3, *L. acidophilus*, *B. longum*, and *L. gasseri*, have the potential to improve CRC by decreasing the size and burden of tumors. Further, co-administration of inulin with *B. longum* and *Bifidobacterium lactis* controlled chemically induced CRC by inducing apoptotic response (Compare & Nardone, 2014). In a study conducted by Kuugbee et al. (2016), it was discovered that a combination of probiotics, specifically *L. acidophilus*, *Bifidobacterium bifidum*, and *Bifidobacterium longum* subsp. *infantis* along with oligofructose and maltodextrin (referred to as LBB), could regulate the composition of the intestinal microbiota and suppress the expression of COX-2 and β-catenin in CRC animal models. This intervention successfully decreased the occurrence, number, and size of tumors, thereby hindering the advancement of CRC (Kuugbee et al., 2016).

Additionally, it has been observed that the consumption of a probiotic mixture produces better effects than the administration of a single probiotic strain since it increases the diversity of the intestinal microbiota and encourages the synergy between probiotic strains for optimal outcomes. Furthermore, studies by Momo et al. (2022) examined a novel pyran derivative from *L. plantarum* H24 with significant antioxidant and anticancer effects, representing it as a promising anticancer drug (Momo et al., 2022). Sheng and colleagues (2022) investigated a novel exopolysaccharide derived from the probiotic bacterium *L. pantheris* TCP102. Their findings indicated that the exopolysaccharide exhibited immune-boosting and anticancer properties, indicating its potential utility in functional foods and natural anti-tumor therapy (Sheng et al., 2022). According to studies by Zhang et al. (2020), *Ligilactobacillus salivarius* Ren successfully prevented mice's colon cancer in treatment along with dimethylhydrazine (DMH) injection-induced changes in colon microbiota (Zhang et al., 2020). Moreover, a study by Pahumunto and Teanpaisan (2023) showed the effective antibacterial efficacy of *L. rhamnosus* SD11 cells and their cell-free supernatants (CFS) by suppressing the pro-inflammatory cytokines in Caco-2 and HIEC-6 cells when exposed to probiotics (Pahumunto & Teanpaisan, 2023). Particularly, *Lacticaseibacillus paracasei* SD1 and *L. rhamnosus* SD11 exhibited substantially greater suppression levels by increasing the expression of IL-10 and hBD (Dikeocha et al., 2021). In the CRC cell line DLD-1, P8, derived from the probiotic bacterium *L. rhamnosus*, exhibits anticancer properties. It was integrated into *Pediococcus pentosaceus*, serving as a vector for intestinal P8 expression and secretion. P8 diminishes the expression of CDK1/Cyclin B1, so effectively inhibiting the proliferation of DLD-1 cells and inducing G2 cell cycle arrest (Khaleel et al., 2023).

3.3.5 Role of Probiotics in Thwarting Liver Cancer

Liver cancer stands out as one of the malignancies among the top five most fatal cancers that sees an annual increase in occurrence. Various factors, including HBV, HCV, NAFLD, cirrhosis due to alcohol consumption, smoking, elevated iron levels, obesity, diabetes, and other dietary factors, contribute to the progression of liver disease. The study by Heydari et al. (2019) has investigated the carcinogenesis-related genes in 38 BALB/c mice. The mice were categorized into four groups, including a control group that received no medication, and a group of mice treated with azoxymethane (AOM) but without any probiotic treatment. The remaining group of mice treated with AOM was divided into two subgroups, each receiving a distinct type of probiotics: *L. acidophilus* and *B. bifidum* (IV). The result suggested significant activity of the probiotic at microRNA and gene expression levels, showing the upregulation of miR-221, miR-155, Bcl-w, and KRAS, and downregulation of miR-122, PTEN, and PU.1 post-treatment (Heydari et al., 2019).

In a retrospective analysis of 1267 HBV-infected individuals, two cohorts were compared for HCC risk, of which one cohort comprised 449 probiotic users with ≥28 cumulative prescribed daily doses (cDDD), while the other included 818 non-users with <28 cDDD. Propensity score matching (PSM) addressed confounding variables, revealing a reduced HCC risk with probiotic use. Adjusted hazard ratios (aHRs) for cDDDs showed decreasing risks: 0.58, 0.28, and 0.12 for cDDDs of 28–89, 90–180, and >180, respectively, while the incidence of HCC decreased with increasing cDDD ranges: 8.7%, 4.7%, and 3.0% for 28–89, 90–180, and >180, respectively. Hence, the result suggests probiotic reduces the HCC risk (Song et al., 2023).

A study investigating the effects of *Bifidobacterium pseudolongum* on NAFLD and HCC utilized two murine models: one subjected to a high-fat, cholesterol-enriched diet and the other to a high-fat, choline-deficient diet. Metabolomic investigations were conducted on germ-free mice using portal vein, fecal, and liver tissue samples. Human NAFLD and HCC cell lines were co-cultured with a conditioned medium from *Bacteroides pseudolongum* and a potential metabolite. Results demonstrated significant depletion of *B. pseudolongum* in mice with NAFLD and HCC, and oral administration inhibited HCC progression in both models. Acetate, a primary metabolite produced by *B. pseudolongum*, showed inhibitory effects on cell proliferation and promoted cell death in HCC cell lines (Song et al., 2023).

Hence, various research has indicated that probiotics may contribute to the treatment and prevention of GI cancers by maintaining gut microbial equilibrium, improving the intestinal barrier, and activating immune responses. Additionally, probiotics have shown their potential to reduce inflammation, improve the efficacy of cancer therapies, and alleviate symptoms associated with GI cancers. Despite the numerous benefits of probiotic therapy, constraints such as reduced viability and off-target effects demand the advancement of probiotic-based nano-formulations. These formulations offer targeted treatment for cancer and thereby enhance the effectiveness of personalized cancer therapy.

3.4 EMERGING PROBIOTIC NANO-FORMULATIONS

Drug delivery methods based on nanoparticles (NPs) have demonstrated numerous benefits in the treatment of cancer, including improved pharmacokinetics, accurate targeting of tumor cells, decreased side effects, and decreased susceptibility to drug resistance (Dadwal et al., 2018). The size and properties of NPs utilized in drug delivery systems are often selected or created to correspond with the pathophysiology of patients' malignancies (Palazzolo et al., 2018; Yao et al., 2020a). Probiotic nano-formulation or nano-probiotics (PNF) refers to the encapsulation of probiotic or probiotics along with NPs or probiotic's bioactive material encapsulated into the NP for increasing the bioavailability of probiotic compounds by enhancing their GI absorption. Concisely, the PNFs are dedicated to enhancing the outcome of cancer treatment by delivering probiotics that were specifically chosen based on the intestinal microbiome of the patient, as represented in **Figure 3.2**.

Screening of the patient's dysbiotic gut, selection of desired probiotics that help in altering the gut microbiome to normal, growth of the desired probiotics, synthesis of probiotic nano-formulation (PNF) for precise drug delivery, and administration of PNFs to patients with particular dysbiosis are personalized cancer treatment.

3.4.1 NEED FOR PROBIOTIC NANO-FORMULATION

As described earlier, probiotics are live microorganisms with beneficial effects on or inside the body. To enhance personalized cancer treatment, an adequate quantity of the desired microbes

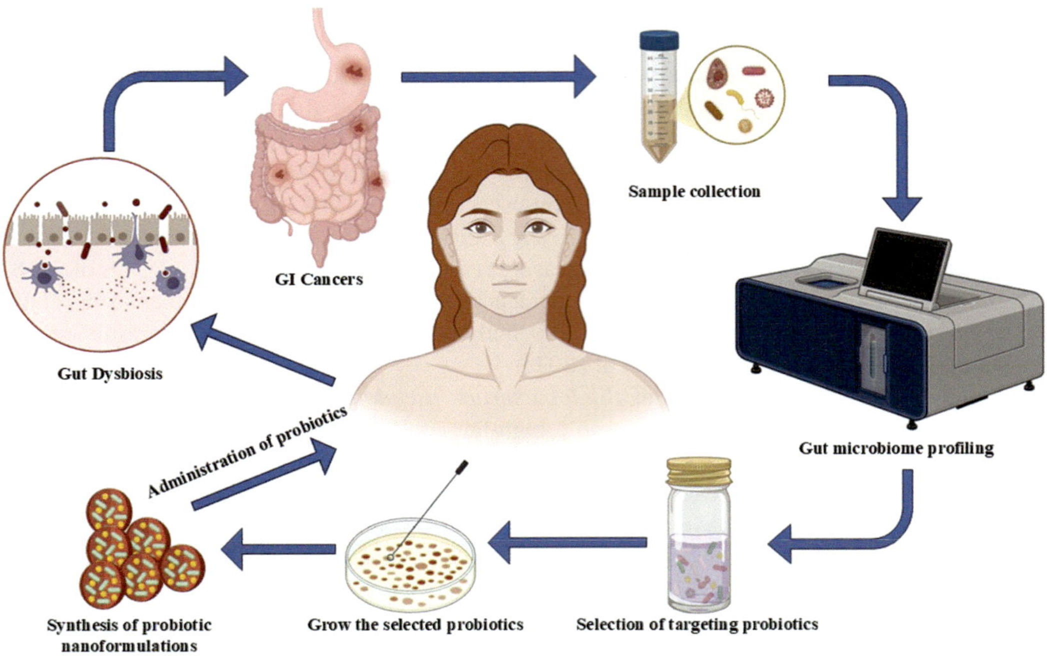

FIGURE 3.2 Role of PNF in personalized cancer therapy.

needs to reach the desired site. Owing to their restricted bioavailability and rapid renal clearance, inadequate quantities of probiotics will reach the targeted site, ultimately diminishing their effectiveness in personalized cancer treatment. In addition, several physicochemical parameters influence the survivability of probiotics, including temperature, oxygen toxicity, and pH, which they encounter during production (Singh et al., 2022). Beyond that, biological factors such as survival in the GI tract play a vital role in determining the viability of probiotics. The bile acid in the liver and small intestine has antimicrobial properties and detergent action, which disrupts the bacterial cell membrane and causes DNA damage, thereby reducing bacterial cell viability (Hamner et al., 2013; Yao et al., 2018, 2020b). Thus, encapsulated probiotic therapy effectively addresses these constraints and provides health advantages to patients and consumers. Most food industries use various techniques, including cryogenic preservation, spray drying, foam drying, freeze drying, and electrospray-coating atomization (EA) technologies, to increase the optimism of the probiotic culture. Among these, EA has proven to be an effective method to enhance the viability of probiotics. Particles with well-controlled sizes, morphologies, structures, and forms can be obtained using the EA approach, which is simple but reliable for various applications.

Also, EA has shown a surge in probiotic viability for up to one year at room temperature compared to the freeze-drying technique (Librán et al., 2017). Since the probiotics are subjected to various physiochemical stresses in the above processes, such as sudden exposure to very high temperatures and switching to very low temperatures to pasteurize the product, their viability was greatly affected. Hence to assure an optimum delivery of desired probiotics, PNF serves as a viable method for enhancing the probiotic delivery (Singh et al., 2022), especially for personalized cancer treatment.

3.4.2 Advantages of Having PNF

PNF has several advantages over conventional probiotic delivery (**Figure 3.3**), such as improved high probiotic load, enhanced cell viability, controlled drug release, and enhanced stability.

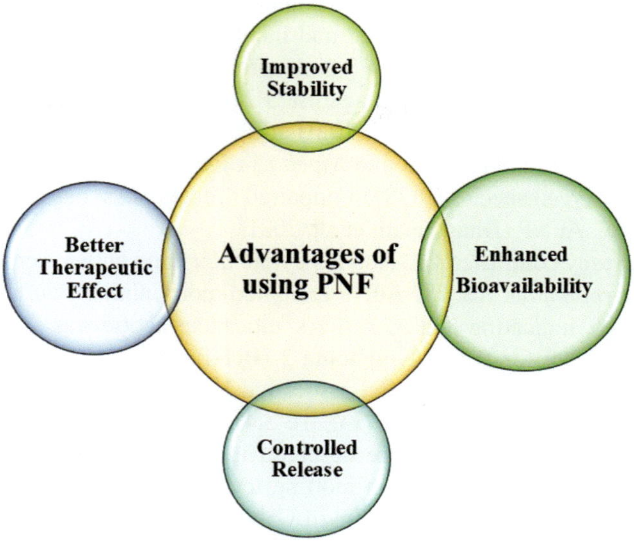

FIGURE 3.3 Advantages of using probiotic nano-formulations (PNF).

Probiotics with the ability to form 10^7 CFU/mL or gram are found to be highly viable. PNF protects the probiotics from exposure to various external factors, such as pressure, temperature changes, and oxidation during food processing and storage, thereby improving their viability. Thus, preservation of viability ensures that probiotics remain metabolically active and effective until they reach the target site. In addition, PNF also ensures controlled probiotic release, which prevents the onset release of probiotics before reaching the target site. PNFs are designed in such a way that they release the probiotics on reaching the lower GI tract so that a higher quantity of probiotics can be released in the desired region, increasing their potential health benefits (Razavi et al., 2021; Sun et al., 2023). Hence, the sustained drug release by PNF facilitates the long-term exposure of the gut or targeted site to the desired probiotic, thereby enhancing the effectiveness of personalized cancer therapy.

3.5 ENCAPSULATED PNF FOR ITS APPLICATION AGAINST GI CANCERS

Several side effects of GI cancer, such as diarrhea, bowel blockage, radiation enteritis, constipation, and fecal impaction, affect both the patients and the duration of therapy. These GI complications often contribute to dose adjustments, treatment delays, and, in severe cases, cessation of anticancer therapy, affecting treatment outcomes (PDQ Supportive and Palliative Care Editorial Board, 2002; Uranga et al., 2023). To surmount these obstacles, probiotics are encapsulated into NPs and directed to augment their anticancer efficacy, as detailed in **Table 3.2**.

3.5.1 PNF as an Effective Medication for Gastric Cancer

The probiotic *Limosilactobacillus fermentum*, as an oral medication transporter, could lead to novel therapeutic strategies for gastric diseases, such as oral cancer medications combined with photothermal therapy and magnetic hyperthermia. This approach involves the simultaneous loading of *L. fermentum* with both magnetic and gold NPs, resulting in AuNP MNP-bacteria systems where both NP types reside within the same layer of bacterial exopolysaccharides (EPS). Another approach involved loading the probiotic with gold NPs first, followed by loading it with magnetic NPs to yield AuNP-bacteria–EPS–MNP with the NPs arranged in two different EPS layers. Both combinations showed prominent anticancer applications when compared with individual compounds. Gold nanoprisms and gold nanorods were too prepared and incubated with *L. fermentum*, resulting in the attachment of aggregated nanoprisms and EPS of the probiotic bacteria with reduced spherical gold NPs that have improved cytotoxic potential against GC (Garcés et al., 2022). Curto-Cumin AuNP (CC-AuNP) was synthesized by Dandapani (2021) utilizing membrane vesicles from the probiotic bacteria *Curtobacterium proimmune* K3 and *Nigella sativa* seed extract. Moreover, the excessive formation of reactive oxygen species (ROS) in impaired mitochondria has been associated with the cytotoxic effects of CC-AuNP (Dhandapani et al., 2021).

Additionally, the study contrasted CC-AuNP's cytotoxicity and anticancer properties with those of *N. sativa* and *C. proimmune* K3. CC-AuNP exhibited more inhibitory effect against AGS cells than the other samples, indicating that *N. sativa*'s anticancer action was amplified by its conversion into gold NPs. Except for B cell lymphoma 2 (Bcl-2), the results showed that the intracellular apoptotic signaling molecules, p53, Bcl-associated X protein (Bax), and caspase-9/caspase-3, were considerably increased in AGS cells (**Figure 3.4**). Moreover, ROS generation and changes in mitochondrial membrane potential were observed in AGS cells treated with CC-AuNP. The expression results from qPCR and Western blotting techniques confirmed the overexpression of autophagy flux-associated biomarkers, including LC3b/a, Beclin-1, p62, and caspase-8. According to this study, CC-AuNP could be a potential therapeutic agent used to treat GC (Dhandapani et al., 2021). To enhance the therapeutic efficacy in treating GC, a possible NP formulation encapsulating the *L. paracasei* GMNL-133 (SGMNL-133) isolate was created. This novel strategy prevented the SGMNL-133 from being broken down by gastric acid, made it easier to pass through the mucous layer, and allowed it to communicate with GC cells. Additionally, studies conducted *in vivo* showed

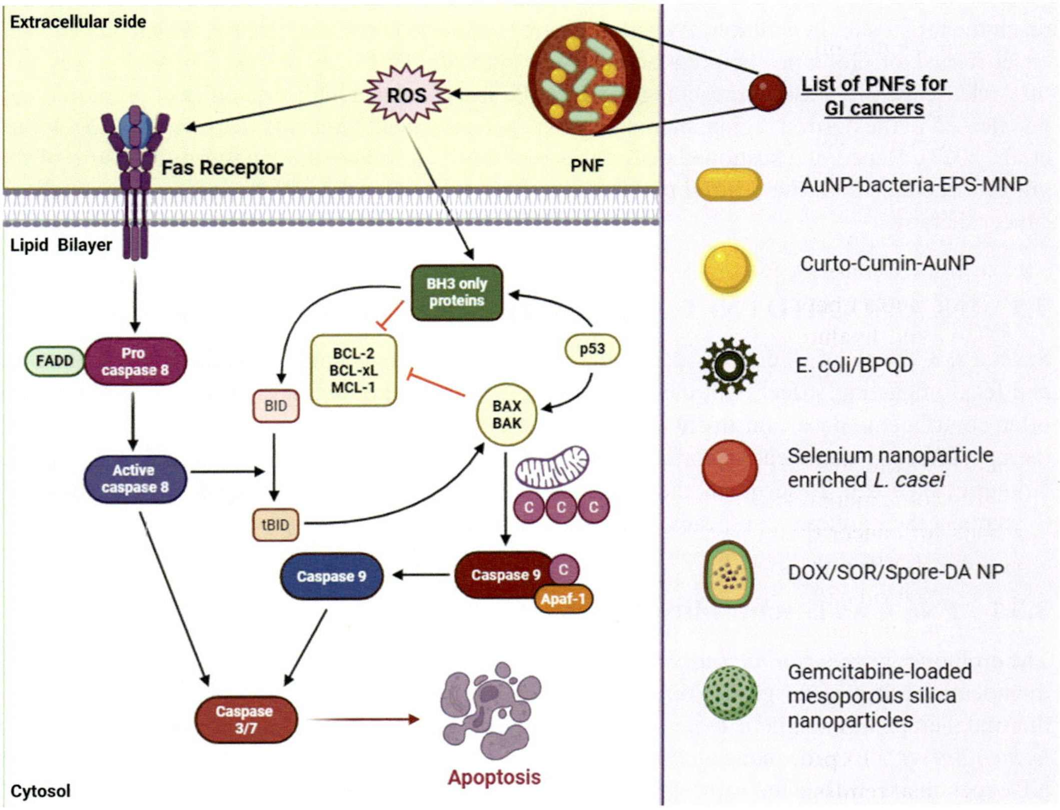

FIGURE 3.4 Mechanism of action of PNF in the induction of apoptosis.

that the addition of SGMNL-133 to NPs significantly increased their efficacy in treating orthotopic gastric tumors while also lowering tissue inflammatory markers (Huang et al., 2024).

Many PNFs are known to trigger apoptosis by generating ROS. The production of ROS simulates the interaction between the Fas ligand and the Fas receptor, which induces the extrinsic apoptosis signaling. Similarly, ROS activates the BH3-only protein, which stimulates the intrinsic signaling pathway by upregulating BAK and BAX. Both pathways activate caspase-3/7 through downstream processes, thereby inducing apoptosis.

3.5.2 Effectiveness of PNF in Combating Colon Cancer

The *E. coli*/BPQDs (EB) system was developed by linking catalase-expressing genetically engineered *E. coli* to black phosphorus quantum dots (BPQDs). This system could target hypoxic tumor tissues on intravenous delivery and facilitate efficient photodynamic treatment. During 660 nm laser irradiation, BPQD-mediated ROS production and bacterial membrane rupture were induced, which led to the release of catalase. By catalyzing the breakdown of hydrogen peroxide to produce oxygen, catalase was able to reduce hypoxia and improve the PDT effectiveness of BPQDs. This treatment approach effectively suppressed tumor growth in both *in vitro* and *in vivo* conditions (Ding et al., 2021).

In the same way, *E. coli* was genetically modified to produce and release nanobodies that target CTLA-4 and PD-L1 under regulated conditions. In animal models, the modified probiotic system showed an improved therapeutic response in comparison to therapeutically relevant antibodies, leading to tumor shrinkage after just one injection. Additionally, there was an improvement in the quantity of activated T cells, memory populations of systemic T cells, and abscopal impact caused by the probiotic delivery of checkpoint inhibitors. Granulocyte-macrophage colony-stimulating factor (GM-CSF), a probiotic-produced cytokine, was used with the platform's flexibility to improve therapeutic efficacy. The probiotic system provides a localized and sustained therapeutic release, minimizing the risk of systemic toxicities (Gurbatri et al., 2020). In the CT26 syngeneic CRC model in BALB/c mice, the anticancer activity of *L. casei*, *L. casei*-derived selenium NPs, and selenium NP–enriched *L. casei*, as well as their anti-tumor potential, demonstrated that, *in vitro*, these substances exhibit cancer-specific antiproliferative activity. In cancer cells, the NPs were also observed to increase ROS levels and cause apoptosis. Oral administration of *L. casei* loaded with selenium NPs diminished the development of colon cancer in mice more successfully than either *L. casei* or the isolated NPs, indicating a possible synergistic impact between the probiotic and the NPs (Spyridopoulou et al., 2021). Deoxycholic acid (DA) and hyaluronic acid (HA) were used to modify *Bacillus coagulans* spores, which were then loaded with chemotherapeutic medicines (doxorubicin and sorafenib, DOX/SOR) to generate an independent NP manufacturing line (NPs). These NPs can shield medications from harm when they travel through the stomach and quickly settle in the intestinal area. Through the bile acid pathway, the DOX/SOR/Spore-DA and DOX/SOR/Spore-HA NPs can effectively enter epithelial cells, increasing basolateral drug release. This biological nanogenerator is a promising approach for cancer therapy because studies have demonstrated that it can produce substantial quantities of NPs on its own in the gut (Song et al., 2019). Another potential treatment involves using a biohybrid called EcNTTVP, which consists of *E. coli* Nissle 1917 (EcN) loaded with an aggregation-induced emission photosensitizer (AIE-PS) called TTVP. This biohybrid is administered along with radiopharmaceutical 18F-fluorodeoxyglucose (18F-FDG) to co-augment the tumor spot and trigger Cerenkov radiation–induced photodynamic therapy (CR-PDT). EcN serves as an immunoadjuvant by enhancing the maturation of dendritic cells (DCs) and cytotoxic T cell (CTL) priming. This synergistic treatment of CR-PDT and immunotherapy results in the efficient remission or prolonged survival of tumor-bearing mice. The suggested medicinal strategy based on EcNTTVP shows potential for clinical translation and may provide considerations for deep-seated tumor therapy (Zhu et al., 2023).

3.5.3 PNF as an Emerging Medication for Treating Pancreatic Cancer

Probiotics have been used to build a new drug delivery method that improves chemotherapy for pancreatic cancer. The medication carriers in this system are *Clostridium butyricum* spores, which are resistant to severe external stress. The spores were coupled with the gemcitabine-loaded mesoporous silicon NPs (MGEM) to increase the efficacy of chemotherapy. The study found that this system resulted in three times higher drug accumulation within the tumor compared to conventional delivery methods, without any side effects (Han et al., 2022). Still, more studies are needed to be performed to confirm the findings of Han et al. (2022).

3.6 FUTURE PERSPECTIVES AND CONCLUSION

Personalized cancer therapy integrated with PNFs, an emerging therapeutic technique with robust anticancer activity. Probiotic-based therapies facilitate understanding of an individual's microbiome and assist in offering customized cancer treatment. Due to the various disadvantages of direct probiotic treatment, PNF can be utilized to enhance personalized cancer therapy. Nanostructured systems can enhance solubility, control the release of bioactive compounds, and protect probiotics during storage and transportation. Additionally, PNFs allow precise delivery of probiotics and can facilitate personalized, targeted therapy to specific sites in the body with *in vivo* investigations demonstrating the safety and efficacy of PNFs. Current studies have shown the apoptosis and autophagy mechanism of anticancer application, while other cancer signaling pathways involved in GI progression need to be explored. Still, many probiotics with significant anticancer applications can be targeted in the future with liver and esophageal cancer, which remains unexplored for PNF treatment. Also, the integration of nanofibers can function as carriers for probiotics, providing advantages such as a large surface area, robust mechanical capabilities, and the ability to regulate the release of probiotics. In brief, the integration of probiotics and nanotechnology has significant prospects for personalized treatment, illness prevention, and enhanced therapeutic results. Many fascinating research breakthroughs still need to be explored with PNF against GI cancers.

REFERENCES

Abbaszadegan, M. R., Riahi, A., Forghanifard, M. M., & Moghbeli, M. (2018). WNT and NOTCH signaling pathways as activators for epidermal growth factor receptor in esophageal squamous cell carcinoma. *Cellular & Molecular Biology Letters*, *23*(1), 42. https://doi.org/10.1186/s11658-018-0109-x

Abraham, B. P., & Quigley, E. M. M. (2017). Probiotics in inflammatory bowel disease. *Gastroenterology Clinics of North America*, *46*(4), 769–782. https://doi.org/10.1016/j.gtc.2017.08.003

Ağagündüz, D., Cocozza, E., Cemali, Ö, Bayazıt, A. D., Nanì, M. F., Cerqua, I., Morgillo, F., Saygılı, S. K., Berni Canani, R., Amero, P., & Capasso, R. (2023). Understanding the role of the gut microbiome in gastrointestinal cancer: A review. *Frontiers in Pharmacology*, *14*. https://doi.org/10.3389/fphar.2023.1130562

Amara, A. A., & Shibl, A. (2015). Role of probiotics in health improvement, infection control and disease treatment and management. *Saudi Pharmaceutical Journal*, *23*(2), 107–114. https://doi.org/10.1016/j.jsps.2013.07.001

Arnold, M., Abnet, C. C., Neale, R. E., Vignat, J., Giovannucci, E. L., McGlynn, K. A., & Bray, F. (2020). Global burden of 5 major types of gastrointestinal cancer. *Gastroenterology*, *159*(1), 335–349.e15. https://doi.org/10.1053/j.gastro.2020.02.068

Ballesteros-Álvarez, J., Nguyen, W., Sivapatham, R., Rane, A., & Andersen, J. K. (2023). Urolithin A reduces amyloid-beta load and improves cognitive deficits uncorrelated with plaque burden in A mouse model of Alzheimer's disease. *GeroScience*, *45*(2), 1095–1113. https://doi.org/10.1007/s11357-022-00708-y

Borruel, N., Casellas, F., Antolin, M., Llopis, M., Carol, M., Espiin, E., Naval, J., Guarner, F., & Malagelada, J. R. (2003). Effects of nonpathogenic bacteria on cytokine secretion by human intestinal mucosa. *The American Journal of Gastroenterology*, *98*(4), 865–870. https://doi.org/10.1111/j.1572-0241.2003.07384.x

Chaib, M., Hafeez, B. B., Mandil, H., Daria, D., Pingili, A. K., Kumari, S., Sikander, M., Kashyap, V. K., Chen, G.-Y., Anning, E., Tripathi, M. K., Khan, S., Behrman, S., Yallapu, M. M., Jaggi, M., Makowski, L., & Chauhan, S. C. (2022). Reprogramming of pancreatic adenocarcinoma immunosurveillance by a microbial probiotic siderophore. *Communications Biology*, *5*(1), 1181. https://doi.org/10.1038/s42003-022-04102-4

Compare, D., & Nardone, G. (2014). The bacteria-hypothesis of colorectal cancer: Pathogenetic and therapeutic implications. *Translational Gastrointestinal Cancer*, *3*(1), 44–53.

Dadwal, A., Baldi, A., & Kumar Narang, R. (2018). Nanoparticles as carriers for drug delivery in cancer. *Artificial Cells, Nanomedicine, and Biotechnology*, *46*(sup2), 295–305. https://doi.org/10.1080/21691401.2018.1457039

Deng, Y., Tang, D., Hou, P., Shen, W., Li, H., Wang, T., & Liu, R. (2021). Dysbiosis of gut microbiota in patients with esophageal cancer. *Microbial Pathogenesis*, *150*, 104709. https://doi.org/10.1016/j.micpath.2020.104709

De Preter, V., Hamer, H. M., Windey, K., & Verbeke, K. (2011). The impact of pre- and/or probiotics on human colonic metabolism: Does it affect human health? *Molecular Nutrition & Food Research*, *55*(1), 46–57. https://doi.org/10.1002/mnfr.201000451

Dhandapani, S., Xu, X., Wang, R., Puja, A. M., Kim, H., Perumalsamy, H., Balusamy, S. R., & Kim, Y. J. (2021). Biosynthesis of gold nanoparticles using *Nigella sativa* and *Curtobacterium proimmune* K3 and evaluation of their anticancer activity. *Materials Science and Engineering C*, *127*. https://doi.org/10.1016/j.msec.2021.112214

Dikeocha, I. J., Al-Kabsi, A. M., Eid, E. E. M., Hussin, S., & Alshawsh, M. A. (2021). Probiotics supplementation in patients with colorectal cancer: A systematic review of randomized controlled trials. *Nutrition Reviews*, *80*(1), 22–49. https://doi.org/10.1093/nutrit/nuab006

Ding, S., Liu, Z., Huang, C., Zeng, N., Jiang, W., & Li, Q. (2021). Novel engineered bacterium/black phosphorus quantum dot hybrid system for hypoxic tumor targeting and efficient photodynamic therapy. *ACS Applied Materials & Interfaces*, *13*(8), 10564–10573. https://doi.org/10.1021/acsami.0c20254

Garcés, V., González, A., Gálvez, N., Delgado-López, J. M., Calvino, J. J., Trasobares, S., Fernández-Afonso, Y., Gutiérrez, L., & Dominguez-Vera, J. M. (2022). Magneto-optical hyperthermia agents based on probiotic bacteria loaded with magnetic and gold nanoparticles. *Nanoscale*, *14*(15), 5716–5724. https://doi.org/10.1039/D1NR08513A

Ge, Y., Shi, S., Deng, J. J., Chen, X. P., Song, Z., Liu, L., Lou, L., Zhang, X., & Xiong, X. F. (2021). Design, synthesis, and evaluation of small molecule Gαq/11 protein inhibitors for the treatment of uveal melanoma. *Journal of Medicinal Chemistry*, *64*(6), 3131–3152. https://doi.org/10.1021/acs.jmedchem.0c01977

Globocon (2024, July 24). *Absolute Numbers, Incidence, Both Sexes, in 2022*. World Health Organization.

Gong, J., Bai, T., Zhang, L., Qian, W., Song, J., & Hou, X. (2017). Inhibition effect of Bifidobacterium longum, Lactobacillus acidophilus, Streptococcus thermophilus and Enterococcus faecalis and their related products on human colonic smooth muscle in vitro. *PLoS One*, *12*, e0172925.

Gupta, V., & Garg, R. (2009). Probiotics. *Indian Journal of Medical Microbiology*, *27*(3), 202–209. https://doi.org/10.4103/0255-0857.53201

Gurbatri, C. R., Lia, I., Vincent, R., Coker, C., Castro, S., Treuting, P. M., Hinchliffe, T. E., Arpaia, N., & Danino, T. (2020). Engineered probiotics for local tumor delivery of checkpoint blockade nanobodies. *Science Translational Medicine*, *12*(530). https://doi.org/10.1126/scitranslmed.aax0876

Hamner, S., McInnerney, K., Williamson, K., Franklin, M. J., & Ford, T. E. (2013). Bile salts affect expression of *Escherichia coli* O157:H7 genes for virulence and iron acquisition, and promote growth under iron limiting conditions. *PLoS ONE*, *8*(9), e74647. https://doi.org/10.1371/journal.pone.0074647

Han, Z.-Y., Chen, Q.-W., Fu, Z.-J., Cheng, S.-X., & Zhang, X.-Z. (2022). Probiotic spore-based Oral drug delivery system for enhancing pancreatic cancer chemotherapy by Gut–Pancreas-axis-guided delivery. *Nano Letters*, *22*(21), 8608–8617. https://doi.org/10.1021/acs.nanolett.2c03131

Heydari, Z., Rahaie, M., & Alizadeh, A. M. (2019). Different anti-inflammatory effects of *Lactobacillus acidophilus* and *Bifidobactrum bifidioum* in hepatocellular carcinoma cancer mouse through impact on microRNAs and their target genes. *Journal of Nutrition & Intermediary Metabolism*, *16*, 100096. https://doi.org/10.1016/j.jnim.2019.100096

Huang, H.-L., Lai, C.-H., Tsai, W.-H., Chen, K.-W., Peng, S.-L., Lin, J.-H., & Lin, Y.-H. (2024). Nanoparticle-enhanced postbiotics: Revolutionizing cancer therapy through effective delivery. *Life Sciences*, *337*, 122379. https://doi.org/10.1016/j.lfs.2023.122379

Iqbal Khan, M. K. (Ed.). (2019). *Advances in Noninvasive Food Analysis*. CRC Press. https://doi.org/10.1201/9780429504877

Iwama, T., Fujiya, M., Konishi, H., Tanaka, H., Murakami, Y., Kunogi, T., Sasaki, T., Takahashi, K., Ando, K., Ueno, N., Kashima, S., Moriichi, K., Tanabe, H., & Okumura, T. (2021). Bacteria-derived ferrichrome inhibits tumor progression in sporadic colorectal neoplasms and colitis-associated cancer. *Cancer Cell International*, *21*(1), 21. https://doi.org/10.1186/s12935-020-01723-9

Jaye, K., Li, C. G., Chang, D., & Bhuyan, D. J. (2022). The role of key gut microbial metabolites in the development and treatment of cancer. *Gut Microbes*, *14*(1). https://doi.org/10.1080/19490976.2022.2038865

Keikha, M., & Karbalaei, M. (2021). Probiotics as the live microscopic fighters against Helicobacter pylori gastric infections. *BMC Gastroenterology*, *21*(1), 388. https://doi.org/10.1186/s12876-021-01977-1

Khaleel, S. M., Shanshal, S. A., & Khalaf, M. M. (2023). The role of probiotics in colorectal cancer: A review. *Journal of Gastrointestinal Cancer*, *54*(4), 1202–1211. https://doi.org/10.1007/s12029-022-00903-2

Kumar, M., Kumar, A., Nagpal, R., Mohania, D., Behare, P., Verma, V., Kumar, P., Poddar, D., Aggarwal, P. K., Henry, C. J. K., Jain, S., & Yadav, H. (2010). Cancer-preventing attributes of probiotics: An update. *International Journal of Food Sciences and Nutrition*, *61*(5), 473–496. https://doi.org/10.3109/09637480903455971

Kumar, S., Metz, D. C., Ellenberg, S., Kaplan, D. E., & Goldberg, D. S. (2020). Risk factors and incidence of gastric cancer after detection of *Helicobacter pylori* infection: A large cohort study. *Gastroenterology*, *158*(3), 527–536. https://doi.org/10.1053/j.gastro.2019.10.019

Kuugbee, E. D., Shang, X., Gamallat, Y., Bamba, D., Awadasseid, A., Suliman, M. A., Zang, S., Ma, Y., Chiwala, G., Xin, Y., & Shang, D. (2016). Structural change in microbiota by a probiotic cocktail enhances the gut barrier and reduces cancer via TLR2 signaling in a rat model of colon cancer. *Digestive Diseases and Sciences*, *61*(10), 2908–2920. https://doi.org/10.1007/s10620-016-4238-7

Lee, S.C., Chua, L.L., Yap, S.H., & Khang, T.F. (2018). *Fusobacterium nucleatum* and colorectal cancer: A review. *World Journal of Gastrointestinal Oncology*, *10*(3), 71–81.

Librán, C. M., Castro, S., & Lagaron, J. M. (2017). Encapsulation by electrospray coating atomization of probiotic strains. *Innovative Food Science & Emerging Technologies*, *39*, 216–222. https://doi.org/10.1016/j.ifset.2016.12.013

Lozupone, C. A., Stombaugh, J. I., Gordon, J. I., Jansson, J. K., & Knight, R. (2012). Diversity, stability and resilience of the human gut microbiota. *Nature*, *489*(7415), 220–230. https://doi.org/10.1038/nature11550

Maleki-Kakelar, H., Dehghani, J., Barzegari, A., Barar, J., Shirmohamadi, M., Sadeghi, J., & Omidi, Y. (2019). *Lactobacillus plantarum* induces apoptosis in gastric cancer cells via modulation of signaling pathways in *Helicobacter pylori*. *BioImpacts*, *10*(2), 65–72. https://doi.org/10.34172/bi.2020.09

Martin-Gallausiaux, C., Salesse, L., Garcia-Weber, D., Marinelli, L., Beguet-Crespel, F., Brochard, V., et al. (2024). *Fusobacterium nucleatum* promotes inflammatory and anti-apoptotic responses in colorectal cancer cells via ADP-heptose release and ALPK1/TIFA axis activation. *Gut Microbes*, *16*(1), 2295384. https://doi.org/10.1080/19490976.2023.2295384

Momo, C. H. K., Mboussaah, A. D. K., François Zambou, N., & Shaiq, M. A. (2022). New pyran derivative with antioxidant and anticancer properties isolated from the probiotic *Lactobacillus plantarum* H24 strain. *Natural Product Research*, *36*(4), 909–917. https://doi.org/10.1080/14786419.2020.1849201

Mozaffari Namin, B., Daryani, N. E., Mirshafiey, A., Yazdi, M. K. S., & Dallal, M. M. S. (2015). Effect of probiotics on the expression of Barrett's oesophagus biomarkers. *Journal of Medical Microbiology*, *64*(4), 348–354. https://doi.org/10.1099/jmm.0.000039

Mu, Q., Tavella, V. J., & Luo, X. M. (2018). Role of *Lactobacillus reuteri* in human health and diseases. *Frontiers in Microbiology*, *9*. https://doi.org/10.3389/fmicb.2018.00757

Nasr, R., Shamseddine, A., Mukherji, D., et al. (2020). The crosstalk between microbiome and immune response in gastric cancer. *International Journal of Molecular Sciences*, 21, 6586. https://doi.org/10.3390/ijms21186586

Nosho, K. (2016). Association of *Fusobacterium nucleatum* with immunity and molecular alterations in colorectal cancer. *World Journal of Gastroenterology*, *22*(2), 557. https://doi.org/10.3748/wjg.v22.i2.557

Palazzolo, S., Bayda, S., Hadla, M., Caligiuri, I., Corona, G., Toffoli, G., & Rizzolio, F. (2018). The clinical translation of organic nanomaterials for cancer therapy: A focus on polymeric nanoparticles, micelles, liposomes and exosomes. *Current Medicinal Chemistry*, *25*(34), 4224–4268. https://doi.org/10.2174/0929867324666170830113755

Pandey, H., Tang, D. W. T., Wong, S. H., & Lal, D. (2023). Gut microbiota in colorectal cancer: Biological role and therapeutic opportunities. *Cancers*, *15*(3), 866. https://doi.org/10.3390/cancers15030866

PDQ Supportive and Palliative Care Editorial Board. (2002). Gastrointestinal Complications (PDQ®): Patient Version. *PDQ Cancer Information Summaries*. https://www.cancer.gov/about-cancer/treatment/side-effects/constipation/gi-complications-pdq

Plummer, M., de Martel, C., Vignat, J., Ferlay, J., Bray, F., & Franceschi, S. (2016). Global burden of cancers attributable to infections in 2012: A synthetic analysis. *The Lancet Global Health*, *4*(9), e609–e616. https://doi.org/10.1016/S2214-109X(16)30143-7

Qiao, Y., Xia, Q., Cao, X., Xu, J., Qiao, Z., Wu, L., Chen, Z., Yang, L., & Lu, X. (2024). Urolithin A exerts anti-tumor effects on gastric cancer via activating autophagy-Hippo axis and modulating the gut microbiota. *Naunyn-Schmiedeberg's Archives of Pharmacology*. https://doi.org/10.1007/s00210-024-03043-5

Razavi, S., Janfaza, S., Tasnim, N., Gibson, D. L., & Hoorfar, M. (2021). Nanomaterial-based encapsulation for controlled gastrointestinal delivery of viable probiotic bacteria. *Nanoscale Advances*, *3*(10), 2699–2709. https://doi.org/10.1039/D0NA00952K

Sexton, R. E., Uddin, M. H., Bannoura, S., Khan, H. Y., Mzannar, Y., Li, Y., Aboukameel, A., Al-Hallak, M. N., Al-Share, B., Mohamed, A., Nagasaka, M., El-Rayes, B., & Azmi, A. S. (2022). Connecting the human microbiome and pancreatic cancer. *Cancer and Metastasis Reviews*, *41*(2), 317–331. https://doi.org/10.1007/s10555-022-10022-w

Sheng, S., Fu, Y., Pan, N., Zhang, H., Xiu, L., Liang, Y., Liu, Y., Liu, B., Ma, C., Du, R., & Wang, X. (2022). Novel exopolysaccharide derived from probiotic *Lactobacillus pantheris* TCP102 strain with immune-enhancing and anticancer activities. *Frontiers in Microbiology*, *13*. https://doi.org/10.3389/fmicb.2022.1015270

Shi, K., Zhang, Q., Zhang, Y., Bi, Y., Zeng, X., & Wang, X. (2023). Association between probiotic therapy and the risk of hepatocellular carcinoma in patients with hepatitis B-related cirrhosis. *Frontiers in Cellular and Infection Microbiology*, *12*. https://doi.org/10.3389/fcimb.2022.1104399

Singh, S., Gupta, R., Chawla, S., Gauba, P., Singh, M., Tiwari, R. K., Upadhyay, S., Sharma, S., Chanda, S., & Gaur, S. (2022). Natural sources and encapsulating materials for probiotics delivery systems: Recent applications and challenges in functional food development. *Frontiers in Nutrition*, *9*. https://doi.org/10.3389/fnut.2022.971784

Singh, T. P., & Natraj, B. H. (2021). Next-generation probiotics: A promising approach towards designing personalized medicine. *Critical Reviews in Microbiology*, *47*(4), 479–498. https://doi.org/10.1080/1040841X.2021.1902940

Song, Q., Zhang, X., Liu, W., Wei, H., Liang, W., Zhou, Y., Ding, Y., Ji, F., Ho-Kwan Cheung, A., Wong, N., & Yu, J. (2023). *Bifidobacterium pseudolongum*-generated acetate suppresses non-alcoholic fatty liver disease-associated hepatocellular carcinoma. *Journal of Hepatology*, *79*(6), 1352–1365. https://doi.org/10.1016/j.jhep.2023.07.005

Song, Q., Zheng, C., Jia, J., Zhao, H., Feng, Q., Zhang, H., Wang, L., Zhang, Z., & Zhang, Y. (2019). A probiotic spore-based Oral autonomous nanoparticles generator for cancer therapy. *Advanced Materials*, *31*(43). https://doi.org/10.1002/adma.201903793

Spechler, S. J. (2013). Barrett's Esophagus. In *Principles of Deglutition* (pp. 723–738). Springer New York. https://doi.org/10.1007/978-1-4614-3794-9_49

Spyridopoulou, K., Tryfonopoulou, E., Aindelis, G., Ypsilantis, P., Sarafidis, C., Kalogirou, O., & Chlichlia, K. (2021). Biogenic selenium nanoparticles produced by: *Lactobacillus casei* ATCC 393 inhibit colon cancer cell growth in vitro and in vivo. *Nanoscale Advances*, *3*(9), 2516–2528. https://doi.org/10.1039/d0na00984a

Sun, Q., Yin, S., He, Y., Cao, Y., & Jiang, C. (2023). Biomaterials and encapsulation techniques for probiotics: Current status and future prospects in biomedical applications. *Nanomaterials*, *13*(15), 2185. https://doi.org/10.3390/nano13152185

Sung, H., Ferlay, J., Siegel, R. L., Laversanne, M., Soerjomataram, I., Jemal, A., & Bray, F. (2021). Global cancer statistics 2020: GLOBOCAN estimates of incidence and mortality worldwide for 36 cancers in 185 countries. *CA: A Cancer Journal for Clinicians*, *71*(3), 209–249. https://doi.org/10.3322/caac.21660

Thilakarathna, W. P. D. W., Rupasinghe, H. P. V., & Ridgway, N. D. (2021). Mechanisms by which probiotic bacteria attenuate the risk of hepatocellular carcinoma. *International Journal of Molecular Sciences*, *22*(5), 2606. https://doi.org/10.3390/ijms22052606

Thirabunyanon, M., Boonprasom, P., & Niamsup, P. (2009). Probiotic potential of lactic acid bacteria isolated from fermented dairy milks on antiproliferation of colon cancer cells. *Biotechnology Letters*, *31*(4), 571–576. https://doi.org/10.1007/s10529-008-9902-3

Uranga, J. A., Nurgali, K., & Abalo, R. (2023). Gastrointestinal Side Effects of Anticancer Therapy. In *Handbook of Cancer and Immunology* (pp. 1–36). Springer International Publishing. https://doi.org/10.1007/978-3-030-80962-1_343-1

Valdovinos-García, L. R., Abreu, A. T., & Valdovinos-Díaz, M. A. (2019). Uso de probióticos en la práctica clínica: resultados de una encuesta nacional a gastroenterólogos y nutriólogos. *Revista de Gastroenterología de México*, *84*(3), 303–309. https://doi.org/10.1016/j.rgmx.2018.05.004

Vogtmann, E., & Goedert, J. J. (2016). Epidemiologic studies of the human microbiome and cancer. *British Journal of Cancer, 114*, 237–242. https://doi.org/10.1038/bjc.2015.465.

Wang, Y., Yang, G., You, L., Yang, J., Feng, M., Qiu, J., Zhao, F., Liu, Y., Cao, Z., Zheng, L., Zhang, T., & Zhao, Y. (2019). Role of the microbiome in occurrence, development and treatment of pancreatic cancer. *Molecular Cancer, 18*(1), 173. https://doi.org/10.1186/s12943-019-1103-2

Yang, J., Liu, X., Cao, S., Dong, X., Rao, S., & Cai, K. (2020). Understanding esophageal cancer: The challenges and opportunities for the next decade. *Frontiers in Oncology, 10*. https://doi.org/10.3389/fonc.2020.01727

Yao, M., Li, B., Ye, H., Huang, W., Luo, Q., Xiao, H., McClements, D. J., & Li, L. (2018). Enhanced viability of probiotics (*Pediococcus pentosaceus* Li05) by encapsulation in microgels doped with inorganic nanoparticles. *Food Hydrocolloids*, *83*, 246–252. https://doi.org/10.1016/j.foodhyd.2018.05.024

Yao, M., Xie, J., Du, H., McClements, D. J., Xiao, H., & Li, L. (2020a). Progress in microencapsulation of probiotics: A review. *Comprehensive Reviews in Food Science and Food Safety*, *19*(2), 857–874. https://doi.org/10.1111/1541-4337.12532

Yao, N., Li, W., Duan, N., Xu, G., Yu, G., & Qu, J. (2024). Exploring the landscape of drug resistance in gastrointestinal cancer immunotherapy: A review. *Medicine*, *103*(2), e36957. https://doi.org/10.1097/MD.0000000000036957

Yao, Y., Zhou, Y., Liu, L., Xu, Y., Chen, Q., Wang, Y., Wu, S., Deng, Y., Zhang, J., & Shao, A. (2020b). Nanoparticle-based drug delivery in cancer therapy and its role in overcoming drug resistance. *Frontiers in Molecular Biosciences*, *7*. https://doi.org/10.3389/fmolb.2020.00193

Yu, L.- X., & Schwabe, R. F. (2017). The gut microbiome and liver cancer: Mechanisms and clinical translation. *Nature Reviews Gastroenterology & Hepatology*, *14*, 527–539. https://doi.org/10.1038/nrgastro.2017.72

Zhang, J., Guo, J., Li, D., Chen, M., Liu, J., Feng, C., He, Q., Zhao, J., Zhang, L., Chen, J., & Shi, Y. (2020). The efficacy and safety of *Clostridium butyricum* and *Bacillus coagulans* in *Helicobacter pylori* eradication treatment. *Medicine*, *99*(45), e22976. https://doi.org/10.1097/MD.0000000000022976

Zhou J., Sun S., Luan S., et al. (2021). Gut microbiota for esophageal cancer: Role in carcinogenesis and clinical implications. *Frontiers in Oncology*, *11*, 717242. https://doi.org/10.3389/fonc.2021.717242

Zhu, Z., Liu, Q., Zhu, K., Wang, K., Lin, L., Chen, Y., Shao, F., Qian, R., Song, Y., Gao, Y., Yang, B., Jiang, D., Lan, X., & An, R. (2023). Aggregation-induced emission photosensitizer/bacteria biohybrids enhance Cerenkov radiation-induced photodynamic therapy by activating anti-tumor immunity for synergistic tumor treatment. *Acta Biomaterialia*, *167*, 519–533. https://doi.org/10.1016/j.actbio.2023.06.009

Zitvogel, L., Daillère, R., Roberti, M. P., Routy, B., & Kroemer, G. (2017). Anticancer effects of the microbiome and its products. *Nature Reviews Microbiology*, *15*(8), 465–478. https://doi.org/10.1038/nrmicro.2017.44

4 Pharmacomicrobiomics and AI Designs in GI Tract Cancers

Naman Kapoor[#], *Harsh Kashyap*[#], *Bhawna Rathi, and Shivani Sharda*
Amity Institute of Biotechnology, Amity University, Noida, India

Pallavi Somvanshi
School of Computational and Integrative Sciences,
Jawahar Lal Nehru University, New Delhi, India

Swarna Kanchan Kesheri
Marshall University, Huntington, United States

CHAPTER LEARNING

- *Cancer Biology*: Differential characterization structuring microbiome affects drug metabolism, efficacy, toxicity, and challenges
- *Algorithm Designs*: ML algorithms analyzing complex microbiome data, identifying patterns, and making predictions about drug interactions and effectiveness
- AI designs integrating data from multi-omics profiling (genomics, proteomics, microbiomics) for deeper insights and accurate predictions
- AI-driven models assisting in drug discovery, optimizing treatment plans, and uncovering novel therapeutic targets

4.1 INTRODUCTION

4.1.1 Conceptualizing Microbiome in Human Physiology and Metabolism

In the gastrointestinal (GI) tract, several varieties of microorganisms and their ecosystem are present in the gut, commonly called gut microbiome. A wide variety of gut microbes reside in the gut, bacteria, fungi, viruses, and archaea (Konstantina et al. 2023; Tiwari et al. 2023). This shows a complex interaction ecosystem with great implications toward human physiology and metabolism, playing a crucial role in maintaining internal balance and other fundamental processes such as immune modulation, digestion, nutrient assimilation, absorption, and neuroendocrine signaling (Senchukova 2023). A gut microbiome is structured by a million bacterial species, occupying different niches throughout the GI tract. Bacteroidetes, actinobacteria, proteobacteria, etc. are dominant phyla, each playing a distinguished role in metabolic activities in

[#] Equivalent First Authors.

DOI: 10.1201/9781003644309-4

the gut. Systems-level ongoing researches indicate that the implication of gut microbiota plays a crucial role not only in the GI functions but also in the systemic processes beyond the gut, such as immune responses and neurological functions (Brian et al. 2023; Tiwari et al. 2023). Microbiome's biodiversity and composition affect the host's general well-being while maintaining the balance of health and dysregulation as a fragile balance, modulating the route of many kinds of disease manifestations (Swer et al. 2022).

A world ruled by microbes unequivocally presents their impactful endorsement of sealing functional fates of inhabiting eco-biosystems. Recent advances in computational algorithms and high-throughput sequencing techniques have radically transformed the understanding of microbiome behavior and effects on human health and disease. Modifications in the constitution and behavior of gut microbiome or dysbiosis have been correlated with etiopathology of not just infectious disorders, but also of metabolic, autoimmune, and non-communicable diseases. The spectrum of gut involvement was significantly addressed, in the past decade, in ailments such as diabetes, obesity, cancer, and inflammatory bowel diseases (IBD). The crosstalk between the gut microbiome and the host cells is mediated by the array of signaling mechanisms, such as pattern recognition receptors, microbial-derived metabolites, and the synthesis of neurotransmitters. Significant repercussions for metabolism, immunological homeostasis, and brain function appear from the mutually beneficial relationship between the microbiome and the host endocrine, immune, and neurological systems (Kaja et al. 2023; Montagnani et al. 2023). Our housed microbes have a major influence on host metabolism, affecting the kinetics and processing of major metabolites in the body, involving bile acids, amino acids, vitamins, and xenobiotics. By donning, these processes relay their role essentially in the energy metabolism, development of bioactive molecules or metabolites, embracing a crosstalk due to multiple factors, such as genetics, diet, immunological status, stress, to align the balance for the host physiology and well-being (María et al. 2023). Initially being directed toward the GI tract, the axis of such balance has been accounted in multiple niches of the human body, configuring the immune-regulation and functioning of the affected system (Sharda et al. 2023).

Study on the molecular relationships between disease conditions and dysbiosis is progressively expanding with many potential applications in precision healthcare and medicines, focused on the microbiome (Brian et al. 2023; Franzosa et al. 2019). Methods that include metagenomic data analysis using bioinformatics pipelines and tools support the functional annotation, taxonomic categorization, and comparative study of microbial populations among samples. Moreover, the artificial intelligence (AI)/machine learning (ML) algorithms are used to pinpoint the microbial biomarkers, anticipate disease consequences, and describe the microbial relationship with the host. The 16S rRNA sequencing provides a targeted and high-throughput approach, replicating and sequencing the hypervariable components of the 16S ribosomal RNA gene, enabling the creation of a profile of bacterial communities with high precision (Garjan et al. 2023). This invigorates the emergence of newer realms of precision sciences involving potential studies, connecting microbiome modulations to drug development and re-purposing. Understanding the influence of the gut microbiota on pharmacokinetics necessitates an awareness of its diversity and functional roles. This is the background of a developing field called pharmacomicrobiomics, where microbial variation interacts with pharmaceutical response.

4.1.2 Pharmacomicrobiomics – Concept and Aspects in Disease

Pharmacomicrobiomics is a rapidly growing field with the convergence of pharmacology, microbiology, and genomics, which investigates how variation in an individual's gut microbiota affects drug metabolism, effectiveness, and toxicity. The gut microbiota actively plays an essential role in the metabolism of drugs, affecting their ADMET actions (absorption, distribution, metabolism, and excretion) for the drugs that are orally administered, tuning metabolism taking place in the liver (Alya et al. 2023; Conti et al. 2022). For example, certain gut bacteria (*Enterococcus faecalis* and *Eggerthella lenta* strains) can metabolize *Warfarin*, an anticoagulant drug, which results in variations in blood-thinning effects among individuals (Mousa et al. 2023). Moreover, it changes the drug efficacy and toxicity by affecting drug activation and inactivation processes and promotes toxicity by metabolizing drugs into toxic compounds and intermediates, which mutate their pharmacokinetic characteristics. In another example similarly observed during cancer chemotherapy, drug *Irinotecan* is metabolized by gut microbiome, the active metabolite of this prodrug Sn-38 is developed in liver and responsible for anticancer action of drug, but a significant amount of drug is eliminated into the colon where it transforms into the toxic form by the microbial *beta-glucuronidase enzymes* present in the gut, resulting in an increase in GI toxicity and reduction in drug efficacy (Mahdy et al. 2023; Rongrong et al. 2023). This concept reflects the dynamic and intricate relationship of human microbiome and pharmacotherapy (drug response), where microbial function and composition might impact the drug action with a variety of methods. By studying the impact of gut microbiota on drug metabolism and elimination, pharmacomicrobiomics would show a promising opportunity for the development of personalized medicine by customizing the patient-specific microbial profile.

In **Table 4.1** several representative types of drugs and their classes show the complex and dynamic interactions with that of gut microbes and how the gut microbiota affects the drug response in the individual; thus understanding the overall gut microbiota can help the researcher and professional to provide the targeted approach toward specific individual to increase overall health outcomes, well-being and increase the efficacy of drug. While pharmacomicrobiomics generally examines how the microbiota influences drug metabolism and effectiveness, it plays a prominent significant role in the field of oncology. This is really important in cancer treatment because cancer is complicated to begin with and has many causes. Pharmacomicrobiomics helps address some of these challenges.

TABLE 4.1
Relationships Between Specific Drug Classes and Their Interactions with Distinct Gut Microbial Species, Shedding Light on the Pharmacomicrobiomics Dynamics, Influencing Drug Metabolism and Efficacy

Drug Name	Drug Class	Gut Microbe	Drug–Microbiome Interactions
Warfarin	Anticoagulants	*Enterococcus faecalis*	Variations in the abundance of *E. faecalis* may influence the efficacy of Warfarin therapy due to its impact on vitamin K production and availability in the gut.
Irinotecan	Chemotherapeutics	*Beta-glucuronidase-producing gut bacteria*	Certain gut bacteria can reactivate glucuronide-conjugated Irinotecan, leading to increased gastrointestinal toxicity and reduced therapeutic efficacy.
Metronidazole	Antibiotics	*Clostridium, Bacteroides, and Fusobacterium*	Involved in activating Metronidazole, affecting its antimicrobial activity against anaerobic microorganisms.
Digoxin	Cardiovascular agents	*Escherichia coli, E. faecalis, Bacteroides thetaiotaomicron*	Linked to potentially influencing the bioavailability and metabolism of digoxin through gut permeability, absorption, and enterohepatic circulation.
Metformin, acarbose	Antidiabetic agents	*Bifidobacterium adolescentis, Akkermansia muciniphila*	Linked to modulating the absorption and metabolism of antidiabetic medications, potentially influencing their effectiveness in managing blood sugar levels.

4.1.3 Cancer – Research Paradigms and Challenges

The investigation of cancer comprises complex paradigms and persistent challenges that have a profound impact on the knowledge of cancer, configuring the spatiotemporal analysis, diagnosis, and therapy. Cancer research consists of a wide spectrum of paradigms that are intended to better understand the causes, varieties, and therapies of cancer (Schneider et al. 2023).

The research paradigms stimulate multi-omics profiling, tumor microenvironment studies, and advancements in immunotherapy toward precision. The genomic profiling has radically transformed cancer studies by identifying the genetic variations that support or promote cancer development and its progression. Tumor microenvironment explores the complicated relationship between cancer cells and surrounding stroma cells, such as immune cells; by focusing on this relationship; thus the development of targeted therapies could be possible for effective treatment. In gradual advancement in immunotherapy by leveraging the immune system and its cells to precisely target and eliminate the cancer cells, such therapy, such as chimeric antigen receptor (CAR) T-cell therapy, has proven exceptional effectiveness in treating the cancer types by isolating and genetically modifying the T cells from the patient's blood and resulting in destruction of cancer cells, thus providing the highly targeted method toward treatment (Ji et al. 2023; Rebecca 2023). Personalized and precision medicine provides specific treatment strategies for a patient by relying on their different molecular, genetic, and clinical attributes and aspects. It focuses on increase in the survival rates, with lowering side effects of an individual (Sandra 2023).

Despite significant advancement, several challenges may be faced, which need to be addressed and overcome. These challenges are fortified in the phenomenon of drug/therapy resistance, metastasis, tumor heterogeneity, and biomarker discovery. A major obstacle is resistance to targeted, chemo, and immunotherapies by cancer cells, restricting the long-term efficacy of traditional treatment. This resistance can be aligned through a variety of mechanisms such as genetic mutations, environmental adaptations, and clonal evolution (Sharma et al. 2017). The primary cause of cancer-related mortality is metastasis, i.e., the dynamic nature of cancer cells spreading to various locations, causing systemic damage. Understanding the mechanisms behind this process can be a vital and important task for the treatment of disease (Turajlic & Swanton 2016). Another substantial challenge is tumor heterogeneity, as it shows intra- and inter-tumoral heterogeneity in genetic alterations, cellular characteristics, and microenvironments. This diversity can result in resistance to therapies. The biggest obstacle in cancer research is the quest for suitable biomarkers for treatment response, rapid detection, and assessment, conforming to biomarkers as highly specific, sensitive, and validated in broad patient groups (Domenic 2023). By overcoming these impasses, novel strategies, research designs, and techniques can be molded, and strategies can be formulated according to the disease conditions, cancer type, and stage of cancer (Srivastav 2024). With the new advancements in cancer research, such as personalized medicine and systems biology, the gut–disease dichotomy becomes very important and has caught researchers' attention. Connecting the gut with diseases may be helpful to understand the exact mechanisms of disease development and treatment efficacy.

4.1.4 Gut – Disease Axis – Correlating the Missing Links of Disease Prognosis (Interaction Between the Microbiome, Drugs, and Cancer Progression)

The gut disease axis is a significant field of research that considers the complex interdependence of the gut microbiota, medication, and the development of cancer. This axis models the dynamics associated with disease prognosis, impacting and emphasizing bi-directional communication between the gut microbiome and the host physiological system. Hence, to better understand the microbiome's role in disease prognosis, tailored treatment, and effective therapeutic solutions, one should be aware of their intricate interconnections (Amer et al. 2023). By connecting all these fragmentary specks of information or links, researchers may uncover novel knowledge and insights that could completely reform how the disease is diagnosed and treated.

Gut flora impacts the pharmacotherapies by altering the drug effectiveness and its bioavailability in the drug metabolism, as these interactions will directly lead to many alterations in the drug metabolic pathways, augmenting adverse side effects with potential complications in therapy. The gut flora is closely intertwined with the immune system function and signaling, exhibiting multiple influences on the immunological responses to pharmacological interventions and the development of cancer (Kouidhi et al. 2023; Mousa et al. 2023). Disruptions in microbiomes can have an impact on cancer development and the treatment outcomes through interference with the inflammatory signals, the activity of immune cells, and the dynamics of the tumor microenvironment or via an associated influence on the development of other diseases, which can act synergistically with cancer (Cátia et al. 2023).

The gut microbiome tweaks the molecular processes associated with the tumor microenvironment by affecting the immune cell infiltration, inflammatory pathways, tumor angiogenesis, and availability of nutrients and metabolites (DiPalma & Blattman 2023). Research conducted in the field has alluded most of the *Bifidobacterium* species toward increased hypo-functioning of the immune checkpoint inhibitors (ICIs), thus promoting anti-tumor immune response. There are other bacterial species, *Fusobacterium nucleatum*, linked to stimulate the growth of cancerous cells and metastases (colorectal cancer) by hampering the activities of 'T cells' and 'NK cells' (Hongyun et al. 2018; Zhao et al. 2022). The investigation of microbiome-targeted therapies has been encouraged by discoveries about the gut–disease axis. Potentially, it involves modifying the microbiome to optimize the outcomes of cancer therapy, where certain adjuvant treatments, involving prebiotics, probiotics, postbiotics, and the FMT, are investigated and studied. In the case of FMT, it shows the potential in restoring and re-establishing the gut microbiome balance. Thus, enhancing the efficacy of ICIs has also shown to reverse the antibiotic-induced dysbiosis in cancer patients and successfully elevate their response toward treatment and decrease the side effects of chemotherapy (Quan & Yu 2023; Kouidhi et al. 2023). Translation in the human mode decodes the gut–disease axis that reveals a very intricate web of relationships that is very complex and complicated for older methods of analysis. This is where AI comes in: it has the computational power to map, analyze, and predict the behavior of cancer with respect to the microbiome.

4.1.5 Magnitude of Studies Pertaining to Microbiome and Artificial Intelligence in Cancer Research

A significant and burgeoning field of study is taking into consideration the fusion of microbiome research and AI, providing novel knowledge and insights into the functions of microbiota in the development, prognosis, and therapeutics of cancer. Incorporation of AI has expanded our understanding of the complex interplay between cancer and microbiome to improve therapeutic innovation, diagnostic precision, and treatment tailoring.

In recent years, a variety of publications studying and investigating the intricate relationship between microbiota research and AI in cancers have been rapidly increasing. Advancements in big data analytics, high-throughput technologies, and AI/ML algorithms such as Support Vector Machines (SVMs), Neural Networks (NMs), and Random Forests in managing the complicated biological data trigger this upsurge of heightened informatics-based knowledge processing (Esteva et al. 2019; Zeller et al. 2014).

Revolutionary applications of the high-throughput sequencing technologies, such as 16s rRNA gene sequencing, metagenome categorization to characterize the human gut microbiota, enable the detection of microbial populations that are correlated with diverse types of cancers to discover their microbial signatures associated with cancer diagnosis, prognosis, and treatment response. ML algorithms are also utilized, such as convolutional neural networks (CNNs), in the analysis of complicated microbiome datasets, also helping the prediction analysis of colorectal cancer with the highest proficiency based on gut microbiota composition. Moreover, ML models utilize the fecal microbiome patterns to identify between healthy and colorectal cancer individuals (Zeller et al. 2014; Zhao et al. 2023).

Gut microbiota influence the pharmacodynamics and pharmacokinetics of cancer drugs and related therapies. AI/ML-driven assessment reveals unique microbial taxa, and their functional pathways correlated with treatment response to enhance the outcomes and overall patient health. Furthermore, by incorporating the multi-omics data, experts can explain the impact of microbial metabolites on cancer pathways, thus providing them personalized therapy plans according to patients unique microbiome profiles. The fusion of AI in microbiome datasets helps one to improve the diagnostic and prognostic tools and can process a large amount of data very accurately and swiftly to enhance early detection and personalized treatment approaches. The scope of research in this matter has shown the importance of collaborative efforts between microbiologists, oncologists, data scientists, and bioinformaticians to comprehend the role of microbiota in cancer and the practical application of findings into clinical practice (Li et al. 2022). The new frontiers in precision oncology are emerging through the convergence of AI with microbiome science. This is nowhere more obvious than in the cancers of the GI tract, where increasingly data-driven intervention is tailored.

4.1.6 Vistas for Precision Medicine – In the Context of AI and GI Tract Cancers

The complexity of discrete diagnostic patterns in cancer studies can be ameliorated by the utilization of AI in the area of precision medicine, most importantly in the aspects of GI tract tumors or cancers, providing a broad range of breakthrough implications. As precision medicine focuses on providing tailored medical treatment options to the individual characteristics of a specific patient, putative work pipelines involving learned data, AI, and its technology will enhance precision medicine by using omics technologies to advance data analysis and AI algorithms. Furthermore, revolutionizing the GI tract cancer diagnosis, treatment approaches, and prognostications hence improve the patient lifestyle and outcomes. The diverse correlations of AI will conclusively include the following parameters of studies:

4.1.6.1 Early Evaluation and Diagnosis

Detection and diagnosis of GI tract cancer in preliminary stages with the help of AI algorithms, especially ML/Deep learning (DL) technique, have shown enormous potential. These AI technologies rapidly examined large datasets from various sources such as genomic sequence, profiles of microbiome, and imaging data in order to detect and diagnose early signs of tumors and cancers that are not overlooked by the conventional or traditional approaches.

For example, in gastric cancer and colorectal polyps, the early detection, and diagnostic rates of have increased by utilizing AI-driven analysis of endoscopic images, especially by training a DL model, i.e., CNNs, to recognize the patterns of endoscopic images effectively and precisely (Vania et al. 2023; Zhang et al. 2019).

4.1.6.2 Prognostications

Prognostications provide the detailed and full profiles for GI tract patients. AI models can incorporate multi-omics data such as genomics, transcriptomics, proteomics, and metabolomics. AI may uncover the molecular signatures and biomarkers associated with the progression of illness and patients' treatment outcomes by understanding the complex relationship among many data layers.

For example, in colorectal cancer, gene expression patterns and microbial fingerprints associated with treatment response and patient survival are examined by the AI-driven analysis for better personalized treatment options and precise risk assessment (Parkash et al. 2022).

4.1.6.3 Predictive Modeling for Treatment Response

By incorporating molecular data, clinical data, imaging data, and electronic health records, AI algorithms use this multimodal approach, which enables the promotion of predictive models that assist physicians to predict a specific patient's response to various treatment options such as chemotherapy, immunotherapy, and targeted therapy. Thus, the area to tailor treatment outcomes can be opened according to the patient's needs and specific profiles.

For example, in immunotherapy, AI algorithms are employed to predict response to ICIs based on characteristics of gut microbiota and tumor microenvironment by utilizing the clinical, molecular, and imaging data. Some microbial species, such as *Akkermansia muciniphila*, are associated with a positive response to this therapy; these AI models evaluate microbiota data and pinpoint individuals who could react to such types of therapy and enhance the outcomes (Hui-Fen 2023; Routy et al. 2018).

4.1.6.4 Drug Research and Repurposing

Drug development and repurposing have been revolutionized by the action of AI by discovering novel drug candidates and inventive applications for preexisting medications. For predicting the safety and efficacy of potential medicinal agents, ML algorithms are used to evaluate a large dataset from clinical trials, biological assays, and chemical libraries.

For example, in colorectal cancer, the Wnt signaling pathways are often dysregulated, and the AI models are employed to screen for drugs that inhibit the important enzymes, playing an essential role in the Wnt signaling pathway. Moreover, repurposing the metformin, an anti-diabetic drug is administered as an adjuvant therapy in colorectal cancer (Zheng et al. 2018).

To operationalize AI-powered precision medicine in GI tract cancers, a holistic workflow has been established that integrates patient data, microbiome profiles, and multi-omics analysis, as depicted in Figure 4.1. The aforementioned primary workflow (**Figure 4.1**) focuses primarily on

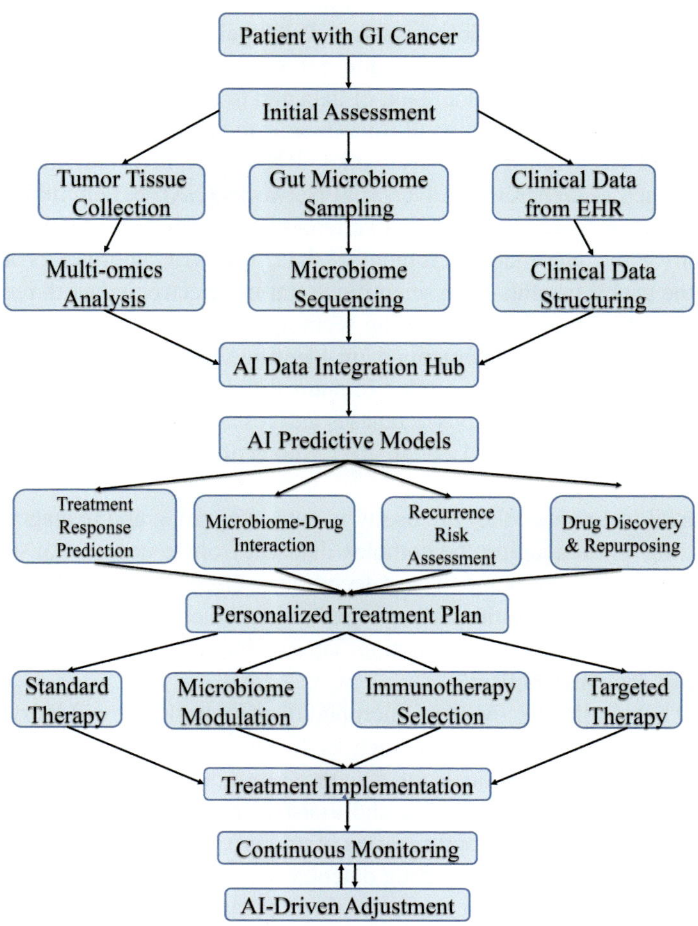

FIGURE 4.1 AI-driven precision medicine workflow in GI cancers.

diagnosis, prognosis, and treatment personalization; drug discovery and repurposing efforts have been synergistically woven into the AI-powered system in parallel.

4.1.7 Role of AI in Analyzing Pharmacomicrobiomics Data for Personalized Therapy

AI translation will reasonably bridge pharmacomicrobiomics, examining and exploring trends of variations in the human microbiota impacting the metabolism, efficacy, and toxicity (MET) processes of the available as well as putative drugs. This area of study holds a practical option for personalized medicines and therapies to patients' microbiome profiles. Due to an increase in the quantity and complexity of pharmacomicrobiomics data, advancement in the data analytical techniques and tools is required; thus, AI comes into the broader picture which is an indispensable tool in the analysis of these data, increasing the ability to interpret these data, discover novel clues and insights, minimize adverse effects, and resulting in more precise and personalized treatment approaches.

There are several AI technologies and techniques used in pharmacomicrobiomics, including ML, DL, and natural language processing (NLP) (Priyanka et al. 2023):

ML: To predict the response of a drug by using the microbial profiles, many algorithms like SVMs, NMs, and Random forests would be developed and trained on designated datasets. Moreover, to identify natural groupings and some patterns within the microbiome data, without labeling, the clustering algorithms (hierarchical clustering and K-means) and dimensionally reduction techniques, such as Principal Components Analysis (PCA) and t-distributed Stochastic Neighbor Embedding (t-SNE), are utilized.

DL: To manage and process, a vast amount of data and to identify intricate, non-linear correlations involved in the composition of microbiome and response of drugs, the DL models, the CNNs, and Recurrent Neural Networks (RNNs) are involved. In addition, generative models, such as Generative Adversarial Networks (GANs), help in the stimulation of microbiome data realistically for model validation and testing of hypotheses.

NLP: To improve the pharmacomicrobiomics data, the NLP approaches are utilized for retrieving the useful insights form scientific literature, electronic health records, and clinical trials reports. Thus, by text mining technique much related research, clinical outcomes and microbiological interactions are identified for the personalized therapy. NLP approaches also aid in the incorporation of many diverse data sources by mapping integration and concepts between various databases and research and assuring an ordered analysis (Arango-Argoty et al. 2018; Li et al. 2017; Luo et al. 2016; Wang et al. 2018).

By using these AI techniques, they are useful in data integration and management processes, by effectively analyzing and managing the complex datasets from genomic, transcriptomics, metabolomic, proteomics, and microbiome. These techniques discover the relationship between drug response and microbiome composition through the integration of sequencing data with that of pharmacokinetic profiles and clinical documentation. This enables a deeper understanding of individual peculiarities toward drug metabolism.

Moreover, they help in the discovery of microbial disease markers by identifying unique microbial signatures that impact drug response such as *Eggerthella lenta*, a bacterial species, linked to Digoxin drug metabolism. AI models analyze these microbiome patterns, predict how changes will affect drug metabolism and response, and assist in recognizing essential microbial agents. Moreover, AI aids in the growth and optimization of pre, pro, and post-biotic therapies that focus on to alter the microbiome and enhance the drug outcomes.

AI will benefit in designing specific strategies that increase the effectiveness of drug and metabolism through modeling various conditions and investigating the effects of diverse microbial populations, such as probiotic *Bifidobacterium longum* administration, that have shown enhanced gut microbiome capabilities to increase the effectiveness and absorption of chemotherapeutic drug 5-fluorouracil by using prediction methods of AI models. Hence, targeted administration, lowering side effects and improved drug outcomes (Haiser et al. 2013; Mousa et al. 2023; Wong et al. 2019).

With the integration of AI technologies, many obstacles and challenges could also occur, including difficulties in pharmacomicrobiomics data integration due to variations in data formats, scales, and sources. Privacy and security of patient information is important and a challenge to maintain. Anonymization technique and encryption method are vital to protect the sensitive information. Certain models of AI mainly DL can be difficult to interpret due to their black box nature or structure. Several ethical and regulatory considerations are raised by implementing AI in healthcare sector, where obtaining regulatory approvals is compulsory, which is difficult (Ali et al. 2023).

4.2 ELEMENTS OF PHARMACOMICROBIOMICS

Pharmacomicrobiomics is a promising field that explores the complex interaction between pharmacology and human microbiome. In this discipline, it delves into the profound influence of the microbiome on disease pathogenesis, therapeutic outcomes, and drug metabolism. Analyzing the exhausative processes of drug–microbe–host processes is connected with thorough processing, using the following designs (**Figure 4.2**).

4.2.1 Diseases Conscription

One of the key aspects of pharmacomicrobiomics is the disease conscription of the microbiome. It generally potentially leads to further disease progression and development of new ailments. Understanding these roles allows us for the identification of microbial signatures that are

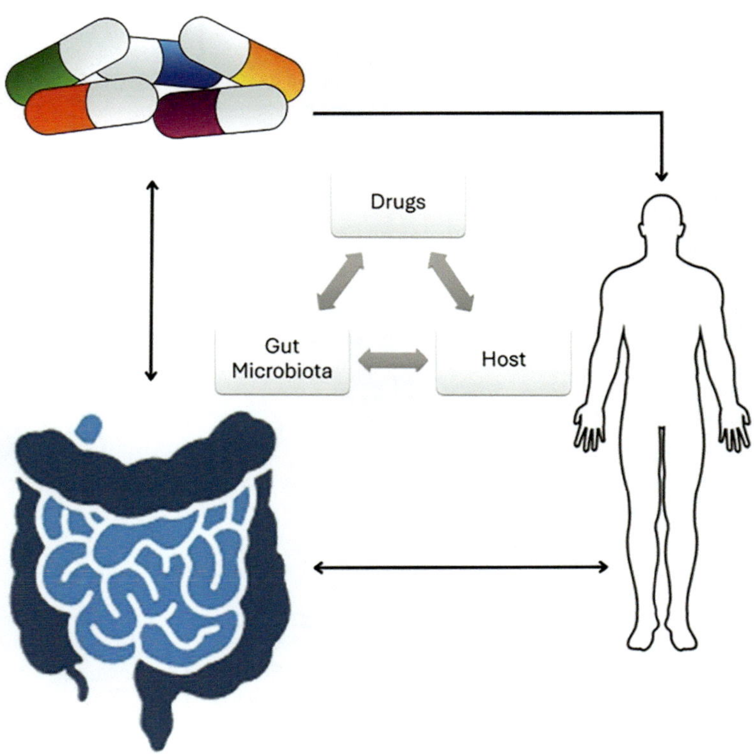

FIGURE 4.2 Pharmacomicrobiomics is the study of drug–host and gut–microbiota interactions.

associated with some specific diseases. This will allow further discovery of possible biomarkers and diagnostic tools in these areas (Curini & Amedei 2021).

Microbial Implications in Disease Development: Several research studies have shown a link between the changes within microbiome and development of various pathologies. For instance, the dysbiosis of the gut has been associated with GI disorders such as IBD and irritable bowel syndrome (IBS) (Kostic et al. 2014).

Microbial Signatures: Some research studies have shown that microbial signatures are associated with some specific diseases. For example, an increased amount of *F. nucleatum* has been linked to colorectal cancer. Hence, it could be related to the tumorigenesis of this condition, whereas a decrease in the amount of *Bifidobacterium* and *Lactobacillus* is generally seen in the patients who have IBS (Cryan & Dinan 2012; Kostic et al. 2014), and these microbial signatures can also be served as disease biomarkers. For example, stool-based microbial tests have been used to diagnose the colorectal cancer and IBD.

Microbial Dysbiosis and Disease States: Dysbiosis is defined as an imbalance within the gut microbiome, which is closely linked possibly resulting in numerous disease states. The gut microbiome plays an important role in maintaining one's overall health. The minute disruptions in this delicate ecosystem can lead to various diseases. This imbalance can be caused by some factors, such as diets, antibiotic use, and the change in lifestyles (Cryan & Dinan 2012).

In GI disorders, IBD dysbiosis can result in increased gut permeability, immune activation, and increased inflammation, all contributing to the pathology of disease states in these disorders. Similarly, in metabolic disorders, such as obesity and diabetes, dysbiosis can change or affect the energy harvest and storage, inflammation, and insulin sensitivity (Baptista et al. 2020; Tremaroli & Bäckhed 2012) (**Figure 4.3**).

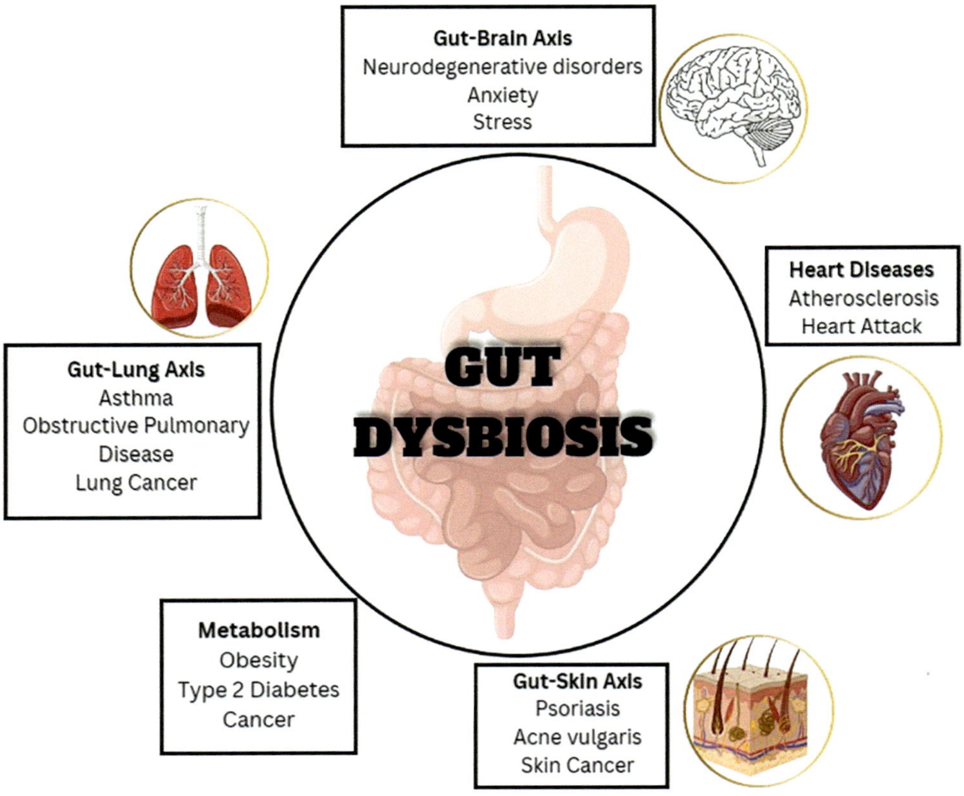

FIGURE 4.3 Connection between gut dysbiosis and various health issues.

Personalized Medicine: Since the human gut microbiome plays an important role in drug metabolism, personalized medicine in pharmacomicrobiomics involves an understanding of connections or links between microbial dysbiosis and disease states. On the basis of this understanding, researchers can make personalized treatment strategies. For example, adjusting the gut microbiota composition through dietary interventions, probiotics, or FMT can enhance the efficacy of therapies for metabolic and GI disorders (Wilson & Nicholson 2017; Zitvogel et al. 2018). Apart from purely theoretical concepts, actual pharmacomicrobiomic application has primary concrete analytical strategies. Microbiomic profiling deconstructs a diseased state that correlates microbes with functional disease markers.

4.2.2 Deconvoluting Disease Analysis and Microbiomics

Disease deconvolution involves the analysis of microbial arrangement and the functional profiles of individuals who have specific diseases. The amalgamation of microbiome information into the analysis of diseases helps researchers in enhancing their understanding of disease pathophysiology. It allows the discovery of microbial markers that are linked to disease gravity and the response for treatment. This is done by utilizing the advanced bioinformatics tools of high-throughput sequencing technologies, complex host genetic–microbiome–drug metabolism interactions.

The intricate relationship of microbiota with disease can only be appreciated if microbiome data can be mapped on traditional disease analysis frameworks (**Table 4.2**). Such integration of other omics data increases the researchers gain in and perception of disease pathophysiology by revealing how the microbes influence the disease course. For example, the integration of immigration with microbiome data supported identifying critical factors in microbial dysbiosis associated with disease flare-ups and remission for IBD research (Goodrich et al. 2014). At the same time, analysis of gut microbiota composition in metabolic diseases, such as obesity and type 2 diabetes, in combination with clinical data, has revealed a clearer picture of how microbial metabolites influence insulin sensitivity and energy balance (Tremaroli & Bäckhed 2012).

Advanced bioinformatics and high-throughput sequencing have to be employed so that it can identify the microbial biomarkers that are associated with disease severity and treatment response. The key approaches that are used in these analyses are metagenomics, transcriptomics, and metabolomics. Similarly, the genetic sequences of microbial communities are analyzed for metagenomic sequencing, which fully describes the microbiome to estimate its diversity and functional potential (Qin et al. 2010). Transcriptome analysis captures active biological processes reflected in patterns of microbiome gene expression (Franzosa et al. 2014). Metabolomics deals with metabolic products

TABLE 4.2
Bioinformatic Techniques for Microbiome-Based Biomarker Discovery

Technique	Description
Machine learning classifiers	Methods, such as random forests, support vector machines, and logistic regression, are used to classify disease status based on microbiome data.
Differential abundance analysis	Identifies bacterial taxa significantly different in abundance between disease and control groups, potential biomarker candidates.
Compositional data analysis	Specialized methods to handle the compositional nature of microbiome data, such as centered log-ratio transformations.
Network analysis	Examines co-occurrence patterns and ecological interactions among microbes, identifying key microbial communities or hub taxa.
Functional profiling	Predicts functional potential of the microbiome from 16S rRNA or shotgun sequencing data, linking functions to disease phenotypes.
Survival analysis	Techniques like Cox proportional hazards models to identify microbiome markers associated with time-to-event outcomes.

which are derived from microbial activity. It also identifies metabolites related to disease states and treatments. Bioinformatic tools allow the integration and interpretation of such large datasets so that the discovery of robust microbial biomarkers can be made.

The complex interactions between host genetics, microbiome, and drug metabolism holds a critical place in pharmacomicrobiomics. The main impact is on the composition and functions of a microbiome, which might influence the host response to the drugs. For instance, genetic variations in drug-metabolizing enzymes can be modulated by the microbiome, altering the pharmacokinetics and pharmacodynamics of drugs. Besides this, there are some microbial species can either convert the drugs into different forms, whether active or inactive, thus influencing therapeutic results. For example, the ability of gut microbiomes to convert a prodrug, irinotecan, to its active ingredient and yet produce severe toxic effects indicates that this gives an action of drug metabolism that necessitates the personalization of dosing strategies based on the composition of the microbiome (Wallace et al. 2010). Understanding these complex interactions is very essential for developing personalized medicine approaches that will consider both the genetic and the microbial factors.

4.2.3 Gaps and New Insights in Disease Analysis

Several gaps remain in comprehending the role in disease development and the treatment outcomes, despite the noteworthy advancement in the understanding of the microbiome. Definitely, by addressing these gaps will generate discoveries and interventions. Many important gaps continue to contradict our understanding that how the microbiome contributes and interacts with disease development and influences outcomes in response to treatments. One primary concern is to separate correlation from causation. Although many studies have been shown a positive correlation between microbial dysbiosis and diseases such as obesity, diabetes, and colorectal cancer, establishing causal relationships is more complex. Longitudinal studies as well as the well-conducted clinical trials are required to identify the microbiome as a cause or consequence of the disease (Blumberg & Powrie 2012). Additionally, the means through microbiota may be used to study the disease processes with immune modulation, metabolic regulation as well as barrier function need more significant understanding.

By leveraging the drug–microbiome interaction, it shows an exciting frontier for novel discoveries and therapeutic interventions. One of the promising areas is the development of microbiome-based diagnostics in which the identification of specific microbial signatures associated with pathological states may even lead to the creation of non-invasive diagnostic tests for the early detection and monitoring of diseases, such as colorectal carcinoma and IBD. Other therapeutic interventions that alter the microbiome are probiotics, prebiotics, and FMT that are being investigated as they have the potential to restore healthy microbial balance and achieve better patient outcomes. For example, FMT had shown effective in treating the recurrent *Clostridium difficile* infection and also being studied for IBD and metabolic states (Zitvogel et al. 2018).

The microbiome can considerably impact drug pharmacokinetics (absorption, distribution, metabolism, and excretion), i.e., ADME and pharmacodynamics (drug's effect on the body). Some intestinal bacteria have developed enzyme systems that can be able to metabolize drugs, changing their efficacy and the safety attributes. For instance, gut microbiota is able to convert the prodrug irinotecan into its active form but also forms some toxic metabolites, which causes adverse side effects, such as diarrhea (Wallace et al. 2010). By analyzing these interactions, experts can make personalized dosing strategies, which can lead to the development of microbiome-modulating therapies toward the maximal efficacy of the drugs and reduction of unwanted effects.

4.2.4 Trends of Progression in Unknown Health Disasters

The human microbiome is critical to the host's response to infectious disease. During a growing health crisis, such as a pandemic, it provides the best insights in disease sensitivity and transmission dynamics. A recent example is the COVID-19 pandemic, where studies established changes within the gut microbiome to be associated with the severity and outcomes of the disease (Yu et al. 2017; Zuo et al. 2020). Furthermore, with microbiome data included, the very patterns of microbes that are associated with increased susceptibility to infection, a severe course of disease, or better recovery could potentially be a basis of forming targets for interventions in the future and public health strategies toward the mitigation of infectious diseases.

Changes in the microbiome can serve as early warning signs for disease outbreaks. Such microbial community can shift often well ahead of clinical incidents and can serve as a precious indicator for early interventions and detections. For example, in *C. difficile* infection, a drastic reduction in microbial diversity with pathogenic bacterial overgrowth was observed before the appearance of symptoms (Seekatz et al. 2014). The healthcare providers can apply the targeted interventions, such as prophylactic treatments or isolation measures, to inhibitor to prevent the spread of infections, by observing these microbiome shifts.

Moreover, the real-time sequencing technologies, such as next-generation sequencing (NGS) and metagenomics, are combined with epidemiological data to enable the tracking of microbial changes during health disasters. These technologies allow for the faster and understandable examination of microbial population. These communities are those that provide the detailed analysis about the composition and the functional potation of the microbiome. For instance, during the Ebola virus epidemic, metagenomic sequencing was used to follow changes in patients' microbiomes, thus helping in specifying the interactions between the virus and the host microbiota (Li et al. 2019). The connection of such kind of sequencing data with epidemiological data, such as clinical outcomes, transmission patterns, and patient demographics, can talk about the factors that diversely influence spread and severity.

4.2.5 Creating the Hub for Drug–Microbiomics Nexus

Pharmacomicrobiomics research depends on the development of a unified platform that integrates medication data, microbiome profiles, and clinical outcomes. In order to pursue personalized therapies, the creation of a hub will enable the storage of numerous datasets and encourage the interdisciplinary collaboration.

Collaborative Platform Integration: Integration of a collaborative platform that extends the research capabilities in pharmacomicrobiomics blends drug data with microbiome profiles and clinical outcomes. After data integration, the collected datasets provide the researcher with a new inclusive insight into how microbiomes influence responses to drugs and the treatment effectiveness. For instance, the understanding of how the gut microbiota communicates with a chemotherapeutic agent could be a way forward to better outcomes for cancer treatments. An open platform to unravel the much-needed biomarkers to anticipate the drug response should support developing and creating such better and personal therapies (Gopalakrishnan et al. 2018).

Repository for Diverse Datasets: The hub would act as a repository or storage for the various datasets. Those are supporting sharing of data on interdisciplinary research. Engagement and collaborative efforts among the researchers within microbiology, pharmacology, genomics, and clinical science would be promoted by active participation and sharing of data. Simplicity in data format and protocol in handling research data through critical procedures that go from collection to sharing with standardization is vital to ensuring the integrity of any repository in use (Quince et al. 2017). Such open access could also be improved in transparency and reproducibility in research despite the current challenges in the field.

Personalized Treatment Development: Drug data combined with microbiome profiles can significantly boost the development of personalized treatments specifically designed according to individual microbiota compositions. Knowledge of distinct microbial communities mediating host drug metabolism and pharmacodynamics would allow treatment tailoring, leading to an optimal therapeutic outcome while decreasing side effects. For instance, in a situation where certain gut bacteria

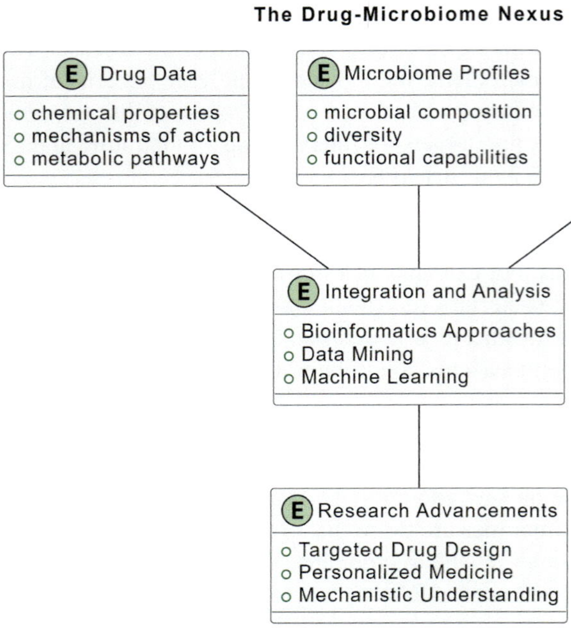

FIGURE 4.4 The drug–microbiome nexus: a collaborative framework.

degrade a drug, the co-administration of probiotics inhibiting these bacteria would assist in improving efficacy of the drug. In addition, personalized treatment strategies might include, on the one hand, the patient's genetic background associated with their lifestyle and environmental exposures for a concerted approach to healthcare (Shreiner et al. 2015) (**Figure 4.4**).

4.3 GI TRACT CANCERS – PARAMOUNT OF MICROBIOME CONTRIBUTION

4.3.1 Prevalence of GI Tract Cancers Worldwide

GI tract cancers or GI tract encompasses various types of cancers such as colorectal, gastric, and esophageal cancers. These cancers account a significant portion of cancer cases and deaths worldwide, with considerable geographical variation. These cancerous malignancies account for a tremendous part of total cancer incidence and death, and the quantity is, of course, quite varied in different regions, owing to lifestyle, dietary habits, genetic predispositions, and environmental factors.

4.3.1.1 Global Burden of GI Tract Cancers

GI tract cancers are a major burden for the world. According to the World Health Organization (WHO), the colorectal cancer is the third most common cancer in the world, while stomach or gastric cancer ranks fifth. Esophageal cancer, although is less prevalent worldwide, has a disastrous prognosis because of its aggressive nature and late-stage (malignancy) appearance. GI tract malignancies are an active global burden. This is added by the fact that the incidence of GI tract cancers is increasing in most parts of the world and emerging as the most typical cancer, even among younger age groups (Hong et al. 2022) (**Figure 4.5**).

4.3.1.2 Incidence and Mortality Rates

Table 4.3 presents the global incidence and mortality rates of major GI tract cancers, highlighting their geographical distribution and notable trends over time.

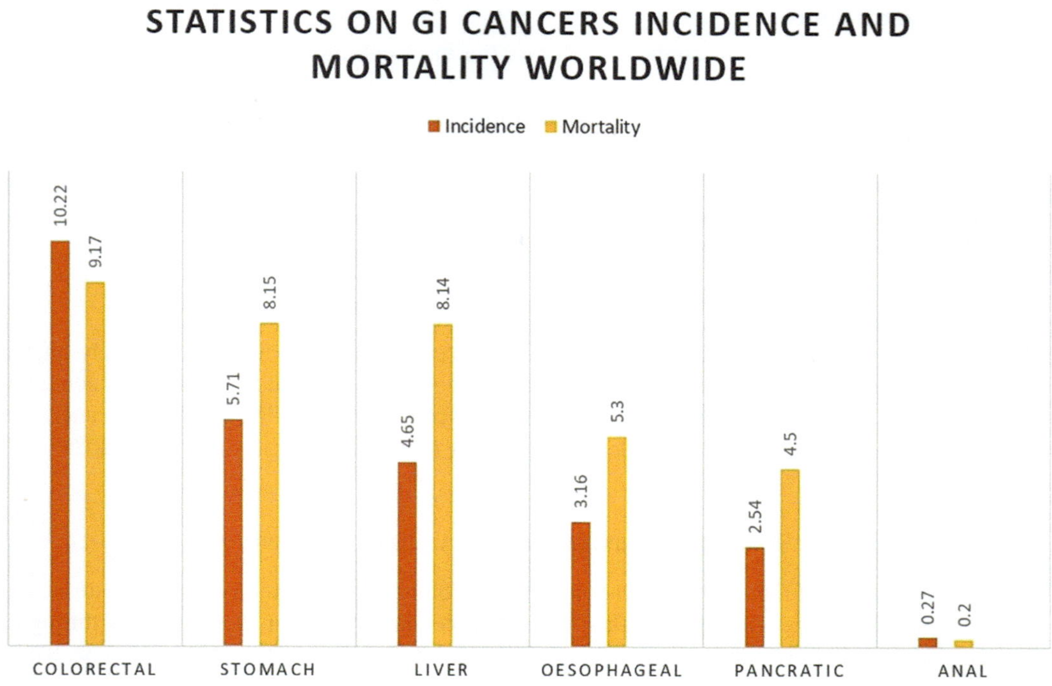

FIGURE 4.5 Contribution of major gastrointestinal cancers to global cancer cases and deaths in 2018.

4.3.1.3 Colorectal Cancer

Colorectal cancer is the third most often diagnosed cancer in worldwide. with estimated 1.9 million additional new cases and 935,000 fatalities in 2020. This colorectal cancer affects both the industrialized and developing countries. The highest rates are seen in the United States and some part of Europe. However, the incidence is increasing in many low- and middle-income nations as they have been influenced by the Western eating and lifestyle practices (Bray et al. 2018).

TABLE 4.3
Global Incidence and Mortality Rates of Major GI Tract Cancers

Cancer Type	Annual Incidence (Cases)	Annual Mortality (Deaths)	Notable Regions	Trends over Time
Colorectal cancer	1.9 million	935,000	High in developed countries (e.g., USA, Australia, Europe)	Increasing in low/middle-income countries due to Westernized lifestyles
Gastric cancer	1.0 million	769,000	High in Eastern Asia (e.g., Japan, Korea, China)	Declining in high-income countries, stable or increasing in low/middle-income countries
Esophageal cancer	604,000	544,000	High in Eastern Asia and Eastern/Southern Africa	Increasing in high-risk regions, stable in Western countries

Sources: Bray et al. (2018), Siegel et al. (2020), and Ferlay et al. (2021).

4.3.1.4 Gastric Cancer

Gastric cancer, also known as stomach cancer, is the most common cancer in the world. These cancer rates are high in East Asia, mainly in Japan, Korea, and China. It is due to their dietary factors, such as consumption of high salt intake and infection with *Helicobacter pylori*. Though the numbers in deaths are decreasing in developed nations because of their better food preservation and their eradication methods, the cases are either stable or increasing in low- and middle-income countries. In 2018, gastric cancer resulted in approximately 1 million new cases and 769,000 deaths globally (Bray et al. 2018).

4.3.1.5 Esophageal Cancer

The Esophageal cancer is the eighth most common cancer in the world, which is relatively high in Eastern Asia and Eastern/Southern Africa. The two major types are squamous cell carcinoma and adenocarcinoma, which are more common in Western countries. In 2018, esophageal cancer has caused 544,000 deaths and 604,000 cancer cases globally (Ferlay et al. 2021; Siegel et al. 2020).

4.3.2 Treatment Approaches Incorporating Pharmacomicrobiomics and AI

Thus, the integration of these two innovations, pharmacomicrobiomics and AI, with its subsequent interpretation of massive datasets, heralds novel therapeutic options for these patients through a detailed understanding of the dynamics between drugs, the host, and the gut microbiome. These approaches can vary from FMT to targeted probiotics or biomarkers derived from microbiome analysis, all set to change the course of cancer treatment drastically.

1. *Fecal Microbiota Transplantation (FMT)*:
   It is defined as taking the healthy, donated fecal bacteria and transplanting them into an ill patient's gut. Some evidence has shown the potential role of FMT in improving response to immunotherapy in colorectal cancer. Modulating gut microbiota through FMT can sensitize and reduce the toxicity of ICIs (Xu et al. 2021).
2. *Targeted Probiotics*:
   Live microorganisms, exerting health benefits to the host, are defined as probiotics. Targeted probiotics are therefore designed toward a beneficial alteration of gut microbiota composition. Targeted probiotic formulations toward specified microbial species can augment the effectiveness of chemotherapy and immunotherapy. For example, *Bifidobacteria* and *Lactobacillus* strains further potentiate anti-tumor immunity while minimizing the GI toxicity of cancer treatment (Matson et al. 2018).
3. *Microbiome-Based Disease Markers*:
   Patient-related biomarkers derived from the microbiome regarding disease progression and treatment response. Molecular definition of microbial signatures of treatment outcome toward therapy personalization. For instance, gut bacteria-related microbial signatures were associated with better responses in patients treated with ICIs for melanoma and colorectal cancer (Matson et al. 2018).

AI technologies, specifically ML and DL, play a very uniquely significant role in the analysis of complex microbiome data and the detection of underlying patterns that can eventually implicate strategies for treatment. The integration of microbiome, genomic, and clinical data by AI will aid in predicting treatment responses, optimizing therapeutic regimens, and developing personalized treatment plans.

AI algorithms should be potent enough to handle enormous datasets resulting from microbiome sequence information in identifying patterns of microbes acting differently under different responses to cancer treatments. An example is the predictive power of AI models for which patients could benefit from FMT or targeted probiotics by their microbiome profile. By the use of AI, it is possible to optimize dosages and combinations of drugs by considering the composition of microbiomes within patients. This approach enhances the drug's effectiveness with a decrease in adverse effects. Therefore, the treatment becomes more effective and safer (Topol 2019).

4.3.3 Role of Microbiome in Treatment Response and Resistance

The GI microbiota plays a fundamental part in determining the therapeutic susceptibility and treatment resilience. Since the gut microbiome contains trillions of microorganisms living in gut, and precise knowledge related to microbial species or profiles has to be acquired in terms of treatment outcomes, it will guide the other goals of attaining treatment optimization and eventually improving patient prognosis in cancers of the alimentary canal.

The gut microbiota is like a dual-edge sword in the realm of chemotherapy as either it can enhance the potency or efficacy of some certain drugs or raise the resistance to their effects. For example, in the case of irinotecan, which is a chemotherapeutic prodrug, it is utilized against the colorectal cancer. Within the gut, some commensal bacteria are present which possess remarkable ability to metabolize irinotecan into its active form and hence support its therapeutic impact (Wallace et al. 2010). Meanwhile, this bacterial group can disrupt the therapeutic efforts by neutralizing drugs, such as gemcitabine, which is a crucial against pancreatic cancer. Certain bacterial species have the ability to deactivate gemcitabine, decreasing its efficacy and contributing to chemoresistance (Geller et al. 2017).

Gut-microbiota-dependent adjustment of the immune system looks like to play a very important role in the efficacy and, in the resistance of immunotherapeutic, specifically the ICIs. For example, patients that host a diverse and balanced gut microbiota mostly respond better to anti-PD-1 and anti-CTLA-4 therapies. A more general microbial dysbiosis in a cancer patient's gut is also known to have the potential for resistance against ICIs. In this regard, a higher baseline abundance of beneficial bacteria, such as *A. muciniphila* and *Bifidobacterium* species, are associated explicitly with enhanced ICI responsiveness (Matson et al. 2018). Intriguingly, some pathogenic bacteria, such as *Enterococcus hirae* and *Barnesiella intestinihominis*, result in better outcomes when treated with cyclophosphamide. This reflects the close and complex crosstalk between the microbiome and immune responses (Routy et al. 2018).

The gut microbiome is an essential factor in the efficacy and resistance of targeted therapies. Among the active biological drugs, tyrosine kinase inhibitors against multiple cancers are most commonly used for these approaches. Some microbial groups can be critical actors in modulating drug metabolism to improve the therapeutic power of tyrosine kinase inhibitors. For instance, different bacterial enzymes can exist in an activating or inactivating state, directly affecting how effective the drug is at that point. On the other hand, a change in the microbiome's composition may result in resistance to target therapies. The degradation of such drugs or their modification by bacterial enzymes ultimately reduces activity and causes therapy failure. This fact underlines that for the development of strategies out of the knowledge achieved in understanding microbial interactions, therapeutics can be improved based on better therapeutic outcomes (Gopalakrishnan et al. 2018) (**Table 4.4**).

4.3.4 Current Challenges in Diagnosing and Treating GI Tract Cancers

Identifying and treating GI tract cancers is difficult as it faces various restrictions and hurdles. As when considering the intricacies of the microbiome, the challenges vary from spotting the disease early and providing the accurate diagnosis to the customized therapies to individuals and effectively tracking disease development. The combination of pharmacomicrobiomics and AI shows promise for addressing these difficulties.

TABLE 4.4
Microbial Influence on Treatment Outcomes in GI Tract Cancers

Therapy Type	Microbial Species	Effect on Treatment	Impact on Outcome
Chemotherapy	*Faecalibacterium prausnitzii*	Enhances efficacy	Improved outcomes with reduced inflammation
	Fusobacterium nucleatum	Reduces efficacy (resistance)	Poor prognosis and reduced response
Immunotherapy	*Akkermansia muciniphila* and *Bifidobacterium* species	Enhances efficacy	Better response to anti-PD-1 therapies and Improved outcomes with checkpoint inhibitors
	Enterococcus hirae	Variable effects	Linked to both positive and negative outcomes
Targeted therapy	Various bacterial enzymes	Modulate drug metabolism	Can enhance or reduce efficacy based on microbial interactions

4.3.4.1 Key Challenges and Potential Solutions

4.3.4.1.1 Early Diagnosis

The significant issue concerning GI tract cancers is the late diagnosis due to the lack of early presenting symptoms and effective screening methods. Early detection of microbiomes for GI system cancers linked to specific microbial signatures will boost the prediction of prognosis and survival rates. For example, changes in gut microbiota composition are known to occur five to ten years before the detection of colorectal cancer due to its contribution to inflammation and fibrosis in the colon (Zup et al. 2017). In this context, AI combined with microbiome datasets will help detect early patterns indicating an initial precancerous process.

4.3.4.1.2 Accurate Diagnosis

One of the problems persists with identifying benign and malignant lesions accurately through traditional diagnostic methods. Endoscopy with biopsy sampling might not be fully diagnostic, while other methods bear more risks than the lesions themselves. These diagnostic techniques can be further improved by integrating microbiome profiles. AI algorithms for deeper diagnostic detail from imaging and biopsy data can detect subtleties that could indicate a malignancy commonly overlooked (Topol 2019).

4.3.4.1.3 Personalized Treatment Selection

Standard treatment protocols will not work optimally for all individuals due to the uniqueness of their microbiome composition. This calls for individualized treatment selection to maximize therapeutic benefit. The microbiome analysis aids the clinicians in developing medicines tailored specifically to a patient's microbial and genetic profile. The AI-driven models that predict therapy responses using such an integrated data help to make more accurate and successful therapeutic decisions (Matson et al. 2018).

4.3.4.1.4 Clinical Disease Monitoring

Tracking changes in the progression of diseases and their response to treatment is an arduous task, one that is usually done by application of invasive techniques. Microbiome-based biomarkers offer an easy way of tracking. Such biomarkers would enable immediate assessment of the patient's state of health; thus, it timely changes in the therapy plan. Longitudinal data from the microbiome may be analyzed thanks to AI technologies for disease progression, as changes are tracked continuously and dynamically (Zitvogel et al. 2018).

4.3.4.1.5 Overcoming Treatment Resistance

Treatment resistance remains a key challenge while combating GI tract cancers with chemotherapeutic and immunotherapeutic modalities. The gut microbiome plays a crucial part in determining the effectiveness of treatment and resistance. The identification of microbes associated with resistance identifies potential ways for altering the microbiota to combat resistance and ultimately conquer it. AI can detect emerging patterns of resistance and adjust the course of treatment to consider such changes, providing patients with the best medicines available (Geller et al. 2017). Chemotherapy and radiotherapy have a negative impact on the gut flora, lowering mucositis, one of the most debilitating side effects for the patient. Such conditions need to be managed such that they optimize the quality of life for the patients' assurance of continuation of treatment of the cancer. Targeted probiotics and FMT provide a promising opportunity for restoring a healthy microbiota balance. AI can hence personalize supportive care by tailoring probiotic treatments based on individual microbiome profiles, thus reducing side effects and improving patient outcomes (Xu et al. 2021).

4.3.5 New Research Avenues in GI Tract Cancers

GI tract cancers, which consists of cancers that affect the esophagus, stomach, small intestine, colon, and rectum, are a major health concern at present. The promising research opportunities in this area that have been shown by recent studies, which might result in improved prevention, diagnosis, and therapy.

Researchers are looking into dysbiosis and are also interested in how the dysbiosis may influence the development of cancers and how they spread. In addition to emphasizing on nutrition, the future research in this field seeks to look into the relationship between factors that can be controlled and the composition of the gut microbiome or microbiota. The researchers are also trying to explore how it may affect and how the body reacts to cancer immunotherapy (Hou et al. 2022).

The cornerstone of a better outcome in GI cancers is early detection and correct diagnosis. On these bases, much investment has been funneled to identify and validate new biomarkers for these malignancies. Concretely, these biomarkers would help in early detection, the selection of treatment options on a personalized basis, and the monitoring of disease progression or response to therapy. GI cancer risk has been associated with a number of ecological and lifestyle variables, which includes nutrition, obesity, and physical activity. In fact, current research concentrates on these correlations in an attempt to figure out the fundamental mechanisms and wants to create successful preventative interventions (Chan et al. 2021).

The imaging and diagnostic modalities of GI carcinomas have shown remarkable progress. Therefore, magnetic resonance imaging related to the GI tract is turning out to be an essential tool for its visualization, motility/investigation, and the function of the GI tract. It will also be a topic of much research in other imaging methods through the availability of new techniques to permit a quicker and better diagnosis (Maccioni et al. 2023). With the onset of the era of personalized medicine, much attention is given to the production of various drugs that target the molecular basis of the tumor of every independent patient. This strategy targets maximum effectiveness with minimal side effects of the treatment (Diamantidis et al. 2021).

4.4 INFORMATION STATISTICS AND PREVENTIVE MEDICINE

4.4.1 Statistical Analysis of Pharmacomicrobiomics Impact on GI Tract Cancers

Statistical analysis in pharmacomicrobiomics includes the application of several statistical techniques to undiscover how the microbiota impacts the drug efficacy, metabolism, and toxicity in GI cancers. Assessing the statistical insights is important for examining the complex relationship, and understanding how pharmacomicrobiomics that affects GI oncology also helps in predicting the therapeutic outcomes and for customizing the personalized treatment approaches. By using the advanced statistical and computational approaches, such as inferential statistics, correlational analysis, regression models, and MetagenomeSeq, scientists can successfully manage the intricacy of microbiota data and retrieve the key insights and meaningful information (Lozupone et al. 2012).

The several key statistical methods and approaches in Pharmacomicrobiomics are as follows:

a. *Descriptive and Inferential Statistics*:

   These statistics methods are used to draw meaningful insights from the pharmacomicrobiomics data, the descriptive statistics, including central tendency (mean, median) and variability, or variance (standard deviation, interquartile range) provides a synopsis of the statistical data. Thus, these statistics help in characterization and identification of microbiome composition and variance among GI cancer individuals. The inferential statistic, including confidence intervals, and hypothesis testing are utilized to make meaningful conclusions about the population and to assess the importance correlations among the microbiome profiles and response of drug (Cassol et al. 2023; Lai et al. 2022).

b. *Microbiome Profiling and Related Analysis*:

   By using the alpha, beta diversity, and differential abundance analysis to provide a better result in understanding of treatment outcomes, microbiota alterations, etc. is essential.

   In alpha diversity (Shannon and Simpson Metric), the abundance distribution and species richness in a sample are estimated and quantified, some statistical tests, like ANOVA or t-tests, help in comparative alpha diversity between treatment categories, such as control and drug for assessment of microbiome alterations.

   In beta diversity (Bray–Curti's dissimilarity and Principal Coordinate Analysis (PCoA)), the differences in microbial community makeup are analyzed, certain statistical test such as permutational multivariate analysis of variance (PERMANOVA) seeks for the major differences in beta diversity carried by on exposure of drug.

   In differential abundance analysis, identification of bacterial taxa, such as higher ranks or species, shows a notable difference in abundance after pharmacological treatment by the use of certain tools such as MaaSL and DESeq2 (Ghosh et al. 2020; Pasolli et al. 2016)

c. *Correlational and Regression Analysis*:

   For correlational analysis, Spearman's rank correlation method, a non-parametric test for understanding the magnitude and direction of association among abundance of microbes and clinical metrics such as response of treatment toward tumor patients, is used.

   In regression analysis, these can evaluate the effects of particular bacterial taxa on efficacy of drug and patient survival and also help in predicting the outcomes based on microbiota data by incorporating the logistic regression, linear regression, etc. (Schloss & Li 2019).

d. *ML and AI algorithms*:

   ML/AI algorithms, such as SVMs, random forests, and NMs, are majorly used for predictive modeling and pattern recognition. These also help in building models that were utilized in predictive analysis of treatment response based on pre-treatment gut microbiota makeup. Moreover, the complex, vast, and the non-linear connections can be managed and solved that are not covered by the conventional techniques (Gopalakrishnan et al. 2018).

e. *Survival Analysis*:

   Certain methods (Kaplan–Meier curves and Cox proportional hazards model) indicate the likelihood of survival over time for several groups of patients thats are stratified or classified according to initial parameters of their gut microbiome. In addition, components that independently impact the patient's survival during medication treatment are analyzed.

Researchers have exemplified this while analyzing the melanoma patient undergoing the treatment that boosts the immune system's ability to fight cancer cells, i.e., anti-PD-1 immunotherapy, the stool as a sample taken from the patient before the treatment process. The gut microbiota composition is analyzed by 16s rRNA gene sequencing method for identifying bacterial species in sample. Patients are broadly divided into responders to immunotherapy and non-responders to immunotherapy.

Statistical methods, such as Microbiome Profiling and Related Analysis and ML algorithms, are employed for analysis. Where alpha diversity (Shannon Metric) was incorporated to compare number of species of gut microbiota among responder and non-responder groups, beta diversity (PCoA) was used to evaluate compositional variations in gut microbiota among groups. Moreover, the differential abundance analysis (DESeq2) evaluates the bacterial taxa with significant different abundances among the broader groups, i.e., responder and non-responders.

Furthermore, the ML algorithm, such as Random Forest, was employed for building predictive models to understand the patient's response to immunotherapy depends upon the pre-treatment gut microbiome composition, the model trained by taking data from subset of patients and evaluated on independent group for examining its accuracy. This model can pinpoint specific taxa of bacteria that will be the potential players in immunotherapy. Scientists can establish microbiome-based therapies to boost the efficacy of specific microbial signatures linked with positive findings (Garland et al. 2016).

4.4.2 Role of Preventive Medicine in Managing GI Tract Cancers

On a worldwide scale, the GI tract cancers that are majorly colorectal, gastric, and esophageal cancers pose a significant health burden and are contributors to the most mortality and disability from cancer. In order to effectively manage, treat, and unfavorable prognosis with these malignancies, preventive medicines and approaches are needed. Great and effective preventive medicines and strategies can potentially be useful in disease prevention, boosting health, and enhancing patient results.

Preventive medicines incorporated a variety of interventions, such as vaccinations, chemoprevention, screenings, and lifestyle modifications for risk reduction, early detection, and effectively managing GI cancers (Schiller & Lowy 2015).

a. *Vaccinations*:

   Several types of vaccinations are currently available in the market and in clinical trials to prevent and decrease the risk of certain types of cancers, such as *human papillomavirus* (*HPV*) vaccine (Gardasil 9 and cervarix), which protects against oropharyngeal and anal cancers. *Hepatitis B virus* vaccine (Recomb Ivax HB and Engerix-B for both pediatric and adolescent, *Helias-B* only for adults) defends against liver cancers and diseases. *H. pylori* vaccine (*EpiVax* and *Helicovaxor* in preclinical and clinical trials) protects us from the peptic ulcer and gastric cancers. And *Cytomegalovirus* (*CMV*) vaccine (CMV-MVA Triplex, CMVpp65-A*0201, CMVPepVax in last phase of clinical trials) provides protection from certain GI tract cancer, including esophageal cancer (Hong et al. 2022; Newman et al. 2023).

b. *Chemoprevention*:

   Non-steroidal anti-inflammatory drugs (NSAIDs), such as ibuprofen, sulindac, and celecoxib, have been linked to reduce the chance of colorectal cancer, working by inhibiting the cyclooxygenase enzymes to reduce inflammation and tumor growth.

   Statins have shown potential in decreasing the risk of colorectal cancer and are often used to lower the level of cholesterols; they block the mevalonate pathway by inhibiting the enzyme HMG-CoA reductase, which is essential for cell survival and division. Moreover, folate supplementation (B vitamin) and minerals (calcium) have been exhibiting the lowering of the risk of colorectal cancer, as they are engaged in the DNA repair and synthesis mechanism. Low levels could show the increased risk of such types of cancers (Jardim et al. 2023).

c. *Screening Programs*:

Frequent GI tract cancer screening facilitates early management and detection, which can enhance the treatment results. Colorectal cancer screening, including the sigmoidoscopy, colonoscopy, and fecal occult blood testing (FOBT) for an early identification of cancers and precancerous polyps at the treatable stage to reduce death rates. Gastric cancer screening, such as endoscopy, is advisable for mass population in regions with a high number of GI incidence rates to diagnose GI-related cancers and pre-cancerous lesions. Screening *H. pylori* is associated with the gastritis by the continuous infection, in which screening can prevent the progression of GI cancer (Jardim et al. 2023).

d. *Lifestyle Modifications*:

Changes in the lifestyle can also impact the risk of GI cancers, by improving the gut health of patient using diet and nutrition, reducing in alcohol and smoking, physical activity, and obesity. By taking care of all these parameters, it can help in lowering the chances of developing colorectal, esophageal, and gastric cancers. Hence, the quality of patient's life improves.

Figure 4.6 depicts the utilization of the several kinds of preventive measures in the case of GI tract cancers for over last five-year, lifestyle modification of such exercise and diet account majority of 40% preventive efforts. Another screening programs include endoscopy, colonoscopy, and more constitute of 30%. Together, vaccinations, such as HBV and HPV, and chemoprevention approaches, make up 15% each of preventive measures. This pie chart is reviewed, which is hypothetical based, in which the actual may vary depending on conditions and research (Ohiagu et al. 2021).

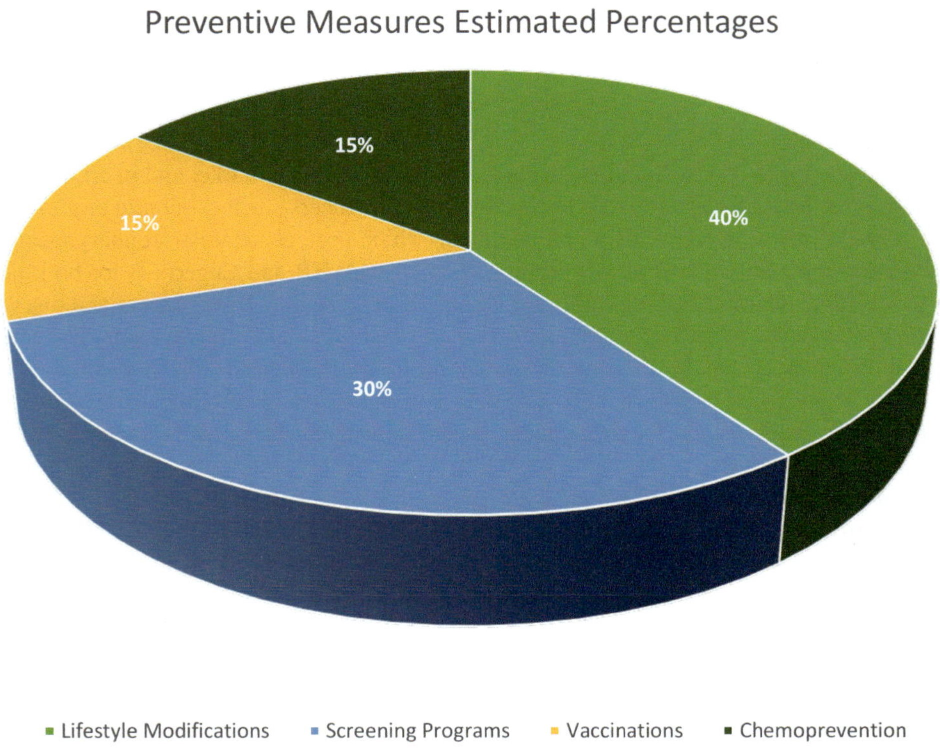

FIGURE 4.6 Pie chart showing the estimated prevalence of several preventive measures for the reduction of GI tract cancers.

4.5 GI TRACT CANCERS AND COMORBIDITIES

4.5.1 Associated Comorbidities in GI Tract Cancers

In GI tract cancers, such as esophageal, gastric, pancreatic, and colorectal cancers, these malignancies are accompanied with many ranges of comorbidities that can cause complications during diagnosis, prognosis, and treatment. Comorbidities mean the coexistence of additional diseases or illnesses in people who are diagnosed with GI cancer. Thus, relationship among the GI tract cancer and comorbidities influences the clinical management and result of individuals with GI tract cancer.

There have been a wide variety of comorbid diseases that are documented, such as diabetes mellitus (DM), cardiovascular disease (CVD), obesity, malnutrition, and depression and anxiety. They also have repercussions on treatment selection, response, and overall survival rates among the individuals with GI tract cancers (Sverdlov et al. 2023).

1. *Metabolic Disorders*

   These disorders include DM and obesity, in which DM is quite common and a significant comorbidity in individuals with GI malignancies in colorectal and pancreatic cancers, which is shown by dysregulation in blood sugar control that negatively influences wound healing and increases the chances of infections. The association among the diabetes and cancer includes an intricate mechanism such as hyperinsulinemia, chronic inflammation, and insulin resistance. DM affects the cancer prognosis and interferes in treatment protocols because in alteration, glucose metabolism can impair the immune system function and lower effectiveness of treatment. On other hand, obesity is a comorbidity in various GI tract cancers, including esophageal and colorectal cancers, which promotes the tumorigenesis due to a connection with chronic inflammation, insulin resistance, and altered levels of adipokines (Chen et al. 2023).
2. *CVD*

   Like heart failure, coronary artery disease, arrhythmias, and hypertension are additional medical conditions in patients with GI cancers. These comorbidities can impact the treatment choices and options because of cardiotoxicity with some chemotherapeutic agents after therapies of cancer (Kari et al. 2022; Zeev 2022).
3. *Chronic Inflammatory and Autoimmune Diseases*

   These disorders, including IBD, chronic hepatitis, and liver cirrhosis, are comorbidities in association with GI tract cancers. Individuals with IBD such as ulcerative colitis (UC) and Crohn's disease have more chances of getting colorectal cancers. IBD contributes to the development of malignancy and dysplasia by prolonged inflammation and immunological dysregulation. On the other hand, chronic hepatitis (both b and c infection) and liver cirrhosis are crucial causes to form liver cancer classified in GI cancer, i.e., hepatocellular carcinoma. Thus, these diseases create a promoted environment for carcinogenesis (Huang et al. 2023; Janus et al. 2010).
4. *Pulmonary Diseases*

   Respiratory conditions, such as chronic obstructive pulmonary disease (COPD) and asthma, are quite common comorbidities with GI cancers, particularly in esophageal cancer. These conditions may render the aesthetic and surgical operations more challenging. Moreover, by the action of certain chemotherapeutic drug and radiation therapy, these comorbidities can be exacerbated (Pressoir et al. 2010).
5. *Renal Dysfunction*

   Abruption in kidney function can impair the excretion process of some chemotherapy drug thus will increase the toxicity in body. Furthermore, it also decreases the treatment choices, dose adjustment, and increases the complications and treatment-related toxicity (Pressoir et al. 2010).

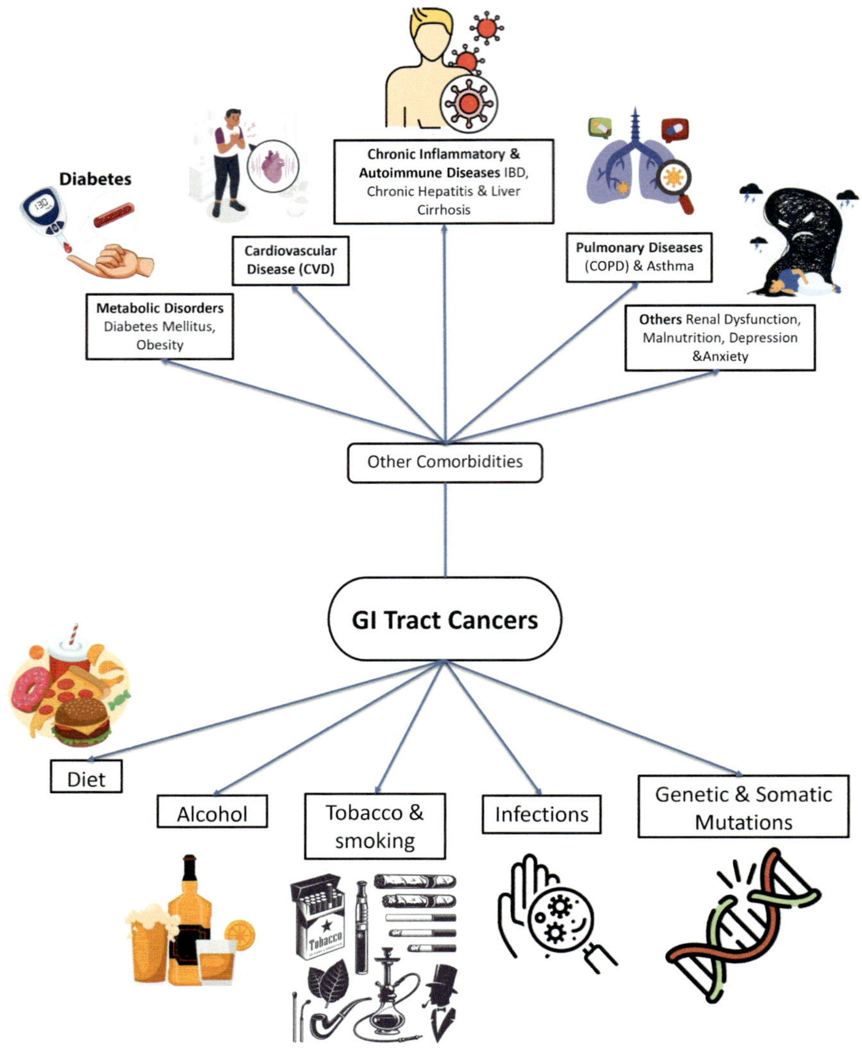

FIGURE 4.7 Schematic representation illustrating the potential association between GI tract cancer, root causes, and comorbidities.

6. *Malnutrition*

   A prevalent effect of GI cancers is malnutrition that is insufficient intake of nutrients, which will result in weakening immune system and decreasing tolerance level to therapy (Walker et al. 2021).
7. *Depression and Anxiety*

   These mental health issues could occur from the emotionally and psychologically exhausting nature of cancer diagnosis and treatment. These have now become very prevalent among cancer individuals, which impacts their life (Walker et al. 2021) (**Figure 4.7**).

4.5.2 Impact of Pharmacomicrobiomics on Managing Comorbid Conditions

As we know, pharmacomicrobiomics is a growing field in which research is performed on the relationship and impact of human gut microbiota in drug metabolism, efficacy, bioavailability, and toxicity. This field has emerged as a solution to the personalized medicine with potential to revolutionize the management of comorbid conditions such as diabetes, CVD, and inflammatory disorders. Healthcare experts can be able to reduce side effects, enhance therapeutic results, and effectively control additional medical conditions that could interfere cancer therapies by modifying and understanding the microbiome and their profiles (Mousa et al. 2023).

In case of managing metabolic disorders such as DM comorbidities with GI cancers, the gut microbiota can affect glucose metabolism and sensitivity of insulin, for example, the utilization of metformin that is the primarily administered drug for type 2 diabetes, which is somehow changed by gut microbiome, thus affecting the pharmacodynamics and pharmacokinetics of drug. Pharmacomicrobiomics field could come as helping hand by providing the customized treatment options; by profiling the gut microbiota, experts can predict which individuals are responding well to drug metformin and enhance the therapeutic effects of metformin, hence improving the glycemic control in patient having diabetic with GI cancer (Anas et al. 2023).

Managing the CVDs comorbidities with GI cancers is very crucial. The gut microbiome can impact the cardiovascular health through alerting metabolism of lipid and systemic inflammation. For example, the gut microbiome reduces the statins that is used in control of hypercholesterolemia. Thus, metabolism of statins reduces their effectiveness, impact on overall bioavailability, and increase in adverse effects. Hence, utilization of personalized microbiome-based adaptions to statin therapy can strengthen lipid-lowering effects and decrease the likelihood of heart diseases and stroke (Longoria et al. 2022; Lu et al. 2022).

In managing the respiratory disorders, such as COPD and asthma, the inhaled corticosteroids were administered. The gut microbiota influences these medication's metabolism and systemic absorption. Pharmacomicrobiomics approaches were used to comprehend the relationship among gut microbiome and inhaled corticosteroids. Finally, it boosts up the therapeutic efficacy, lowering the side effects, and helps experts in the implementation of microbiome-modifying approaches and tailoring dosages system (Shi et al. 2023).

In case of managing the chronic inflammatory and autoimmune diseases such as IBD, chronic hepatitis, and liver cirrhosis, drugs such as, infliximab, anti-viral therapies (direct-acting antivirals) and rifaximin, respectively, are used. Numerous studies have shown that gut microbiota can degrade and modify these medications and therapies, thus reducing their potential therapeutic effects, influencing absorption, and increasing the production of toxin compounds. The pharmacomicrobiomics field resolves these concerns by offering precision approaches based on microbiome profiles to improve the efficacy of drugs and overall treatment outcomes (Lorenzo 2022; Ning et al. 2023).

REFERENCES

Ali O, Abdelbaki W, Shrestha A, Elbasi E, Abdallah M, Dwivedi YK. A systematic literature review of artificial intelligence in the healthcare sector: Benefits, challenges, methodologies, and functionalities. J Innov Know. 2023;8(1):100333.doi: 10.1016/j.jik.2023.100333.

Alya H, Moossavi S, Arrieta M-C, Coburn B. Principles and terminology for host–microbiome–drug interactions. Open Forum Infect Dis. 2023. doi: 10.1093/ofid/ofad195.

Anas M, Begg M, Al Tarhuni M, Gonzalez N, Sanivarapu R, Mohammed L. Understanding the role of the gut microbiome in diabetes and therapeutics targeting leaky gut: A systematic review. Cureus. 2023. doi: 10.7759/cureus.41559.

Arango-Argoty G, Garner E, Pruden A, Heath LS, Vikesland P, Zhang L. DeepARG: A deep learning approach for predicting antibiotic resistance genes from metagenomic data. Microbiome. 2018;6(1):23. doi: 10.1186/s40168-018-0401-z.

Asseri AH, Bakhsh T, Abuzahrah SS, Ali S, Rather IA. The gut dysbiosis-cancer axis: Illuminating novel insights and implications for clinical practice. Front Pharmacol. 2023. doi: 10.3389/fphar.2023.1208044.

Baptista LC, Sun Y, Carter CS, Buford TW. Crosstalk between the gut microbiome and bioactive lipids: Therapeutic targets in cognitive frailty. Front Nutr. 2020;7:17. doi: 10.3389/fnut.2020.00017.

Blumberg R, Powrie F. Microbiota, disease, and back to health: A metastable journey. Sci Transl Med. 2012 Jun 6;4(137):137rv7. doi: 10.1126/scitranslmed.3004184.

Bray F, Ferlay J, Soerjomataram I, Siegel RL, Torre LA, Jemal A. Global cancer statistics 2018: GLOBOCAN estimates of incidence and mortality worldwide for 36 cancers in 185 countries. CA Cancer J Clin. 2018. doi: 10.3322/caac.21492.

Brian B, Liebert A, Borody TJ, Herkes GK, McLachlan CS, Kiat H. Neurodegenerative and neurodevelopmental diseases and the gut-brain axis: The potential of therapeutic targeting of the microbiome. Int J Mol Sci. 2023. doi: 10.3390/ijms24119577.

Cassol I, Ibañez M, Pablo J. Unraveling key features of microbial alpha-diversity metrics and their practical applications. Res Sq. 2023. doi: 10.21203/rs.3.rs-2595260/v1.

Cátia D, Cabral C, Jarak I, Veiga F, Dourado M, Figueiras A. The debate between the human microbiota and immune system in treating aerodigestive and digestive tract cancers: A review. Vaccines. 2023. doi: 10.3390/vaccines11030492.

Chen M, Jian X, Maoling W, Junyao Y, Chen T. Cardiovascular complications of pan-cancer therapies: The need for cardio-oncology. Cancers. 2023. doi: 10.3390/cancers15113055.

Ching Chan W, Millwood IY, Kartsonaki C, Du H, Guo Y, Chen Y, Bian Z, Walters RG, Lv J, He P, Hu C, Li L, Yang L, Chen Z, China Kadoorie Biobank (CKB) Collaborative Group. Spicy food consumption and risk of gastrointestinal-tract cancers: Findings from the China Kadoorie Biobank. Int J Epidemiol. 2021 Feb;50(1):199–211. doi: 10.1093/ije/dyaa275.

Conti G, Federica D, Fabbrini M, Brigidi P, Barone M, Turroni S. Pharmacomicrobiomics in anticancer therapies: Why the gut microbiota should be pointed out. Genes. 2022. doi: 10.3390/genes14010055.

Cryan JF, Dinan TG. Mind-altering microorganisms: The impact of the gut microbiota on brain and behaviour. Nat Rev Neurosci. 2012 Oct;13(10):701–12. doi: 10.1038/nrn3346.

Curini L, Amedei A. Cardiovascular diseases and pharmacomicrobiomics: A perspective on possible treatment relevance. Biomedicines. 2021;9(10):1338. doi: 10.3390/biomedicines9101338.

Diamantidis MD, Papaioannou M, Hatjiharissi E. Primary gastric non-Hodgkin lymphomas: Recent advances regarding disease pathogenesis and treatment. World J Gastroenterol. 2021 Sep 21;27(35):5932–45. doi: 10.3748/wjg.v27.i35.5932. PMID: 34629810; PMCID: PMC8475005.

DiPalma MP, Blattman JN. The impact of microbiome dysbiosis on T cell function within the tumor microenvironment (TME). Fron Cell Dev Biol. 2023. doi: 10.3389/fcell.2023.1141215.

Esteva A, Robicquet A, Ramsundar B, Kuleshov V, DePristo M, Chou K, …, Dean J. A guide to deep learning in healthcare. Nat Med. 2019;25(1):24–29.

Ferlay J, Colombet M, Soerjomataram I, Parkin DM, Piñeros M, Znaor A, Bray F. Cancer statistics for the year 2020: An overview. Int J Cancer. 2021 Apr 5. doi: 10.1002/ijc.33588. Epub ahead of print. PMID: 33818764.

Franzosa EA, Morgan XC, Segata N, Waldron L, Reyes J, Earl AM, Giannoukos G, Boylan MR, Ciulla D, Gevers D, Izard J, Garrett WS, Chan AT, Huttenhower C. Relating the metatranscriptome and metagenome of the human gut. Proc Natl Acad Sci USA. 2014 Jun 3;111(22):E2329–E2338. doi: 10.1073/pnas.1319284111.

Franzosa EA, et al. Gut microbiome structure and metabolic activity in inflammatory bowel disease. Nat Microbiol. 2019.doi: 10.1038/s41564-019-0442-5

Garjan HS, Yadollah O, Poursheikhali AM, Ferdousi R. In-silico computational approaches to study microbiota impacts on diseases and pharmacotherapy. Gut Pathogens. 2023. doi: 10.1186/s13099-023-00535-2.

Garland SM, Kjaer SK, Muñoz N, Block SL, Brown DR, DiNubile MJ, …, Study FP. Impact and effectiveness of the quadrivalent human papillomavirus vaccine: A systematic review of 10 years of real-world experience. Clin Infect Dis. 2016;63(4):519–27.

Geller LT, Barzily-Rokni M, Danino T, Jonas OH, Shental N, Nejman D, Gavert N, Zwang Y, Cooper ZA, Shee K, Thaiss CA, Reuben A, Livny J, Avraham R, Frederick DT, Ligorio M, Chatman K, Johnston SE, Mosher CM, Brandis A, Fuks G, Gurbatri C, Gopalakrishnan V, Kim M, Hurd MW, Katz M, Fleming J, Maitra A, Smith DA, Skalak M, Bu J, Michaud M, Trauger SA, Barshack I, Golan T, Sandbank J, Flaherty KT, Mandinova A, Garrett WS, Thayer SP, Ferrone CR, Huttenhower C, Bhatia SN, Gevers D, Wargo JA, Golub TR, Straussman R. Potential role of intratumor bacteria in mediating tumor resistance to the chemotherapeutic drug gemcitabine. Science. 2017 Sep 15;357(6356):1156–60. doi: 10.1126/science.aah5043. PMID: 28912244; PMCID: PMC5727343.

Ghosh TS, Das M, Jeffery IB, O'Toole PW. Adjusting for age improves identification of gut microbiome alterations in multiple diseases. eLife. 2020;9:e50240. doi: 10.7554/eLife.50240.

Goodrich JK, Waters JL, Poole AC, Sutter JL, Koren O, Blekhman, R, …, Ley RE. Human genetics shape the gut microbiome. Cell. 2014;159(4):789–99. doi: 10.1016/j.cell.2014.09.053.

Gopalakrishnan V, Spencer CN, Nezi L, Reuben A, Andrews MC, Karpinets TV, Prieto PA, Vicente D, Hoffman K, Wei SC, Cogdill AP, Zhao L, Hudgens CW, Hutchinson DS, Manzo T, Petaccia de Macedo M, Cotechini T, Kumar T, Chen WS, Reddy SM, Szczepaniak Sloane R, Galloway-Pena J, Jiang H, Chen PL, Shpall EJ, Rezvani K, Alousi AM, Chemaly RF, Shelburne S, Vence LM, Okhuysen PC, Jensen VB, Swennes AG, McAllister F, Marcelo Riquelme Sanchez E, Zhang Y, Le Chatelier E, Zitvogel L, Pons N, Austin-Breneman JL, Haydu LE, Burton EM, Gardner JM, Sirmans E, Hu J, Lazar AJ, Tsujikawa T, Diab A, Tawbi H, Glitza IC, Hwu WJ, Patel SP, Woodman SE, Amaria RN, Davies MA, Gershenwald JE, Hwu P, Lee JE, Zhang J, Coussens LM, Cooper ZA, Futreal PA, Daniel CR, Ajami NJ, Petrosino JF, Tetzlaff MT, Sharma P, Allison JP, Jenq RR, Wargo JA. Gut microbiome modulates response to anti-PD-1 immunotherapy in melanoma patients. Science. 2018 Jan 5;359(6371):97–103. doi: 10.1126/science.aan4236.

Haiser HJ, Gootenberg DB, Chatman K, Sirasani G, Balskus EP, Turnbaugh PJ. Predicting and manipulating cardiac drug inactivation by the human gut bacterium *Eggerthella lenta*. Science. 2013;341(6143):295–8. doi: 10.1126/science.1235872.

Hong M-Z, Li J-M, Chen Z-J, Lin X-Y, Pan J-S, Gong L. Global burden of major gastrointestinal cancers and its association with socioeconomics, 1990–2019. Front Oncol. 2022. doi: 10.3389/fonc.2022.942035.

Hong SW, Byeon J-S. Endoscopic diagnosis and treatment of early colorectal cancer. Intest Res. 2022. doi: 10.5217/ir.2021.00169.

Hou K, Wu ZX, Chen XY, et al. Microbiota in health and diseases. Sig Transduct Target Ther. 2022;7:135. doi: 10.1038/s41392-022-00974-4.

Hongyun W, Chen L, Lian G, Yang J, Li F, Zou Y, Lu F, Yin Y. Antitumor mechanisms of bifidobacteria (review). Oncol Lett. 2018. doi: 10.3892/OL.2018.8692.

Huang R, Hammelef E, Sabitsky M, Ream C, Khalilieh S, Zohar N, Lavu H, Bowne WB, Yeo CJ, Nevler A. Chronic obstructive pulmonary disease is associated with worse oncologic outcomes in early-stage resected pancreatic and periampullary cancers. Adv Cardiovasc Dis. 2023. doi: 10.3390/biomedicines11061684.

Hui-Fen S. Machine learning and AI in cancer prognosis, prediction, and treatment selection: A critical approach. J Multidiscip Healthc. 2023. doi: 10.2147/JMDH.S410301.

Janus N, Launay-Vacher V, Byloos E, et al. Cancer and renal insufficiency results of the BIRMA study. Br J Cancer. 2010. 103:1815–21. doi: 10.1038/sj.bjc.6605979.

Jardim SR, de Souza LMP, de Souza HSP. The rise of gastrointestinal cancers as a global phenomenon: Unhealthy behavior or progress? Int J Environ Res Public Health. 2023. doi: 10.3390/ijerph20043640.

Ji N, Tiwari AK, Yang, D-H. Unraveling immunotherapy's role in propelling cancer outcomes. Cancer Rep. 2023. doi: 10.1002/cnr2.1862.

Kaja K, Cudnoch-Jędrzejewska A, Czarzasta K. Communication of gut microbiota and brain via immune and neuroendocrine signaling. Front Microbiol. 2023. doi: 10.3389/fmicb.2023.1118529.

Kari H, Sundquist K, Lundquist J, Försti A, Liska V, Hemminki A, Li X. Personal comorbidities and their subsequent risks for liver, gallbladder and bile duct cancers. Int J Cancer. 2022. doi: 10.1002/ijc.34308.

Konstantina A, Adamopoulos PG, Scorilas A. Unveiling the human gastrointestinal tract microbiome: The past, present, and future of metagenomics. Adv Cardiovasc Dis. 2023. doi: 10.3390/biomedicines11030827.

Kostic AD, Xavier RJ, Gevers D. The microbiome in inflammatory bowel disease: Current status and the future ahead. Gastroenterology. 2014 May;146(6):1489–99. doi: 10.1053/j.gastro.2014.02.009.

Kouidhi S, Zidi O, Belkhiria Z, Rais H, Ayadi A, Ayed FB, Mosbah A, Cherif A, El Gaaied ABA. Gut microbiota, an emergent target to shape the efficiency of cancer therapy. Explor Targeted Antitumor Ther. 2023. doi: 10.37349/etat.2023.00132.

Lai J, Ferdous T, Dinu I, Groizeleau J, Danska J, McCoy KD, Arrieta M-C, Kozyrskyj AL, Greenwood CMT. Beta-diversity distance matrices for microbiome sample size and power calculations—How to obtain good estimates. Comput Struct Biotechnol J. 2022. doi: 10.1016/j.csbj.2022.04.032.

Li H, Xia J, Zhang Y, Xu L. Microbiome-based machine learning prediction of clinical outcomes in infectious diseases: A review. Brief Bioinform. 2017;21(5):1649–63. doi: 10.1093/bib/bbx118.

Li T, Mbala-Kingebeni P, Naccache SN, Thézé J, Bouquet J, Federman S, Somasekar S, Yu G, Sanchez-San Martin C, Achari A, Schneider BS, Rimoin AW, Rambaut A, Nsio J, Mulembakani P, Ahuka-Mundeke S, Kapetshi J, Pybus OG, Muyembe-Tamfum JJ, Chiu CY. Metagenomic next-generation sequencing of the 2014 Ebola virus disease outbreak in the democratic republic of the Congo. J Clin Microbiol. 2019 Aug 26;57(9):e00827–19. doi: 10.1128/JCM.00827-19.

Li W, Chen T. An insight into the clinical application of gut microbiota during anticancer therapy. 2022. doi: 10.1155/2022/8183993.

Longoria CR, Guers JJ, Campbell SC. The interplay between cardiovascular disease, exercise, and the gut microbiome. Rev Cardiovasc Med.2022. doi:10.31083/j.rcm2311365

Lorenzo B. Treatment and management of chronic inflammatory bowel diseases: Optimizing present and future therapeutic choices. Stomatology. 2022. doi: 10.3390/jcm11185267.

Lozupone CA, Stombaugh JI, Gordon JI, Jansson JK, Knight R. Diversity, stability and resilience of the human gut microbiota. Nature. 2012;489(7415):220–30. doi: 10.1038/nature11550.

Lu W, Wang S, Zhang Q, He C, Fu C, Wei Q. The role of the gut microbiota in health and cardiovascular diseases. Mol Biomed. 2022. doi: 10.1186/s43556-022-00091-2.

Luo Y, Thompson WK, Herr TM, Zeng Z, Berendsen MA, Jonnalagadda SR, …, Liao KP. Natural language processing for EHR-based pharmacovigilance: A structured review. Drug Safety. 2016;39(11):785–99. doi: 10.1007/s40264-017-0558-6.

Maccioni F, Busato L, Valenti A, Cardaccio S, Longhi A, Catalano C. Magnetic resonance imaging of the gastrointestinal tract: Current role, recent advancements and future prospectives. Diagnostics (Basel). 2023 Jul 19;13(14):2410. doi: 10.3390/diagnostics13142410.

Mahdy MS, Azmy AF, Dishisha T, Mohamed WR, Ahmed KA, Hassan A, Aidy SE, El-Gendy AO. Irinotecan-gut microbiota interactions and the capability of probiotics to mitigate Irinotecan-associated toxicity. BMC Microbiol. 2023. doi: 10.1186/s12866-023-02791-3.

María José M-L, Mangalam AK, Regaldiz A, González-Madrid E, Rangel-Ramírez MA, Vallejos OP, Méndez C, Bueno SM, Melo-Gonzalez F, Duarte Y, Opazo MC, Kalergis AM, Riedel CA. Gut microbiota short-chain fatty acids and their impact on the host thyroid function and diseases. Front Endocrinol. 2023. doi: 10.3389/fendo.2023.1192216.

Matson V, Fessler J, Bao R, Chongsuwat T, Zha Y, Alegre M-L, Luke JJ, Gajewski TF. The commensal microbiome is associated with anti-PD-1 efficacy in metastatic melanoma patients. Science. 2018. doi: 10.1126/science.aao3290.

Montagnani M, Lucrezia B, Potenza MA, Charitos IA, Skender T, Colella M, Santacroce L. The crosstalk between gut microbiota and nervous system: A bidirectional interaction between microorganisms and metabolome. Int J Mol Sci. 2023. doi: 10.3390/ijms241210322.

Mousa S, Sarfraz M, Mousa WK. The interplay between gut microbiota and oral medications and its impact on advancing precision medicine. Metabolites. 2023. doi: 10.3390/metabo13050674.

Newman P, Joshua M. Potential role of non-steroidal anti-inflammatory drugs in colorectal cancer chemoprevention for inflammatory bowel disease: An umbrella review. Cancers. 2023. doi: 10.3390/cancers15041102.

Ning L, Zhou YL, Sun H, et al. Microbiome and metabolome features in inflammatory bowel disease via multi-omics integration analyses across cohorts. Nat Commun. 2023;14:7135. doi: 10.1038/s41467-023-42788-0.

Ohiagu FO, Chikezie PC, Chikezie CM. Pathophysiology of diabetes mellitus complications: Metabolic events and control. Biomed Res Ther. 2021. doi: 10.15419/BMRAT.V8I3.663.

Parkash O, Saleha Siddiqui AT, Jiwani U, Rind F, Padhani ZA, Rizvi A, Hoodbhoy Z, Das JK. Diagnostic accuracy of artificial intelligence for detecting gastrointestinal luminal pathologies: A systematic review and meta-analysis. Front Med. 2022. doi: 10.3389/fmed.2022.1018937.

Pasolli E, Truong DT, Malik F, Waldron L, Segata N. Machine learning meta-analysis of large metagenomic datasets: Tools and biological insights. PLoS Comput Biol. 2016;12(7):e1004977. doi: 10.1371/journal.pcbi.1004977.

Pressoir M, Desné S, Berchery D, Rossignol G, Poiree B, Meslier M, Traversier S, Vittot M, Simon M, Gekiere JP, Meuric J, Serot F, Falewee MN, Rodrigues I, Senesse P, Vasson MP, Chelle F, Maget B, Antoun S, Bachmann P. Prevalence, risk factors and clinical implications of malnutrition in French Comprehensive Cancer Centres. Br J Cancer. 2010;102(6):966–71. doi: 10.1038/sj.bjc.6605578.

Priyanka B, WanjulParshuram M, Laxman G. Future directions of AI in pharma: Innovation in pharmaceutical industry. Int J Multidiscip Res. 2023;5(3). https://www.ijfmr.com/papers/2023/3/3098.pdf

Qin J, Li R, Raes J, et al. A human gut microbial gene catalogue established by metagenomic sequencing. Nature. 2010;464:59–65. doi: 10.1038/nature08821.

Quan L, Yu H. Immuno-oncology-microbiome axis of gastrointestinal malignancy. World J Gastrointest Oncol. 2023. doi: 10.4251/wjgo.v15.i5.757.

Quince C, Walker A, Simpson J, et al. Shotgun metagenomics, from sampling to analysis. Nat Biotechnol. 2017;35:833–44. doi: 10.1038/nbt.3935.

Rebecca, M-M. Targeting cancer cell signaling using precision oncology towards a holistic approach to cancer therapeutics. 2023. doi: 10.31219/osf.io/w2uy8.

Rongrong W, Chen J, Jia Y, Chen Y, Li Y, Yan R. Fecal microbial SN-38G metabotypes in colorectal cancer patients are associated with irinotecan-induced delayed diarrhea. 2023. doi: 10.1124/jpet.122.221890.

Routy B, Le Chatelier E, Derosa L, Duong CPM, Alou MT, Daillère R, Fluckiger A, Messaoudene M, Rauber C, Roberti MP, Fidelle M, Flament C, Poirier-Colame V, Opolon P, Klein C, Iribarren K, Mondragón L, Jacquelot N, Qu B, Ferrere G, Clémenson C, Mezquita L, Masip JR, Naltet C, Brosseau S, Kaderbhai C, Richard C, Rizvi H, Levenez F, Galleron N, Quinquis B, Pons N, Ryffel B, Minard-Colin V, Gonin P, Soria JC, Deutsch E, Loriot Y, Ghiringhelli F, Zalcman G, Goldwasser F, Escudier B, Hellmann MD, Eggermont A, Raoult D, Albiges L, Kroemer G, Zitvogel L. Gut microbiome influences efficacy of PD-1-based immunotherapy against epithelial tumors. Science. 2018 Jan 5;359(6371):91–97. doi: 10.1126/science.aan3706. Epub 2017 Nov 2. PMID: 29097494.

Sandra G. Advancements in precision medicine for cancer treatment: Personalizing the fight against cancer. 2023. doi: 10.31219/osf.io/v68kw.

Schloss PD, Li JZ. Predicting cancer treatment response using the microbiome. Genome Biol. 2019;20(1):139. doi: 10.1038/s41467-022-30512-3.

Schneider KA, Chittenden A, Shannon KM. Cancer diagnosis and treatment. ResearchGate. 2023, Feb; unknown. https://www.researchgate.net/publication/368993761_CANCER_DIAGNOSIS_AND_TREATMENT

Seekatz AM, Aas J, Gessert CE, Rubin TA, Saman DM, Bakken JS, Young VB. Recovery of the gut microbiome following fecal microbiota transplantation. mBio. 2014 Jun 17;5(3):e00893–14. doi: 10.1128/mBio.00893-14.

Senchukova MA. Microbiota of the gastrointestinal tract: Friend or foe? World J Gastroenterol. 2023. doi: 10.3748/wjg.v29.i1.19.

Schiller, JT, Lowy DR. Virus infection and human cancer: An overview. Recent Results in Cancer Res. 2015;193: 1–10. doi: 10.1007/978-3-319-18851-1_1.

Sharda S, Avasthi A, Kaur N. Structuring Inflammasome-Epigenome – Phenotypic Axis in Gynecological Cancers. 2023. 1–15. doi: 10.1007/978-981-99-2196-6_25-2.

Sharma P, Hu-Lieskovan S, Wargo JA, Ribas A. Primary, adaptive, and acquired resistance to cancer immunotherapy. Cell. 2017;168(4):707–23.

Shi H, Zhao T, Geng R, Sun L, Fan H. The associations between gut microbiota and chronic respiratory diseases: A Mendelian randomization study. Front Microbiol. 2023. doi: 10.3389/fmicb.2023.1200937.

Shreiner AB, Kao JY, Young VB. The gut microbiome in health and in disease. Curr Opin Gastroenterol. 2015 Jan;31(1):69–75. doi: 10.1097/MOG.0000000000000139.

Siegel RL, Miller KD, Jemal A. Cancer statistics, 2020. CA Cancer J Clin. 2020 Jan;70(1):7–30. doi: 10.3322/caac.21590.

Srivastav S, Singh L, Avasthi A, Kaur N, Gaertner W, Kesheri M, Kanchan S, Sharda S. Integromics: Tracking the multi-omic expanse in theragnostics. 2024. 135–173. doi: 10.1007/978-981-97-1769-9_6.

Sverdlov AL, Koczwara B, Cehic DA, Clark RA, Hunt L, Nicholls SJ, Thomas L, Thornton-Benko E, Kritharides L. When cancer and cardiovascular disease intersect: The challenge and the opportunity of cardio-oncology. Heart Lung Circ. 2023. doi: 10.1016/j.hlc.2023.04.301.

Swer NM, Venkidesh BS, Murali TS, Mumbrekar KD. Gut microbiota-derived metabolites and their importance in neurological disorders. Mol Biol Rep. 2022. doi: 10.1007/s11033-022-08038-0.

Tiwari P, Dwivedi R, Bansal M, Tripathi M, Dada R. Role of gut microbiota in neurological disorders and its therapeutic significance. Stomatology. 2023. doi: 10.3390/jcm12041650.

Topol EJ. High-performance medicine: The convergence of human and artificial intelligence. Nat Med. 2019;25:44–56. doi: 10.1038/s41591-018-0300-7.

Tremaroli V, Bäckhed F. Functional interactions between the gut microbiota and host metabolism. Nature. 2012 Sep 13;489(7415):242–9. doi: 10.1038/nature11552.

Turajlic S, Swanton C. Metastasis as an evolutionary process. Science. 2016;352(6282):169–75.

Vania M, Tama BA, Maulahela H, Lim S. Recent advances in applying machine learning and deep learning to detect upper gastrointestinal tract lesions. IEEE Access. 2023;11:66544–67. doi: 10.1109/access.2023.3290997.

Walker ZJ, Xue S, Jones MP, Ravindran AV. Depression, anxiety, and other mental disorders in patients with cancer in low- and lower-middle-income countries: A systematic review and meta-analysis. JCO Glob Oncol. 2021;7:1233–50. doi: 10.1200/GO.21.00056.

Wallace BD, Wang H, Lane KT, Scott JE, Orans J, Koo JS, Venkatesh M, Jobin C, Yeh LA, Mani S, Redinbo MR. Alleviating cancer drug toxicity by inhibiting a bacterial enzyme. Science. 2010 Nov 5;330(6005):831–35. doi: 10.1126/science.1191175.

Wang Z, Lian W, Zhang Y. Generative adversarial networks in microbiome research. bioRxiv. 2018. doi: 10.1101/393900.

Wilson ID, Nicholson JK. Gut microbiome interactions with drug metabolism, efficacy, and toxicity. Transl Res. 2017 Jan;179:204–22. doi: 10.1016/j.trsl.2016.08.002.

Wong CY, Yusoff WFMW, Iqbal HA, Loke MF, Tan LTH. Probiotics for the treatment of chemotherapy-induced diarrhea: A comprehensive review. Nutrients. 2019;11(6):1283. doi: 10.3390/nu11061283.

Xu HM, Huang HL, Zhou YL, Zhao HL, Xu J, Shou DW, Liu YD, Zhou YJ, Nie YQ. Fecal microbiota transplantation: A new therapeutic attempt from the gut to the brain. Gastroenterol Res Pract. 2021 Jan 16;2021:6699268. doi: 10.1155/2021/6699268.

Yu J, Feng Q, Wong SH, Zhang D, Liang QY, Qin Y, …, Wu WKK. Metagenomic analysis of faecal microbiome as a tool towards targeted non-invasive biomarkers for colorectal cancer. Gut. 2017 Jan;66(1):70–78. doi: 10.1136/gutjnl-2015-309800

Zeev E. Cancer and autoimmune diseases: A tale of two immunological opposites? Front Immunol. 2022. doi: 10.3389/fimmu.2022.821598.

Zeller G, Tap J, Voigt AY, Sunagawa S, Kultima JR, Costea PI, …, Bork P. Potential of fecal microbiota for early-stage detection of colorectal cancer. Mol Syst Biol. 2014;10(11):766.

Zhang R, Zheng Y, Mak TW, Yu J, Luo H, Wong SH. Deep learning model for the automated detection of polyps in colonoscopy: A systematic review and meta-analysis. Gastroenterology. 2019;158(4):1020–32.

Zhao L, Walkowiak S, Dilantha Fernando WG. Artificial intelligence: A promising tool in exploring the phytomicrobiome in managing disease and promoting plant health. Plants. 2023. doi: 10.3390/plants12091852.

Zhao T, Wang, X, Liwu F, Yang K. *Fusobacterium nucleatum*: Anew player in regulation of cancer development and therapeutic response. Cancer Drug Resist. 2022. doi: 10.20517/cdr.2021.144.

Zheng S, Li Y, Chen H, Xu R, Xie L. Deep learning-based drug discovery and development. Nat Rev Drug Discov. 2018;17(6):478–98. doi: 10.1038/nrd.2018.37.

Zitvogel L, Ma Y, Raoult D, Kroemer G, Gajewski TF. The microbiome in cancer immunotherapy: Diagnostic tools and therapeutic strategies. Science. 2018;359(6382):1366–70. doi: 10.1126/science.aar6918.

Zuo T, Zhang F, Lui GCY, Yeoh YK, Li AYL, Zhan H, Wan Y, Chung ACK, Cheung CP, Chen N, Lai CKC, Chen Z, Tso EYK, Fung KSC, Chan V, Ling L, Joynt G, Hui DSC, Chan FKL, Chan PKS, Ng SC. Alterations in gut microbiota of patients with COVID-19 during time of hospitalization. Gastroenterology. 2020 Sep;159(3):944–55.e8. doi: 10.1053/j.gastro.2020.05.048.

5 Gut Microbiome

A Novel Screening Tool for Colorectal Cancer

Rayvathy Balasubramanian and Sudhasri Ganeshan
Dr. ALM PG Institute of Basic Medical Sciences, University of Madras, Taramani, Chennai, Tamil Nadu, India

Globally, 10% of all cancer cases diagnosed are found to be CRC, making it the third most prevalent type of cancer and the second most frequent cause of cancer-related deaths [Siegel et al., 2023]. The emergence of early onset colorectal cancer (EOCRC) in individuals under 50 has become a growing concern in recent times. In terms of epidemiology, pathology, anatomy, metabolism, and biology, EOCRC differs from late-onset colorectal cancer (LOCRC). By 2030, the incidence of EOCRC is predicted to rise by more than 140% [Hofseth et al., 2020]. Obesity, increased body mass index, and early exposure to carcinogenic factors as well as other external factors, such as diet with less fibre content and excessive intake of preserved food, may result in an increased incidence of EOCRC. Obesity in early childhood can result in dysbiosis and inflammation, which can induce EOCRC [Hofseth et al., 2020]. The incidence of EOCRC is influenced by a number of external and internal environmental factors. External environmental factors include general factors such as stress, education, socioeconomic status, and climate changes, and specific factors such as infections, radiation, drugs, alcohol, tobacco, food, and exercise. Hormones, oxidative stress, inflammation, gut microbiota, and metabolic factors are some of the internal environmental factors.

The gut microbiome plays a crucial role in the pathogenesis of chronic diseases, particularly cancers, by influencing immune regulation, inflammation, and metabolic processes. Dysbiosis, or an imbalance in the gut microbial community, can lead to chronic inflammation, oxidative stress, and immune dysregulation, all of which promote carcinogenesis. Additionally, microbial metabolites and toxins can affect cellular signaling pathways, DNA integrity, and epigenetic modifications, thereby contributing to disease progression and tumor development. The complex interactions between the gut microbiota and host cells underscore its significant impact on the initiation and advancement of various chronic conditions, including cancer.

In colorectal cancer (CRC), the gut microbiome significantly impacts tumor initiation, progression, and overall disease outcome. Specific bacterial species can induce chronic inflammation, disrupt the integrity of the intestinal barrier, and produce carcinogenic metabolites, thereby promoting colorectal carcinogenesis through multiple pathways. These microbial alterations can also modulate host immune responses and influence gene expression in epithelial cells. Alterations in the gut microbiota composition have been strongly linked to early-onset colorectal cancer, highlighting its role as a key internal environmental factor influencing CRC risk, development, and potentially patient prognosis.

DOI: 10.1201/9781003644309-5

5.1 GUT MICROBIOME

Several bacterial populations that coexist in mutualistic relationships within the epithelial barriers of various organs of a host make up the microbiota. The microbiota is an ecosystem with a metabolic activity that interacts with stromal and epithelial cells and is vital to human health. It performs a variety of tasks, including the synthesis of several vital metabolites, pathogen avoidance, regulation of overgrowth of harmful bacteria, and activation of host immunity (Rubinstein et al., 2013). In the gastrointestinal tract, the richest microbiota is seen in the colon. The colonic microbiome is abundant in number and also performs more metabolic functions (Rooks and Garrett, 2016). There is a lot of variation in the composition of microbiota among individuals, driven by external environmental factors such as diet, chemical exposure, and antibiotic/medication consumption. It has been demonstrated that dietary modifications have a major impact on gut microbiota.

Pathogenic alterations in the profile and functions of the microbiome are known as dysbiosis. Changes in the quantity of beneficial gut bacteria can exacerbate long-term inflammatory diseases and increase the synthesis of carcinogenic compounds, which can result in neoplasia. Recent studies have observed a direct link between dysbiosis of gut flora and pathophysiology of many non-communicable diseases such as obesity, type 2 diabetes mellitus, non-alcoholic fatty liver disease, autoimmune disorders, and various malignancies (Gagnière et al., 2016). In addition to the variations in the gut flora, the products of their metabolism also can prove either beneficial or harmful to the host. Examples of such microbiome-derived metabolites that play role in human diseases are short-chain fatty acids (SCFAs), polyphenols, vitamins, tryptophan catabolites, and polyamines. The role of certain microbial metabolites such as SCFAs and polyamines has been studied previously, and the results show that abnormalities in these metabolites are significantly associated with the development and spread of a variety of tumour types (Jahani-Sherafat et al., 2018).

Chronic inflammation is considered to be the primary pathology in the initiation of CRC. Progression of carcinogenesis happens when immature myeloid cells or pro-inflammatory helper T cells are drawn to the malignant cells. This recruitment of immune cells happens under the influence of inflammatory cytokines and chemokines produced by the malignant cells. A pro-tumorigenic milieu consisting of growth and angiogenic factors, tissue remodelling enzymes, and suppressed anti-tumour T-cell response promotes tumour progression (Francescone et al., 2014).

The probable association of gut microbiome in the pathogenesis of CRC was perceived in the early 1970s. In a germ-free mouse model, when the colon was exposed to the carcinogen 1,2-dimethylhydrazine, it was observed that the incidence of CRC formation was greatly reduced (Reddy et al., 1975). The study could not identify the specific microorganism causing this condition at the time. Nonetheless, a related study employing different colon cancer models demonstrated that gut microorganisms' existence or absence had a major impact on the development of colon cancer (Son et al., 2015) (**Figure 5.1**).

5.2 BACTERIA INDICATED IN CRC PATHOGENESIS

5.2.1 Streptococcus bovis/gallolyticus

One of the earliest bacteria with a proven link to CRC is *Streptococcus bovis*. It is a Gram-positive bacterium and is also known as Group D Streptococci. There have been descriptions of this association dating back to 1966, and many important studies have been done to prove this. Adenomas and carcinomas seem to occur more frequently in cases with *S. bovis* bacteramia. Notably, Burns *et al.* demonstrated a unique correlation between *S. bovis* in the stool and a higher incidence of villous and tubulovillous adenomas (Burns et al., 1985). The likelihood of concurrent CRC in patients with *S. bovis* bacteramia varies widely between studies, with estimates ranging from 6 to 71% (Gold et al., 2004). Regarding the subtypes, it was found that *S. bovis* biotype I, *S. gallolyticus*, was

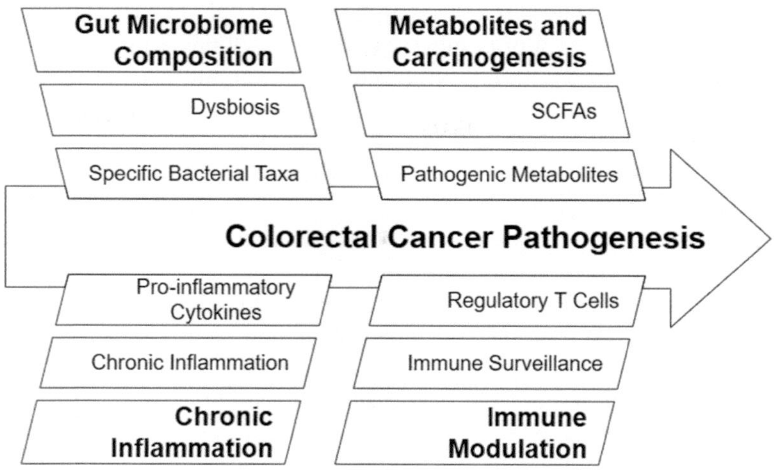

FIGURE 5.1 Understanding the role of gut microbiome in colorectal cancer.

found to be predominantly associated with CRC. In a study of septicaemic patients, blood cultures of 71% grew CRC, developed by *S. gallolyticus*, whereas very few patients (17%) are infected with that developed by other *S. bovis* subtypes (Abdulamir et al., 2011). When biopsy tissue specimens from CRC patients were analysed for the presence of *S. gallolyticus* DNA, approximately half of the specimens were found to be positive. However, when normal colon tissue from healthy controls was evaluated, less than 10% had *S. gallolyticus* DNA. Individuals with seropositivity for *S. gallolyticus* IgG antibodies were linked to higher risks of colorectal adenomas and carcinomas even in the absence of detectable bacteramia. The study done by Abdulamir *et al.* reported that 68% of patients with CRC, 78% of patients with adenoma, and 17% of control patients had positive serum antibodies for *S. gallolyticus* (Abdulamir et al., 2009). In light of these findings, serum antibody testing for *S. gallolyticus* may play a part in CRC screening algorithms in the future. There is a less hope for stool testing because a 17-year longitudinal research found no link between faecal *S. bovis* and an increased risk of colorectal neoplasia (Boltin et al., 2015).

Due to its affinity to collagen I and IV, *S. gallolyticus* has a greater biofilm-forming capacity than other *S. bovis* subtypes. The bacterial pathogen's propensity to produce endocarditis can be explained by the abundance of collagen I found in heart valves. Basement membrane of colonic mucosa is rich in collagen IV. In case of CRC, colonization of *S. bovis* is increased due to its affinity towards the collagen-rich environment of colon. Besides colonization, *S. bovis* favours tumorigenesis by supporting abnormal proliferation of cells and inhibiting apoptosis. *S. bovis* causes upregulation of COX-2 and generation of pro-inflammatory cytokines such as IL-1, IL-8, and NF-κB, which all promote angiogenesis and cellular proliferation while lowering apoptosis in cancerous cells (Abdulamir et al., 2010). The primary component involved in this process of malignant transformation is *S. bovis* cell wall antigen. This was proved by a study done on carcinogen-treated rats that had pre-neoplastic colon lesions. The rats were divided into three groups: one group received live *S. bovis*, the second group received cell wall antigen alone, and the third group was maintained as a control. The pre-cancerous lesions were more pronounced in the rats in the first and the second groups in contrast to the control group, and 50% of the rats which received cell wall antigen developed adenomas (Ellmerich et al., 2000).

5.3 SULPHIDOGENIC BACTERIA

The synthesis of hydrogen sulphide by sulphidogenic bacteria, including *Desulfovibrio*, *Fusobacterium*, and *Bilophila wadsworthia*, has been linked to the development of CRC. It has been demonstrated that the genotoxic substance hydrogen sulphide damages DNA, resulting in chromosomal or genomic instability (Attene-Ramos et al., 2006). More than 80% of sporadic CRCs have genomic instability with high frequency of mutations in genome (Lindblom, 2001). Significant genotoxicity is observed at colonic sulphide concentrations in colonocyte cell lines where DNA repair capability is inhibited (Attene-Ramos et al., 2006). This implies that hydrogen sulphide produced by sulphidogenic bacteria in the colon plays a role in the formation of CRC. It is presumed that hydrogen sulphide enters into colonic epithelial cells by diffusion and affects the mitochondria, resulting in uncontrolled proliferation of cells mediated by the Ras/MAPK pathway.

Apart from CRC patients, sulphidogenic bacteria are also found in abundance in people who are on high-fat diet. It is already a proven fact that people on high-fat diet are at high risk for developing CRC (Magalhães et al., 2012). In another study, African-Americans with CRC exhibited higher amounts of sulphidogenic bacteria than non-Hispanic whites. This may be attributed to the variations in the dietary pattern of these two races [Yazici et al., 2017].

5.3.1 Fusobacterium nucleatum

It is a Gram-negative anaerobe commonly linked to periodontal disease. Numerous investigations on the gut microbiome have revealed that, in comparison to controls, patients with CRC had significantly higher concentrations of *F. nucleatum* and lower overall microbial community diversity (Ahn et al., 2013). Research has proved that *F. nucleatum* can also act as a prognostic indicator for CRC patients. An increased likelihood of lymph node involvement is particularly predicted by higher tissue and faecal concentrations of this bacterium (Suehiro et al., 2017). According to other studies, moderate to high *F. nucleatum* concentrations were linked to worse CRC survival (Flanagan et al., 2014, Mima et al., 2016). Furthermore, *F. nucleatum* might play a more important role in the hyperplastic polyp pathway, thereby favouring CRC development. The prevalence of *F. nucleatum* varies based on the position and histological type of the lesion – e.g., Yu *et al.* observed that *F. nucleatum* are more prevalent in sessile serrated adenomas and hyperplastic polyps located in the proximal part of colon (Yu et al., 2016).

Numerous theories have been put out to explain *F. nucleatum*'s involvement in the pathophysiology of CRC. By creating a pro-inflammatory milieu, attaching to the surface of the host cell, invading the host cell, and transporting other bacteria to the afflicted tissue, these bacteria are able to facilitate immune cell migration. It has also been demonstrated that like the sulphidogenic bacteria this bacterium also produces hydrogen sulphide. *F. nucleatum* uses a unique surface virulence factor, FadA which by attaching to E-cadherin present on CRC cell membrane infiltrates into these cells [Rubinstein et al., 2013]. E-cadherin ordinarily functions as a tumour suppressor; however, this activity is reduced by FadA binding and receptor modification. By attaching and invading the host colonic epithelial cells, *F. nucleatum* produces chronic inflammation. Apart from this, *F. nucleatum* also creates a pro-inflammatory milieu outside of the tumour cell by enlisting immune cells that infiltrate tumours (Kostic et al., 2013). Research has focused on the role of diet in *F. nucleatum*-induced CRC. A large prospective cohort study compared the presence of *F. nucleatum* in CRC tissue samples from individuals following Western diet versus a healthy high-fibre diet rich in fruits, vegetables, and whole grains. A lower risk of CRCs with *F. nucleatum* was linked to high-fibre diet (Mehta et al., 2017).

5.3.2 Helicobacter pylori

The World Health Organisation has classified the tiny, spiral, Gram-negative bacteria *Helicobacter pylori* as a known carcinogen because of its clear link to the emergence of stomach cancer. Though the data is still more debatable, there is evidence to show a possible link between *H. pylori* and CRC. According to Zumkeller et al. (2006) people with *H. pylori* infection had a 1.4-fold higher risk of CRC. *H. pylori* infects host gastric epithelial cells and produces chronic gastritis. The *cagA* oncoprotein, which is exclusive to some *H. pylori* strains, is a virulence factor of the bacterium and is involved in inflammation and development of cancer. According to another study, there is a correlation between *cagA* seropositivity and a higher risk of colon and stomach cancer. The risk of developing cancer was found to be ten times higher in infection caused by *H. pylori* strains with *cagA*-gene than strains that do not have this gene (Shmuely et al., 2001). However, this study was retrospective in nature, and rather than focusing on tissue biopsies or urease breath tests, it examined the subjects' blood IgG antibodies alone. Thus, it is unclear if *cagA* encouraged the development of CRC or if its presence in the patient's serum was accidental. Research is still determining the precise mechanism by which *H. pylori* cause stomach carcinogenesis and, consequently, whether this might be linked to CRC. The processes by which *H. pylori* may cause CRC are still up for debate and require more research.

5.3.3 Bacteroides fragilis

It is a Gram-negative anaerobic bacterium found as a normal flora in the human colon. It has two molecular subtypes: enterotoxigenic [enterotoxigenic *B. fragilis* (ETBF)] and nontoxigenic. The enterotoxigenic strain causes diarrhoea in humans. The *bft* gene encodes the ETBF-specific toxin, *B. fragilis* toxin (BFT). It has been demonstrated that ETBF affects the development of CRC in murine models by producing the metalloprotease toxin. This toxin increases the permeability of colonic epithelial cells by breaking down the intercellular adhesion protein E-cadherin. This results in the activation of β-catenin/Wnt signalling (Toprak et al., 2006). *B. fragilis* makes up less than 1% of the gut microbiota in a healthy person. In case of terminal-stage CRC, this bacterium becomes more abundant in the malignant tissue. The presence of this bacterium in the cancer tissue is assessed and quantified to calculate survival rate of the CRC patients (Wei et al., 2016). The abundance of this bacterium in the cancer tissue samples indicates worst prognosis as indicated by the study of Boleij *et al.* This study reported that *bft* gene was positive in the tissue specimens of all terminal-stage CRC patients (Boleij et al., 2015). Using stool samples, Toprak *et al.* discovered large variations in the presence of the *bft* gene. PCR revealed the presence of the *bft* gene in 38% of the samples from CRC patients and 12% of the control group's samples (Toprak et al., 2006). Many studies are focusing on creating screening methods that use ETBF in the CRC diagnosis.

5.3.4 Clostridium septicum

Clostridium septicum is a Gram-positive and obligatory anaerobic bacillus that produces spores. From its original habitat, the gastrointestinal tract, *C. septicum* migrates to colon and rectum in case of an inflammation or ulceration. The systemic spread of *C. septicum* results in a fatal condition called gas gangrene which has a 48-hour fatality rate of up to 79% (Forrester et al., 2016). Patients with gas gangrene are at high risk of developing colon cancer. CRC patients with abundant *C. septicum* in their gut flora were found to have advanced cancers with significant tumour invasion which breaks the mucosal integrity and paves way for further spread of the bacteria. Overall, 57% of CRCs that are linked to *C. septicum* start in the caecum. Caecum has ideal conditions for the selective growth of *C. septicum* because of the highly acidic pH (5.7) (Larson et al., 1995).

5.3.5 Enterococcus faecalis

Enterococcus faecalis is a facultative anaerobic Gram-positive commensal bacterium. Research has verified that people with CRC have higher concentrations of *E. faecalis* in their faeces (Balamurugan et al., 2008). The contribution of *E. faecalis* to the development of CRC is still debatable, though. Numerous investigations have revealed that it has the capacity to produce extracellular superoxide and reactive oxygen species (ROS), which can harm colonic epithelial cell DNA and cause mutations resulting in CRC (Huycke and Moore, 2002; Wang et al., 2008). Additionally, *E. faecalis* produces metalloprotease, which has the ability to incite inflammation and alter the intestinal epithelial barrier (Steck et al., 2011). In contrast, some research suggests that *E. faecalis* is a significant probiotic microbe and might help prevent CRC (Gong et al., 2017).

5.3.6 Peptostreptococcus anaerobius

It is a member of the normal gut and oral flora. It grows in anaerobic culture conditions and takes up Gram-negative stain. It binds to the α2/β1 integrins of the colonic epithelial cells with the help of its surface receptor, namely, putative cell wall binding repeat 2 (PCWBR2). This binding stimulates the PI3K–Akt pathway. Activation of this pathway induces proliferation of cells and initiates inflammatory reaction (Long et al., 2019). In addition, it alters the innate immune function by interacting with colon cell pattern-recognizing receptors TLR-2 and TLR-4, stimulates ROS production, and promotes carcinogenesis (Tsoi et al., 2017).

5.3.7 Parvimonas micra

Parvimonas micra is a component of the common microflora of the oral cavity and gastrointestinal tract. It has been implicated as a pathogen in diseases associated with oral cavity such as endodontic abscesses, odontogenic infections, and periodontitis lesions. It is identified as a rare aetiology in chronic sinusitis, otitis media, and arthritis involving prosthetic joints. The role of *P. micra* in CRC pathogenesis has been demonstrated recently by a study which used a strain isolated from a patient with CRC in vitro and proved that carcinoma was produced by inflammation cascade induced by Th17 cells and activation of oncogenic Wnt signalling pathway, leading to uncontrolled colonocyte proliferation (Zhao et al., 2022).

5.3.8 *Salmonella* spp.

Chronic colonization and infections with *Salmonella* spp. can raise the chance of developing chronic cholecystitis as well as other gastrointestinal disorders, including malignancies. The *Salmonella*-derived multi-functional protein called AvrA protein apart from regulating inflammation and apoptosis also promotes intestinal cell proliferation, resulting in malignancy. Studies done on animal models of colon cancer have proved that the AvrA-mediated cell proliferation occurs by activation of Wnt/β-catenin and STAT3 signalling pathways (Lu et al., 2016). Typhoid toxin, another genotoxin produced by *Salmonella*, causes damage to DNA in colonic epithelial cells by activating the phosphoinositide 3-kinase (PI3K) pathway (Martin et al., 2019).

5.3.9 Campylobacter jejuni

Campylobacter jejuni is a Gram-negative, microaerophilic bacterium often known as a food-borne pathogen producing gastroenteritis in humans. Apart from gastroenteritis, this bacterium can also produce extra-intestinal diseases such as inflammatory bowel disease and Guillain–Barre syndrome. It has a capability to produce inflammatory reaction in intestine and in systemic circulation. The carcinogenic potential of this bacterium is implicated in the production of a genotoxin called cytolethal distending toxin (CDT). This toxin causes enlargement of the infected enterocytes and damages the DNA by producing nicks. Ultimately it ceases the division of infected cells, resulting in death of the cells. Animal studies using nude mice have studied the effect of CDT in colorectal tumorigenesis (He et al., 2019). The dysbiosis associated with CRC is not restricted to bacterial species alone but also involves fungi and viruses, leading to altered mycobiome and virome.

5.4 DYSBIOSIS OF MYCOBIOME AND VIROME IN CRC

Different mycobiome patterns were found in patients with early stage versus late-stage CRC compared to controls. Research has observed the presence of a balanced coexistence of bacteria and fungi in the gut of healthy controls. On the contrary, this balance was disturbed in case of CRC patients. The dysbiosis in mycobiome in CRC patients was found to be linked with altered gut bacterial composition in CRC patients. Also bacterial-fungal co-occurrences were also reduced in CRC patients when compared to controls (Coker et al., 2019; Malik et al., 2018). There is apparently a connection between CRC and the enteric virome. Increased diversity in bacteriophage viromes was observed in CRC cases when compared to controls. This was linked to a decrease in bacterial diversity and a slight enrichment of certain viral taxa, whose bacterial hosts (such as ETBF, *F. nucleatum*, and *Escherichia coli*) have been linked to CRC. These results suggest a relationship between the bacteriome and virome in CRC risk (Nakatsu et al., 2018). As the studies are very limited, still more research has to be done and more data are needed to decipher the role of the complex interactions happening between gut microbiota – bacteriome, virome, and mycobiome – in the development of CRC.

5.5 GUT MICROBIAL METABOLITES AND CRC

The gut microbiome is a rich source of metabolites and secretory proteins, known as the "secretome". Growth factors, cytokines, proteases, and oncometabolites – which are linked to the advancement of cancer – are all included in this metabolic pool. Metabolic products of microbiota such as L-2-hydroxyglutarate, succinate, fumarate, D-2-hydroxyglutarate, and lactate that accumulate in cancer cells after metabolism are called oncometabolites. Recent studies have demonstrated that intramucosal carcinomas and multiple polypoid adenomas have significantly elevated levels of microbial metabolites, such as phenylalanine, bile acids, and branched-chain amino acids. These findings raise the possibility that microbial metabolites could be used as markers for early CRC screening (Louis et al., 2014). Research has shown that dysbiosis in gut microbiota disrupts bile acid metabolism and results in their accumulation; in turn these toxic bile acid metabolites alter gut microbial composition, favouring CRC development. Among the bile acid metabolites, deoxycholic acid (DCA) was found to have a greater link with CRC. Compared to healthy controls, DCA levels were found to be higher in the gut, serum, and faeces of people with CRC and those at high risk for the disease (Bayerdorffer et al., 1993). DCA mediates inflammation and carcinogenesis in the gut by two mechanisms – inhibiting the nuclear translocation of nuclear transcription factor RelA and blocking the activation of the NF-κB signalling pathway. DCA induces β-catenin signalling activation and ROS-induced DNA damage to host cells, both of which aid in the development of CRC (Muhlbauer et al., 2004). Additionally, DCA has the ability to alter the composition of the gut microbiota to a dysbiotic state, which promotes the growth of tumours in the gut.

Conversely, several bacterial metabolites offer CRC protection and anti-tumorigenic properties. The primary metabolites obtained from the fermentation of indigestible carbohydrates such as fibre and resistant starch are saturated fatty acids (SCFAs), which include propionate and butyrate. Butyric acid is an anti-inflammatory chemical that prevents immune cells and colonocytes from producing histone deacetylases, which leads to the hyperacetylation of certain transcription factors and signal transduction-related proteins. Consequently, pro-inflammatory factors are down-regulated, cell proliferation is inhibited, and CRC cells are selectively induced to undergo apoptosis. Butyrate also has significant anti-tumorigenic properties, such as preventing angiogenesis and reducing the growth of harmful microorganisms in the digestive system (Fung et al., 2012). Additionally, indole-derived metabolites, generated by *Clostridium* and *Bacteroides* species during their metabolism of tryptophan, exhibit a protective effect against CRC by producing anti-inflammatory effect (Gao et al., 2018) (**Figure 5.2**).

Characteristic	Deoxycholic Acid (DCA)	Butyric Acid	Indole-derived Metabolites
Effect on CRC	Promotes CRC development	Inhibits CRC development	Protective effect against CRC
Mechanism	Blocks NF-κB signalling Induces β-catenin signalling and ROS-induced DNA damage to host cells	Prevents histone deacetylases production by immune cells and colonocytes	Anti-inflammatory effect
Gut Microbiota	Alters to dysbiotic state	Reduces harmful microorganisms	Generated by Clostridium and Bacteroides

FIGURE 5.2 Role of gut microbial metabolites in CRC development.

5.6 MICROBIOME-BASED BIOMARKERS FOR CRC DIAGNOSIS

Finding innovative biomarkers that are trustworthy and non-invasive is ideal for CRC diagnosis. The discovery of microbial biomarkers aids in the development of non-invasive CRC diagnostic methods. The incidence and mortality of CRC can be decreased by using accurate tests to screen people who are at average risk. The sensitivity of current clinical diagnostic techniques, such as the faecal occult blood test (FOBT), to identify CRC is limited. Despite faecal immunochemical testing (FIT) being sensitive in detecting CRC, it may miss tumours that do not bleed or bleed less.

Microbial signatures that potentially predict CRC in a variety of populations have been found through extensive investigations on faecal metagenomes. A study done in 2017 found a group of 22 genes linked to CRC. RNA polymerase subunit (rpoB) from *P. micra*, two transposases from *Peptostreptococcus anaerobius*, and butyryl-CoA dehydrogenase from *F. nucleatum* were the four significant CRC-related genes detected in different populations [Yu et al., 2017]. Numerous recent investigations have found microbial indicators linked to CRC. A total of 17 bacterial genera and families were found by Huo *et al.* to be promising biomarkers for CRC recurrence and patient prognosis [Huo et al., 2022]. *Fusobacterium*, *Gemella*, *Campylobacter*, *Peptostreptococcus*, *Alloprevotella*, and *Parvimonas* were the six major genera that Li *et al.* found to be consistently over-represented in tumour mucosa [Li et al., 2022]. Out of this, *F. nucleatum* was found to be useful for screening CRC by detecting antibodies against it in serum samples; also, it had a prognostic role as its abundance indicates a poor survival rate in CRC patients. Likewise, antibodies against *S. gallolyticus* have been investigated as possible indicators for CRC.

Biomarkers for early CRC screening may also be microbial metabolites, such as bile acids and SCFAs, that have been linked to the progression of CRC. Numerous investigations have documented varying concentrations of microbiological metabolites, such as ursodeoxycholic acid, reduced butyrate levels, and elevated acetate levels, in the faecal samples of patients suffering from CRC (Mohseni et al., 2020). A preliminary CRC diagnosis marker could be derived from the analysis of CRC metagenomes, which indicate a decrease of carbohydrate degradation genes, and an enrichment of genes related to protein and mucin catabolism. *Peptostreptococcus* and *Parvimonas* are linked to CRC stage I, while *Fusobacterium*, *Streptococcus*, *Parvimonas*, Burkholderiales,

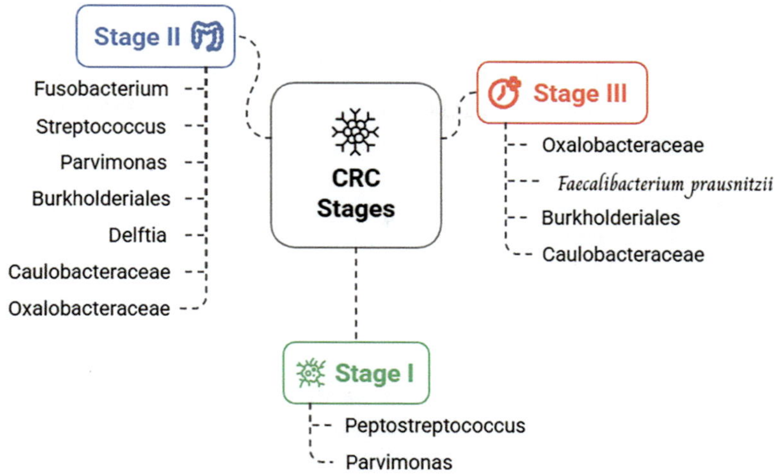

FIGURE 5.3 Microbial prognostic markers linked to stages of colorectal cancer.

Delftia, Caulobacteraceae, and Oxalobacteraceae are linked to stage II, and Oxalobacteraceae, *Faecalibacterium prausnitzii*, Burkholderiales, and Caulobacteraceae are linked to stage III of the disease (Zhang et al., 2021).

Important members of the gut microbiota, fungi, and viruses may also serve as CRC biomarkers. The gut mycobiome was found to be disrupted in CRC patients in metagenome-wide association research that included 204 control people, 197 patients with adenoma, and 184 patients with CRC. In particular, the class Malasseziomycetes was enriched, and the classes Saccharomycetes and Pneumocystidomycetes were depleted in CRC patients as compared to healthy controls, resulting in a larger Basidiomycota:Ascomycota ratio. Thus, this work clarified for the first time that fungal markers may be utilized to diagnose CRC and that the enteric fungal profile is linked to CRC (Coker et al., 2019). In a similar vein, examination of the viral profiles in faecal samples revealed a notable rise in gut phage diversity in CRC. The quantities of 22 viral indicators could be used to differentiate CRC patients from healthy individuals (Nakatsu et al., 2018) (**Figure 5.3**).

5.7 TECHNIQUES TO CHARACTERIZE GUT MICROBIOME

The composition of the gut microbiome was poorly studied until the 1990s as the only method available to study gut microbiome was microbiological culture. Majority of the organisms in gut microbiome are uncultivable. Culture-independent methods have contributed to our understanding of the intricacy of this milieu. The most recent methods for identifying and characterizing microorganisms that cannot be cultured are quick, precise, and comfortable with a high throughput. These methods enable bacterial species identification and illustrate the diversity of the gut microbiota. They are based on sequence divergences of the small subunit ribosomal RNA (16S rRNA), which are highly conserved across different species of bacteria. Additionally, they offer quantitative and qualitative data on the types of bacteria and changes happening in the gut microbiota in relation to diseases (Fraher et al., 2012).

Although the use of 16S rRNA technology has greatly advanced our understanding of the diversity and composition of the gut microbiota, it has not shed light on the important correlation between microbial patterns and the development or progression of disease. Instead of just sequencing certain DNA fragments, this method may sequence every DNA fragment present in the sample. The technique's strength lies in its ability to detect novel, functioning genes. However, the technique's drawback is that it is unable to differentiate between the DNA of living and dead cells, offer gene expression profiles, or forecast how certain conditions would affect it.

An extensively utilized technique for determining the metagenomic makeup of gut microbiome samples is whole-genome shotgun metagenomic sequencing. Although whole-genome shotgun metagenomic sequencing data provides gene-level information, it can also serve as motivation for analysing the millions of microbial genes that are commonly identified in microbiome studies. In this method, DNA fragments are broken randomly, sequenced, and then reassembled into a continuous sequence by reconstructing overlapping sequences. The benefit of this method is that the data regarding the genetic diversity of the gut microbiota is gathered. It is possible to draw correlations between the gut microbiota and disease status using data on the genetic diversity and makeup of the microbiome. Shotgun metagenomics sequencing has a number of drawbacks, including high cost and the computational burden of large-scale data analysis that is difficult for typical laboratories to handle (Ranjan et al., 2016).

Next-generation sequencing, a high-throughput method, has transformed research on the human gut microbiota and made it possible to investigate the diversity of uncultured gut microbe populations in an adequate and economical manner. With the use of next generation sequencing (NGS) technology, amplicon sequencing of the 16S-seq is specifically targeted, and when the amplicons are sequenced, bioinformatics analysis is carried out to characterize the samples' relative taxonomical abundances. Over the next few years, there will be a lot of potential for translation of this technique into the clinic thanks to the speedy sequencing of human genomes and the very low cost of generating genome-wide data, including genetic, transcriptomic, and epigenetic information (Finotello et al., 2018). In addition to metagenomics, metabolomics, proteomics, transcriptomics, and phenomics are critical for examining the characteristics, roles, metabolites, proteins, and RNA of the gut microbiome. Understanding the mechanisms underlying the host–microbiome interaction will depend on the integrated study of these omics data (**Figure 5.4**).

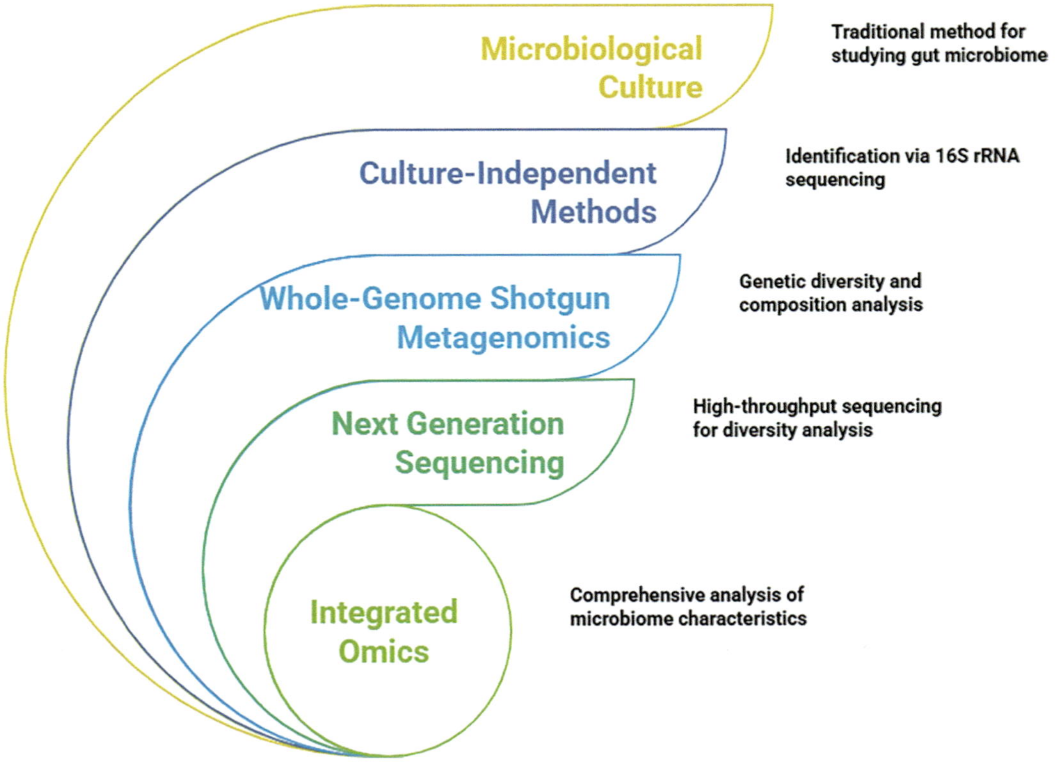

FIGURE 5.4 Methods to explore gut microbiome.

REFERENCES

Abdulamir AS, Hafidh RR, Abu Bakar F. (2011) The association of *Streptococcus bovis/gallolyticus* with colorectal tumors: the nature and the underlying mechanisms of its etiological role. J Exp Clin Cancer Res. 30(1):11.

Abdulamir AS, Hafidh RR, Bakar FA. (2010) Molecular detection, quantification, and isolation of *Streptococcus gallolyticus* bacteria colonizing colorectal tumors: inflammation-driven potential of carcinogenesis via IL-1, COX-2, and IL-8. Mol Cancer. 9:249.

Abdulamir AS, Hafidh RR, Mahdi LK, et al. (2009) Investigation into the controversial association of *Streptococcus gallolyticus* with colorectal cancer and adenoma. BMC Cancer. 9:403.

Ahn J, Sinha R, Pei Z, et al. (2013) Human gut microbiome and risk for colorectal cancer. J Natl Cancer Inst. 105:1907–1911.

Attene-Ramos MS, Wagner ED, Plewa MJ, et al. (2006) Evidence that hydrogen sulfide is a genotoxic agent. Mol Cancer Res. 4:9–14.

Balamurugan R, Rajendiran E, George S, et al. (2008) Real-time polymerase chain reaction quantification of specific butyrate-producing bacteria, *Desulfovibrio* and *Enterococcus faecalis* in the feces of patients with colorectal cancer. J. Gastroenterol. Hepatol. 23:1298–1303.

Bayerdorffer E, Mannes GA, Richter WO, et al. (1993) Increased serum deoxycholic acid levels in men with colorectal adenomas. Gastroenterology. 104:145–151.

Boleij A, Hechenbleikner EM, Goodwin AC, et al. (2015) The *Bacteroides fragilis* toxin gene is prevalent in the colon mucosa of colorectal cancer patients. Clin Infect Dis. 60:208–215.

Boltin D, Goldberg E, Bugaevsky O, et al. (2015) Colonic carriage of *Streptococcus bovis* and colorectal neoplasia: a prospective 17-year longitudinal case-control study. Eur J Gastroenterol Hepatol. 27:1449.

Burns CA, McCaughey R, Lauter CB. (1985) The association of *Streptococcus bovis* fecal carriage and colon neoplasia: possible relationship with polyps and their premalignant potential. Am J Gastroenterol. 80:42–46.

Coker OO, Nakatsu G, Dai RZ, et al. (2019) Enteric fungal microbiota dysbiosis and ecological alterations in colorectal cancer. Gut. 68:654–662.

Ellmerich S, Schöller M, Duranton B, et al. (2000) Promotion of intestinal carcinogenesis by *Streptococcus bovis*. Carcinogenesis. 21:753–756.

Finotello F, Mastrorilli E, Di Camillo B. (2018) Measuring the diversity of the human microbiota with targeted next–generation sequencing, Brief Bioinform. 19:679–692.

Flanagan L, Schmid J, Ebert M, et al. (2014) *Fusobacterium nucleatum* associates with stages of colorectal neoplasia development, colorectal cancer and disease outcome. Eur J Clin Microbiol Infect Dis. 33:1381–1390.

Forrester J, Shkolyar E, Gregg D, et al. (2016) Nontraumatic *Clostridium septicum* myonecrosis in adults: case report and a 15-year systematic literature review. Infect Dis Clin Pract. 24:318.

Fraher MH, O'Toole PW, Quigley EM. (2012) Techniques used to characterize the gut microbiota: a guide for the clinician. Nat Rev Gastroenterol Hepatol. 9:312–322.

Francescone R, Hou V, Grivennikov SI. (2014) Microbiome, inflammation, and cancer. Cancer J. 20(3):181–189.

Fung KY, Cosgrove L, Lockett T, et al. (2012) A review of the potential mechanisms for the lowering of colorectal oncogenesis by butyrate. Br J Nutr. 108:820–831.

Gagnière J, Raisch J, Veziant J, et al. (2016) Gut microbiota imbalance and colorectal cancer. World J. Gastroenterol. 22:501–518.

Gao J, Xu K, Liu H, et al. (2018) Impact of the gut microbiota on intestinal immunity mediated by tryptophan metabolism. Front Cell Infect Microbiol. 8:13.

Gold JS, Bayar S, Salem RR. Association of *Streptococcus bovis* bacteremia with colonic neoplasia and extracolonic malignancy. *Arch Surg*. 2004 Jul;139(7):760–765. doi: 10.1001/archsurg.139.7.760. PMID: 15249410.

Gong J, Bai T, Zhang L, et al. (2017) Inhibition effect of *Bifidobacterium longum, Lactobacillus acidophilus, Streptococcus thermophilus* and *Enterococcus faecalis* and their related products on human colonic smooth muscle in vitro. PLoS One. 12(12):e0189257.

He Z, Gharaibeh RZ, Newsome RC, et al. (2019) *Campylobacter jejuni* promotes colorectal tumorigenesis through the action of cytolethal distending toxin. Gut. 68(2):289–300.

Hofseth LJ, Hebert JR, Chanda A, et al. (2020) Early-onset colorectal cancer: initial clues and current views. Nat Rev Gastroenterol Hepatol. 17(6):352–364.

Huo R.X, Wang Y.J, Hou S.B, et al. (2022) Gut mucosal microbiota profiles linked to colorectal cancer recurrence. World J Gastroenterol. 28:1946–1964.

Huycke MM, Moore DR. (2002) In vivo production of hydroxyl radical by *Enterococcus faecalis* colonizing the intestinal tract using aromatic hydroxylation. Free Radic Biol Med. 33:818–826.

Jahani-Sherafat S, Alebouyeh M, Moghim S, et al. (2018) Role of gut microbiota in the pathogenesis of colorectal cancer; a review article. Gastroenterol Hepatol Bed Bench. 11:101–109.

Kostic AD, Chun E, Robertson L, et al. (2013) *Fusobacterium nucleatum* potentiates intestinal tumorigenesis and modulates the tumor-immune microenvironment. Cell Host Microbe. 14:207–215.

Larson CM, Bubrick MP, Jacobs DM, et al. (1995) Malignancy, mortality, and medicosurgical management of *Clostridium septicum* infection. Surgery. 118:592–597.

Li Y, Cao H, Fei B, et al. (2022) Gut microbiota signatures in tumor, para-cancerous, normal mucosa, and feces in colorectal cancer patients. Front Cell Dev Biol. 10:916961.

Lindblom A. (2001) Different mechanisms in the tumorigenesis of proximal and distal colon cancers. Curr Opin Oncol. 13:63–69.

Long X, Wong CC, Tong L, et al. (2019) *Peptostreptococcus anaerobius* promotes colorectal carcinogenesis and modulates tumour immunity. Nat Microbiol. 4:2319–2330.

Louis P, Hold GL, Flint HJ. (2014) The gut microbiota, bacterial metabolites and colorectal cancer. Nat Rev Microbiol. 12:661–672.

Lu R, Wu S, Y-g Z, et al. (2016) *Salmonella* protein AvrA activates the STAT3 signaling pathway in colon cancer. Neoplasia. 18(5):307–316.

Magalhães B, Peleteiro B, Lunet N. (2012) Dietary patterns and colorectal cancer: systematic review and meta-analysis. Eur J Cancer Prev. 21:15.

Malik A, Sharma D, Malireddi RKS, et al. (2018) SYK-CARD9 signaling axis promotes gut fungi-mediated inflammasome activation to restrict colitis and colon cancer. Immunity. 49:515–530.

Martin OC, Bergonzini A, d'Amico F, et al. (2019) Infection with genotoxin-producing *Salmonella enterica* synergises with loss of the tumour suppressor APC in promoting genomic instability *via* the PI3K pathway in colonic epithelial cells. Cell Microbiol. 21(12):e13099.

Mehta RS, Nishihara R, Cao Y, et al. (2017) Association of Dietary Patterns With Risk of Colorectal Cancer Subtypes Classified by *Fusobacterium nucleatum* in Tumor Tissue. JAMA Oncol. 3:921–927.

Mima K, Nishihara R, Qian ZR, et al. (2016) *Fusobacterium nucleatum* in colorectal carcinoma tissue and patient prognosis. Gut. 65:1973–1980.

Mohseni A.H, Taghinezhad S.S, Fu X. (2020). Gut microbiota-derived metabolites and colorectal cancer: New insights and updates. Microb Pathog. 149:104569.

Muhlbauer M, Allard B, Bosserhoff AK, et al. (2004) Differential effects of deoxycholic acid and taurodeoxycholic acid on NF-kappa B signal transduction and IL-8 gene expression in colonic epithelial cells. Am J Physiol Gastrointest Liver Physiol. 286:G1000–G1008.

Nakatsu G, Zhou H, Wu WKK, et al. (2018) Alterations in enteric virome are associated with colorectal cancer and survival outcomes. Gastroenterology. 155:529–541.

Ranjan R, Rani A, Metwally A, et al. (2016) Analysis of the microbiome: Advantages of whole genome shotgun versus 16S amplicon sequencing, Biochem Biophys Res Commun. 469:967–977.

Reddy BS, Narisawa T, Wright P, et al. (1975) Colon carcinogenesis with azoxymethane and dimethylhydrazine in germ-free rats. Cancer Res. 35(2):287–290.

Rooks MG, Garrett WS. (2016) Gut microbiota, metabolites and host immunity. Nat Rev Immunol. 16:341–352.

Rubinstein MR, Wang X, Liu W, et al. (2013) *Fusobacterium nucleatum* promotes colorectal carcinogenesis by modulating E-cadherin/β-catenin signaling via its FadA adhesin. Cell Host Microbe. 14:195–206

Shmuely H, Passaro D, Figer A, et al. (2001) Relationship between *Helicobacter pylori* CagA status and colorectal cancer. Am J Gastroenterol. 96:3406–3410.

Siegel RL, Wagle NS, Cercek A, et al (2023) Colorectal cancer statistics, 2023. CA Cancer J Clin. 73(3):233–254.

Son JS, Khair S, Pettet DW III, et al. (2015) Altered interactions between the gut microbiome and colonic mucosa precede polyposis in APCMin/+ mice. PLoS One. 10(6):e0127985.

Steck N, Hoffmann M, Sava IG, et al. (2011) *Enterococcus faecalis* metalloprotease compromises epithelial barrier and contributes to intestinal inflammation. Gastroenterology. 141:959–971.

Suehiro Y, Sakai K, Nishioka M, et al. (2017) Highly sensitive stool DNA testing of *Fusobacterium nucleatum* as a marker for detection of colorectal tumours in a Japanese population. Ann Clin Biochem. 54:86–91.

Toprak NU, Yagci A, Gulluoglu BM, et al. (2006) A possible role of *Bacteroides fragilis* enterotoxin in the aetiology of colorectal cancer. Clin Microbiol Infect. 12:782–786.

Tsoi H, Chu ESH, Zhang X, et al. (2017) *Peptostreptococcus anaerobius* induces intracellular cholesterol biosynthesis in colon cells to induce proliferation and causes dysplasia in mice. Gastroenterology. 152:1419–1433.

Wang X, Allen TD, May RJ, et al. (2008) *Enterococcus faecalis* induces aneuploidy and tetraploidy in colonic epithelial cells through a bystander effect. Cancer Res. 68:9909–9917.

Wei Z, Cao S, Liu S, et al. (2016) Could gut microbiota serve as prognostic biomarker associated with colorectal cancer patients' survival? A pilot study on relevant mechanism. Oncotarget. 7:46158–46172.

Yazici C, Wolf PG, Kim H, et al. (2017) Race-dependent association of sulfidogenic bacteria with colorectal cancer. Gut. 66:1983–1994.

Yu J, Chen Y, Fu X, et al. (2016) Invasive *Fusobacterium nucleatum* may play a role in the carcinogenesis of proximal colon cancer through the serrated neoplasia pathway. Int J Cancer. 139:1318–1326.

Yu J, Feng Q, Wong S.H, et al. (2017) Metagenomic analysis of faecal microbiome as a tool towards targeted non-invasive biomarkers for colorectal cancer. Gut. 66:70–78.

Zhang M, Lv Y, Hou S, et al. (2021) Differential mucosal microbiome profiles across stages of human colorectal cancer. Life. 11:831.

Zhao L, Zhang X, Zhou Y, et al. (2022) *Parvimonas micra* promotes colorectal tumorigenesis and is associated with prognosis of colorectal cancer patients. Oncogene. 41:4200–4210.

Zumkeller N, Brenner H, Zwahlen M, et al. (2006) *Helicobacter pylori* infection and colorectal cancer risk: a meta-analysis. Helicobacter. 11:75–80.

6 The Intersection of Oncology and Infectious Diseases in Human Health

The Battle between Pathogens

Anu Shibi Anilkumar, Sheena Mariam Thomas, and Ramakrishnan Veerabathiran
Chettinad Hospital and Research Institute,
Chettinad Academy of Research and Education,
Kelambakkam, Tamil Nadu, India

6.1 INTRODUCTION

Any condition that affects the normal functioning of a body organ or system, the psyche, or the organism as a whole and is accompanied by particular signs and symptoms is considered a "disease" (Nii-Trebi, 2017). An infection-driven disease is any illness brought on by pathogens or their toxic byproducts and spread to a susceptible host by an infected person, animal, or contaminated object. Infectious diseases are a significant global health burden that puts a strain on economies and public health systems while disproportionately affecting vulnerable populations (GBD 2013 Mortality and Causes of Death Collaborators, 2015).

Infectious diseases accounted for the majority of the world's premature mortality and disability burden. Global pandemics of contagious illnesses such as smallpox, cholera, and influenza have occasionally challenged the survival of entire nations in past centuries (Holmes et al., 2017). Microorganisms are usually the cause of infectious diseases, which become significant depending on the type and extent of harm that the agents causing them do to organs or systems after entering a host. Pathogens typically enter the host by the nose, skin, genital openings, eyes, or mouth. The major cause of tissue damage is these infectious agents' development and metabolic activity in bodily fluids or cells. This results in releasing toxins or enzymes that interfere with the regular operation of organs or systems (Nii-Trebi, 2017). It is necessary to identify the source and transmission routes to develop preventive measures to combat an infection (Pallavi et al., 2023).

The prevalence of newly emerging infectious diseases is increasing, leading to a substantial loss of life for both humans and animals as well as high costs to society (Lindahl and Grace, 2015). Infectious diseases can cause worldwide outbreaks and can be unpredictable. Despite their transmissibility, they can develop immunity to reinfection (McArthur, 2019). Managing infectious disease risk is complex due to several complicated circumstances, with multiple current demographic trends indicating a heightened possibility of pathogen transmission (Chew et al., 2020). Despite improvements in prevention and control, infectious diseases still represent a serious risk to the health of both humans and animals. It is becoming increasingly clear that

 DOI: 10.1201/9781003644309-6

when several agents infect host communities and individuals simultaneously, the public health burden is greatly increased, and preventative and control measures are made more difficult (Heesterbeek et al., 2015).

According to epidemiological studies, numerous transmissible agents contribute to the genesis of different cancer forms. Infectious pathogens are key environmental factors that contribute to cancer (Oluwasola and Adeoye, 2005). For about 15% of cancers, infectious organisms have been implicated in the etiology (Alibek et al., 2012). Infectious agents, primarily bacteria and viruses, are responsible for several malignancies worldwide and are one of the few recognized causes of cancer (Pagano et al., 2004). The biogeography of human infectious diseases is relatively understudied compared to other biological taxa, and biogeographic insights have been minimally applied to public and global health initiatives (Murray et al., 2015).

In contrast to malignancies that are solely caused by genetic or environmental factors, infection-driven tumors frequently entail intricate interactions between the host and the virus. Chronic inflammation, immune system evasion, and direct genetic or epigenetic changes in host cells are some of these interactions that result in unchecked growth and carcinogenesis (Ofoezie et al., 2025). Tumors often start in inflammatory tissues due to infection with pathogens, some of which can directly or indirectly cause cancer or other aseptic reasons that compromise tissue integrity (Trinchieri, 2015).

There are several similarities between cancer and infectious disorders. Numerous proteins recognized by host T cells are expressed by cancer cells and pathogenic organisms, and both cause inflammation mediated by T cells (Hotchkiss and Moldawer, 2014). Pathogen invasiveness is a critical component affecting disease onset probability and results (Engering et al., 2013). The host's immune response is a crucial environmental factor influencing an invading pathogen's establishment, survival, and reproduction (Bradley and Jackson, 2008).

There are now many infectious agents known to either cause or contribute to certain types of cancer in humans. Therefore, it is vital to address the understanding of these factors and how they interact with cancer (Masrour-Roudsari and Ebrahimpour, 2017). Infectious diseases continue to present a formidable challenge to global health. The increasing incidence of emerging infections, the intricate interplay of host and environmental factors, and the significant social and economic impact highlight the urgent need for sustained efforts to prevent, control, and research various diseases, including cancers. Addressing these challenges necessitates a collaborative approach, combining advancements in medicine, biotechnology, and public health. Thus, the continuous battle of infectious pathogens in cancer impacting human health is covered in detail in this chapter.

6.2 THE NATURE OF PATHOGENS: THE ADVERSARIES IN THE BATTLE

A breakthrough came in the nineteenth century with the germ theory of disease, which transformed medical knowledge by proving that germs are the source of human illness. This revolutionary concept replaced earlier beliefs that diseases were caused by miasmas, or "bad air," and personal moral failings. Instead, it identified life forms in the environment as the actual agents of disease (Cockerill et al., 2017).

An organism is considered a pathogen when it causes disease in its host, and virulence represents the severity of disease symptoms. Pathogens encompass a wide range of organisms, including both unicellular and multicellular eukaryotic life forms. The ability of pathogens to produce diseases depends on virulence factors, genes encoding proteins essential for host colonization, immunoevasion, immunosuppression, nutrient acquisition, and intracellular entry and exit (Balloux and van Dorp, 2017). Numerous species can infect humans, but the most common ones include bacteria, fungi, viruses, protozoa, and helminths (Bartlett et al., 2022). The key pathogens, associated diseases, and their characteristics are mentioned in **Table 6.1**.

TABLE 6.1
Key Pathogens, Associated Diseases, and Their Characteristics

Pathogen	Organism	Disease(s)	Characteristics
Bacteria	*Escherichia coli*	Diarrhea, urinary tract infections, sepsis	Toxins, adhesion molecules, secretion systems
	Staphylococcus aureus	Skin infections, pneumonia, sepsis, endocarditis	Toxins, surface proteins, antibiotic resistance
	Mycobacterium tuberculosis	Tuberculosis	Acid-fast cell wall, immune evasion
Viruses	*Human Immunodeficiency Virus* (HIV)	Acquired immunodeficiency syndrome (AIDS)	Antigenic variation, immune suppression
	Influenza virus	Influenza (Flu)	Antigenic shift, antigenic drift
	Hepatitis B virus	Hepatitis B, liver cancer	Antigenic variation, immune evasion
	Hepatitis C virus	Hepatitis C, liver cirrhosis, liver cancer	Immune evasion, chronic infection potential
	SARS-CoV-2	COVID-19	Spike protein, immune suppression, latency
Protozoa	*Plasmodium falciparum, P. vivax*, etc.	Malaria	Intracellular life cycle, immune evasion
	Entamoeba histolytica	Amoebiasis	Trophozoite form, tissue invasion
Fungi	*Cryptococcus neoformans*	Cryptococcosis, meningitis	Capsule, resistance to antifungal drugs
	Aspergillus fumigatus	Aspergillosis (lung infections)	Conidia (spores), immune evasion, biofilm formation
	Candida albicans	Candidiasis (oral thrush, systemic infections)	Biofilm formation, hyphal growth
Zoonotic Pathogens	*Rabies virus*	Rabies	Neurotropism, transmission through bites
	Ebola virus	Ebola virus disease	Immune suppression, hemorrhagic fever
	Borrelia burgdorferi	Lyme borreliosis	Surface proteins, immune evasion
	Avian influenza virus	Avian influenza (bird flu)	Antigenic variation, zoonotic transmission

6.2.1 Bacteria: Resistance and Infectious Agents

Bacteria are among the most diverse and widespread pathogens, capable of causing various human diseases. These unicellular prokaryotic organisms rapidly adapt to environmental changes, enabling them to evade host defenses and develop resistance to antibiotics. Pathogenic bacteria such as *Escherichia coli*, *Staphylococcus aureus*, and *Mycobacterium tuberculosis* employ various virulence factors—including toxins, adhesion molecules, and secretion systems—to invade and damage host tissues. A significant challenge in treating bacterial infections is the emergence of multidrug-resistant (MDR) strains. The overuse and misuse of antibiotics in clinical and agricultural settings have accelerated the selection of bacteria resistant to multiple antibiotic classes, complicating treatment options. The rise of MDR bacteria is recognized as a significant public health concern, with broad-spectrum antibiotic usage closely linked to their increased prevalence (van Duin and Paterson, 2016).

Beyond their role as infectious agents, certain bacteria have also been implicated in cancer development. It has been well established that specific bacterial species can contribute to tumor formation through direct and indirect mechanisms. Bacteria may enter tumors via the vasculature and persist due to the availability of nutrients in hypoxic regions, allowing their replication within the tumor microenvironment. This localized bacterial proliferation can significantly influence tumor progression (Cummins and Tangney, 2013).

Bacteria and bacterial infections contribute to cancer development by promoting chronic inflammation, disrupting cell cycle regulation, and interfering with key signaling pathways. Various bacterial components including enzymes, oncogenic peptides, and toxins can facilitate tumor growth through these mechanisms (Yusuf et al., 2023). Strong evidence links *Helicobacter pylori* to gastric cancer and mucosa-associated lymphoid tissue (MALT) lymphoma (Crowe, 2005). Similarly, *Salmonella typhi* has been related to gallbladder cancer (Vaishnavi et al., 2005), *Streptococcus bovis/gallolyticus* with colorectal tumors (Abdulamir et al., 2011), and *Chlamydia pneumoniae* with lung cancer (Premachandra and Jayaweera, 2022). Immunological evasion, immune suppression, and chronic infection are key mechanisms by which bacterial agents contribute to carcinogenesis (Mager, 2006).

Addressing bacterial infections and their role in disease requires a multifaceted approach. Strategies such as developing novel antibiotics, implementing bacteriophage therapy, and improving antibiotic stewardship are critical to controlling bacterial infections and limiting their impact on human health (Liu et al., 2022; Strathdee et al., 2023).

6.2.2 Viruses: Multifaceted Microbial Invaders

Viruses are obligate intracellular pathogens that rely on the host's cellular framework for replication. Despite their simple structure, consisting of genetic material encased in a protein coat, viruses have evolved highly sophisticated mechanisms to infect host cells and evade immune responses (Eisenreich et al., 2019). Notable human viruses include HIV, influenza, hepatitis B and C, and SARS-CoV-2 (Miranda et al., 2022). Viruses utilize diverse strategies such as antigenic variation, latency, and suppression of host immune responses to ensure their survival and replication. The emergence of viral diseases such as COVID-19 has highlighted the global health risks posed by viral pathogens and underscored the urgent need for vaccine development, antiviral medications, and robust surveillance networks to prevent and control outbreaks (Thomas et al.,2025; Han et al., 2023; Iannello et al., 2006).

The role of viruses in cancer development has been well established through extensive experimental research. Oncogenic viruses can alter healthy cells by inducing genomic instability, evading growth suppressors, resisting apoptotic signals, promoting replicative immortality, and facilitating angiogenesis. Their capacity to integrate into the host genome further highlights the significant impact of viral infections on carcinogenesis (Ameya et al., 2023).

Several human oncoviruses have been identified as causative agents in different types of cancer (Schiller and Lowy, 2021). Hepatitis viruses, including hepatitis B virus (HBV), hepatitis C virus (HCV), and hepatitis D virus (HDV), are among the significant risk factors for hepatocellular carcinoma (HCC) (Shen et al., 2023). Epstein–Barr virus (EBV) has been linked to a variety of malignancies, including nasopharyngeal carcinoma (NPC), lymphoepithelial-like carcinomas (LELCs), gastric cancer (GC), T cell and natural killer (NK) cell lymphomas (TNKL), Hodgkin lymphoma (HL), diffuse large B cell lymphoma (DLBCL), and lymphomas associated with immunosuppressed individuals (Solares et al., 2024). Kaposi sarcoma herpesvirus (KSHV) is the causative agent of Kaposi Sarcoma and other related malignancies (Goncalves et al., 2017). Understanding how viruses contribute to cancer development is essential for targeted therapies, vaccines, and preventive strategies. Continued research into viral oncogenesis will provide critical insights into practical intervention approaches to mitigate the burden of virus-associated cancers.

6.2.3 Protozoa and Fungi: Rare but Dangerous Threats

Although bacterial and viral infections are more commonly associated with cancer, fungal and protozoan pathogens can also cause severe diseases, particularly in individuals with weakened immune systems (Ferreira and Borges, 2002; Wahab et al., 2024). Pathogenic fungi, such as *Cryptococcus neoformans*, *Aspergillus fumigatus*, and *Candida albicans*, can lead to life-threatening infections, often exhibiting intrinsic resistance to many antifungal agents, posing significant treatment challenges (Garvey et al., 2022).

Narunsky-Haziza et al. (2022) discovered a fungal microbiome atlas spanning 35 cancer types and demonstrated fungi's presence in every tumor type they analyzed. Notably, different malignancies exhibit distinct fungal profiles, such as *Candida* species, which contribute to the pathophysiology of colorectal cancer (Dohlman et al., 2022). Other fungal species, including *C. albicans*, *Malassezia globosa*, *Blastomyces gilchristii*, and *Malassezia restricta*, have been implicated in various forms of human cancer (Zong et al., 2023).

Invasive fungal infections (IFIs) further complicate cancer progression, as they are associated with high disease severity and fatality rates. The most prevalent fungal genera and species linked to cancer are *Aspergillus flavus*, *Aspergillus parasiticus*, *Fusarium verticillioides*, *C. albicans*, *Candida glabrata*, *Candida tropicalis*, and *Fusarium proliferatum* (Hosseini et al., 2022). Fungal infections can contribute to various types of cancer, such as esophageal cancer (Koo et al., 2017), gastric cancer (Nucci and Anaissie, 2001), colorectal cancer (Coker et al., 2019), lung cancer (Ching-López and Rodríguez Pavón, 2020), cervical cancer (Moradi et al., 2017), skin cancer (Ferrándiz-Pulido et al., 2019), and ovarian cancer (Banerjee et al., 2017).

Beyond fungal pathogens, protozoan parasites also impose a significant disease burden in many world regions. *Plasmodium* species, the causative agents of malaria, and *Entamoeba histolytica*, responsible for Amebiasis, have complex life cycles involving multiple hosts and developmental stages, complicating treatment and prevention strategies (Sutrave and Richter, 2021). Advances in antifungal and antiparasitic therapies, along with improved diagnostics, are crucial for mitigating the impact of these infections (Ferreira and Borges, 2002; Wahab et al., 2024).

Chronic inflammation induced by parasitic infections also plays a key role in helminth-induced carcinogenesis. Inflammatory cells such as macrophages and eosinophils generate free radicals in response to parasites, leading to oxidative stress and DNA damage. This can result in genetic instability, mutations, and malignant transformation (El-Gayar and Mahmoud, 2014). Specific helminths are strongly associated with cancer, such as *Schistosoma haematobium*, which is linked to bladder cancer, and *Opisthorchis* and *Clonorchis* flukes, which are associated with cholangiocarcinoma (de Martel and Franceschi, 2009).

6.2.4 Pathogen Emergence and Re-Emergence

Emerging pathogens have recently entered a population or have existed but are rapidly increasing in incidence or geographic range (McArthur, 2019). Examples include the *Zika virus*, *Nipah virus*, and novel strains of *influenza*. Re-emerging pathogens, such as *M. tuberculosis* and *dengue virus*, represent diseases that were previously under control but are now resurging due to factors such as antimicrobial resistance (AMR), climate change, and increased human mobility (Wang et al., 2021).

Pathogen emergence and re-emergence can cause cancer by impairing the immune system, causing persistent inflammation, and having direct oncogenic effects that result in tumor formation and unchecked cell growth (Khabbaz et al., 2015). The rise of emerging and re-emerging pathogens highlights the critical need for robust public health infrastructure, global research collaborations, and investments in pathogen genomics, vaccine development, and outbreak preparedness. The One Health initiative, which integrates environmental, animal, and human health, is crucial in tackling this growing threat.

6.2.5 Zoonotic Diseases: Human–Animal Transmission of Pathogens

Zoonotic diseases are infections transmitted from animals to humans, either through direct interaction with infected animals or indirectly by way of vectors such as mosquitoes and ticks. Examples include *rabies*, *Ebola*, *Lyme*, and *avian influenza*. Many newly emerging infectious diseases are zoonotic, underscoring the interconnectedness of human and animal health (Rahman et al., 2020).

The growing human–wildlife interface, driven by urbanization, deforestation, and agricultural expansion, has increased the risk of zoonotic spillover events (Roberts et al., 2021). Mitigating zoonotic disease risks requires surveillance of animal populations, vector control, promoting safe agricultural practices, and strengthening veterinary and public health collaboration under the One Health framework (Sharan et al., 2023).

Although humans commonly encounter animal viruses and bacteria, their potential contribution to human cancer is still unknown. The majority of animal oncoviruses are species-specific and difficult to infect in people. Animal viruses could still be dangerous, though, just like human and simian polyomaviruses can cause tumors in rats (Efird et al., 2014).

6.3 THE HUMAN IMMUNE SYSTEM: DEFENDING THE BODY AGAINST INFECTION

Organs of a human body use defensive mechanism, which are vital for defending against diseases and maintaining overall health. In addition to defending against infections, the immune system is indispensable in protecting the body from hazardous substances and abnormal cell changes, such as neoplasms (tumors). The primary players in the immune system are leukocytes, which circulate all over the body via the vascular channels. These white blood cells work to detect and combat disease agents, such as bacteria, viruses, and other pathogens. The body exchanges cells and bodily fluids between the lymphatic vessels and blood to detect and respond to invading pathogens. This exchange facilitates the function of the lymphatic system. Immune cells and foreign particles enter the lymphatic nodes through incoming lymphatic vessels. Upon entering the bloodstream, immune cells are brought to various tissues all across the body, where they continue to detect foreign antigens. Over time, these cells gradually return to the lymphatic system, repeating the surveillance cycle. In the lymph nodes and the spleen, immune cells gather, interact, and work together to confront and eliminate pathogens (Chowdhury et al., 2020).

The immune system has two distinct mechanisms of response to invading microbes: natural (innate) and acquired (adaptive) immunity. Innate immune responses (IIR) are activated whenever an infectious agent is encountered, regardless of the frequency of its occurrences. These responses provide an immediate defense. On the other hand, acquired immune reactions intensify with repetitive exposure to a specific infection, becoming more efficient and effective over time. This adaptive immunity is the body's ability to "remember" a pathogen after the first exposure. IIR involve various cells and molecular components. These responses are carried out by phagocytic cells, such as neutrophils, macrophages, and monocytes, which engulf and digest foreign particles. Other cells, including basophils, mast cells, and eosinophils, release inflammatory mediators that help initiate immune responses. Also, NK cells are responsible for recognizing and killing cells affected by infection. The molecular elements of natural immunity include cytokines such as interferons, complement proteins, and acute-phase proteins, which help coordinate immune responses and fight infections (Turvey and Broide, 2010).

Acquired immune responses, in contrast, rely on the initiation and production of antigen-reactive B and T cells. These cells are initiated when their surface receptors bind to specific antigens. Antigen-presenting cells (APCs) exhibit these antigens to the lymphoid cells, which helps coordinate the immune response. Key players are B cells in the acquired immune response that produce immunoglobulins, antibodies that selectively target and neutralize extracellular disease agents, such as bacteria and viruses. T cells aid B cells in generating antibodies and can eradicate infected cells directly or activate macrophages to clear intracellular pathogens (Alberts et al., 2002).

Thus, innate and acquired immune responses cooperate to get rid of infections. The natural defense system contributes to the initial defense mechanism, while the acquired immune system enhances the body's defense mechanisms against infections upon subsequent exposures. Both responses are necessary to defend the body effectively. All immune cells originate from pluripotent stem cells found in the fetal bone marrow and liver. These stem cells give rise to various immune cells, which travel throughout the extracellular fluid, including the blood and lymph. B cells undergo maturation in the bone marrow, whereas T cells travel to the thymus to complete their maturation and become fully functional.

Adaptive immune responses develop in secondary lymphoid organs, encompassing lymph nodes, spleen, and MALT. These are critical sites where the body's immune responses are initiated and coordinated. In the lymph nodes and spleen, lymphocytes are activated by antigens, and this activation occurs in distinct compartments dedicated to B and T cells (Ruddle and Akirav, 2009).

6.3.1 The Influence of the Inborn Immune System in Early Defense

As a result of evolutionary pressures from pathogens, all multicellular organisms have evolved the proficiency to effectively distinguish and eliminate incurring pathogens while minimizing damage to their cells. Innate immune cells, which are equipped with a confined group of germline-encoded receptors and molecules, can sense an array of diverse pathogens despite the vast molecular diversity these invaders present. These highly diverse pathogens are delivered to innate immune defense cells via general molecules that are commonly possessed by many infectious agents, called pathogen-associated molecular patterns (PAMPs). PAMPs are conserved molecular features produced by different microorganisms. These molecular patterns are not structurally specific or vary in antigenicity. Furthermore, host cells do not possess PAMPs, which enables the innate immune system (IIS) to discern between self and nonself (Uthaisangsook et al., 2002).

Pathogens display several PAMPs, such as peptidoglycan (PGN), lipoteichoic acid (LTA), lipopolysaccharide (LPS), the unmethylated CpG motif in DNA, double-stranded RNA from RNA viruses, and mannan from yeast cell walls. LPS is a common characteristic factor of Gram-negative bacterial cell walls, while PGN is found within the cell membrane walls of Gram-positive and Gram-negative bacteria, along with mycobacteria. LTA is located in the cell walls of many Gram-positive bacteria. The unmethylated CpG motif is prevalent in microbial DNA but not in mammalian DNA (Mogensen, 2009).

The IIS ascertains PAMPs through a series of nonclonal, germline-encoded receptors known as pattern-recognition molecules or receptors (PRMs/PRRs). These receptors have broad specificity and are found on vertebrate cells, including epithelial cells and immune effector cells, which are typically the first to encounter pathogens during an infection. PRMs/PRRs are divided into three functional categories: (i) endocytic receptors, (ii) secreted proteins, and (iii) signaling receptors. A key group of signaling receptors is the Toll receptor family, initially discovered in *Drosophila*. It was later demonstrated that Toll-like receptors (TLRs) also play a significant role in mammals, including human cells. When Toll proteins and TLRs interact with their respective ligands, they trigger intracellular signaling networks that activate immune response genes (Gulati et al., 2018).

The signals triggered by PAMPs initiate the synthesis of inflammatory cytokines such as TNF-α, IL-6, IL-1, and IFNs, and a range of effector cytokines and chemokines. APCs detect pathogens by binding their PRRs to PAMPs. Following this binding, APCs process the pathogens to their specific antigens and display them through MHC molecules to T cells. T cells activate upon recognizing the pathogen-derived MHC-bound antigens and the co-stimulatory molecules on APCs. PAMPs and pathogen components induce the expression of co-stimulatory molecules such as CD80 and CD86 on APCs. Since self-molecules do not possess these pathogen-associated structures, they cannot trigger the expression of co-stimulatory molecules on APCs, thus preventing T-cell activation against self-antigens and maintaining immune tolerance. Consequently, regulating co-stimulatory molecule expression using the IIS is critical for controlling adaptive immune responses. Moreover, the IIS produces various effector cytokines in response to different pathogens. These cytokines, including IL-4, IL-5, IL-10, IL-12, TGF-β, and IFN-γ, influence the nature of both innate and adaptive immune responses. For instance, IL-12, produced by macrophages, and IFN-γ, produced by NK cells, promote differentiation of T cells into Th1 effector cells. In contrast, IL-10, churned out by macrophages, and IL-4, generated by mast cells and basophils, foster the differentiation of Th2-type cells (Yi et al., 2024).

Complement is a key component of the IIS and serves as the frontline protection. This cascade-like system provides an immediate barrier against invading microorganisms and is integral to coordinating both innate and adaptive immune functions. Complement activation generates new products that attach to the surface of various disease agents, including Gram-negative and Gram-positive bacteria, helminths, fungi, and viruses. This binding leads to the destruction and removal of the invading microbes. Consequently, the complement system significantly contributes to the host's health by eliminating most foreign invaders early in the infection process. As a fundamental aspect of the immune defense system, the complement system is activated almost immediately within seconds following the introduction of a pathogen into the human body. This highly efficient defense mechanism comprises more than 60 distinct proteins and their activation products, which initiate a cascade of reactions. Activating this cascade results in potent and reactive products with various biological activities, including chemokinetic, inflammation-inducing, and cytolytic activities, and, in some cases, antimicrobial and antifungal properties. The key effector roles of the activated complement system consist: (i) the release of inflammatory mediators, such as C3a and C5a, which act as anaphylatoxins; (ii) antimicrobial effects exerted by C3a and C4a; (iii) the opsonization of foreign surfaces by C3b, promoting their recognition and clearance via phagocytosis; (iv) the synthesis of the membrane attack complex (MAC), also known as the terminal complement complex, which disrupts the target membrane by creating pores and inducing cytotoxicity; (v) supporting and directing the adaptive immune response; and (vi) facilitating the anti-inflammatory, silent elimination of cellular debris, altered self-cells, apoptotic or necrotic cells, and immune complexes (Zipfel, 2009).

Complement activation occurs either spontaneously or through antibodies. The alternative pathway is activated spontaneously and continuously, initiated by a conformational change in C3. This activation starts a cascade of reactions that generate immune activation products designed to wreck and eliminate extraneous particles or virulent agents. Complement activation can also occur via the lectin pathway, which is initiated by carbohydrate structures found on bacterial surfaces. Additionally, a thrombin-mediated activation pathway has been recently discovered, which bypasses the initial C3 activation step (Gros et al., 2008).

The alternative pathway functions as a central defense mechanism for immune surveillance. Its beginning phases are spontaneous and indiscriminate, not distinguishing between self and foreign cells. Activation begins in the fluid phase, with lately activated C3 components depositing indiscriminately on nearby surfaces. Once activated, the complement system amplifies on any surface. However, these early reactions are slow, allowing time for regulation. Self-specific regulators intervene at this stage to prevent additional unfolding of the cascade. Regulation and inhibition of the complement cascade occur rapidly in the liquid form but are most effective on the surfaces of healthy native-cells. These self-cells are provided with membrane-bound regulatory proteins and acquire inhibitors attached to their surfaces. This combination of surface-bound and membrane-associated regulators prevents further activation of the cascade on self-cells, helping to maintain homeostasis within the host. In contrast, regulation does not occur on foreign particles, infectious agents, or altered self-cells, as they lack these complement regulators. Consequently, the complement cascade continues on these surfaces, leading to opsonization, cellular damage, and removal by phagocytosis (Schmidt et al., 2016). The IIS and its pathogen evasion mechanism are depicted in **Figure 6.1**.

Given the potent damaging capacity of complement effector products, their generation and targeting are tightly regulated. Under normal physiological conditions, complement activation results in the destruction of infectious agents while simultaneously protecting host surfaces and cells. However, pathogenic microbes can evade complement recognition or debilitate their

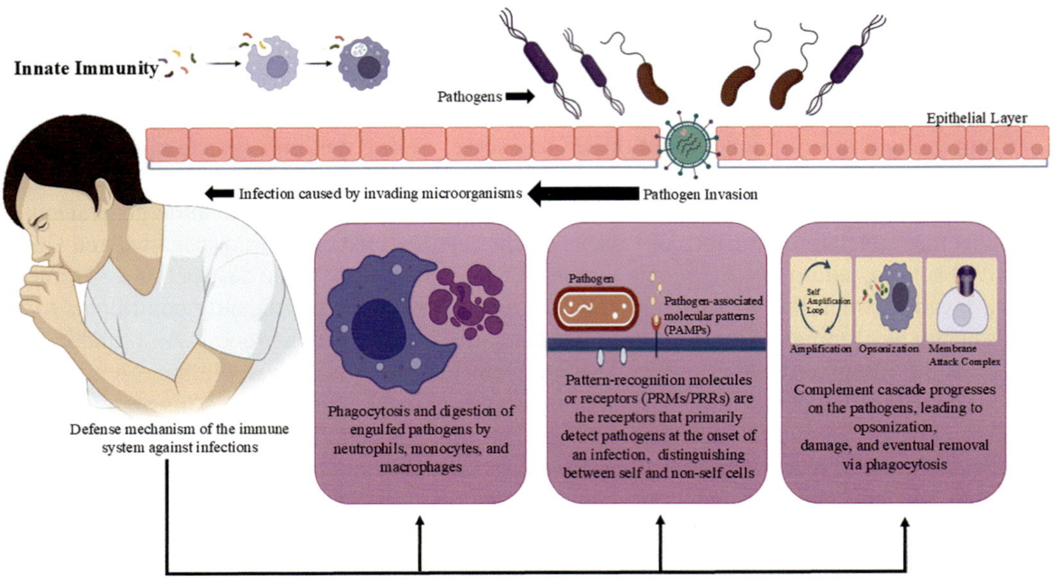

FIGURE 6.1 Innate immune response to pathogen invasion.

effector products, making the complement system dysregulated. This impaired control can increase and intensify local complement activity, potentially damaging the host's surfaces and structures.

6.3.2 Adaptive Immunity: Tailored and Specific Responses

The later phase of the immune response, known as acquired immunity, is also called adaptive or specific immunity. The immune system adapts to detect and respond to particular antigens. Antigens provoke an immune response consisting of proteins, carbohydrates, lipids, or smaller molecules (such as dinitrophenol when linked to a carrier). These infectious agents can be derived from external invaders or the body's cells, which are termed self-antigens. The range of potential antigens is vast. Unlike the innate defense system, which uses receptors with general specificity, the acquired immune system is tailored to identify a wide variety of specific antigens through specialized receptors expressed on immune cells, each designed to recognize just one antigen. This precise recognition mechanism is the result of evolutionary pressures and plays a key role in the formation of immunological memory, enabling the defense system to "remember" pathogens it has previously encountered. It is defined by a vast array of receptors produced through somatic gene recombination and immune memory formation. The two main elements of adaptive immunity are lymphocytes and soluble mediators (Merlo and Mandik-Nayak, 2013). Lymphocytes, essential for antigen recognition, are divided into T and B cells. Another aspect of acquired immunity is humoral immunity, derived from the Latin word "humor," meaning fluid. This immune response component involves soluble molecules such as antibodies, which bind to antigens or immune cells. Antibodies, or "antikorpers," as first termed by German scientist Paul Ehrlich in 1891, are one of the primary components. Cellular and humoral immune responses can recognize between 10^9 and 10^{11} distinct antigenic determinants. The extraordinary characteristic of the acquired defense system is its potential to efficiently target new pathogens while minimizing harm to the host's tissues.

Once the immune system detects a pathogen, specific T and B cells undergo a rapid clonal selection and expansion process. Within days, a few cells with receptors that recognize the pathogen multiply into thousands of cells capable of responding to the threat (Langefeld et al., 2009; Liongue et al., 2011; Shanker, 2010). A key outcome of this rapid expansion is the establishment of immune memory. After the pathogen is cleared, most of the activated effector cells die off. Yet, a small subset of these cells, known as memory cells, persists for years or even decades. These memory cells facilitate the immune system to elicit a quicker and more robust response if the pathogen is reencountered in the future. This mechanism forms the foundation of immunization, a prominent, influential, and effective medical measure that saves millions of lives annually (Farber et al., 2016).

The key elements of the adaptive immune system include T cells, cytokines, B cells, and antibodies. T cells mature in the thymus and travel to the spleen and lymph nodes. They are classified into two primary types: helper T cells (Th cells) and cytotoxic T cells (CTLs). Helper T cells release cytokines that help regulate the activity of other kinds of immune cells, also from the IIS, while cytotoxic T cells are responsible for eliminating infected cells, especially those infected by viruses. T cells are differentiated by the surface proteins they carry: Th cells typically express CD4, while CTLs express CD8. All T cells also express CD3, a protein complex essential for recognizing antigens and activating T cells (Vallejo et al., 2004).

Cytokines are small signaling molecules, mainly generated by helper T cells, though innate immune cells, APCs, and B cells also form them. They regulate immune responses by interacting with target cells with specific receptors. Often, cytokines work together to shape the behavior of effector cells. Key cytokines, such as IL-2 and IFN-γ, play crucial roles in steering immune responses. B cells are formed in the bone marrow and resemble T cells in size and shape. However, B cells have an enlarged nucleus and minimal cytoplasm in their resting state. B cells' membrane-associated surface receptor form of an antibody sets B cells apart. Following activation via antigen binding, B cells differentiate into plasma cells that produce immunoglobulins, which are soluble versions of the B cell receptor. These antibodies are high-molecular-weight (~250 kDa), Y-shaped proteins produced by plasma cells. They have strong binding affinity sites designed to detect and bind to antigens. Antibodies are crucial in marking pathogens for destruction or neutralizing their harmful effects. The dynamics of adaptive immunity are complex, with immune mediators working individually or in combination and sometimes even antagonistically. As an illustration in viral infections, the initial immune response may prioritize cytotoxic T cells, whereas the later stages see B cells producing antibodies to neutralize viral particles present in the extracellular environment. However, unchecked inflammation can cause tissue damage, and the immune system must regulate this inflammation carefully. This regulation is mainly controlled by a specific group of helper T cells, which release biochemical signals to inhibit inflammation following its initial activation (Keselowsky et al., 2020). **Figure 6.2** represents the adaptive immune response to pathogen invasion.

6.3.3 Immune Evasion Mechanisms of Pathogens and Cancer

Immune evasion strategies are essential for the survival and persistence of pathogens and are closely linked to the molecular mechanisms that regulate immune responses. These strategies can be broadly categorized into passive and active forms.

Passive evasion involves mechanisms that allow pathogens to conceal themselves or modify their surface structures to avoid detection by the immune system. For example, *Plasmodium* shields its surface to evade immune recognition and employs antigenic variation, altering its surface antigens to escape detection. *Plasmodium falciparum* has over 60 surface variants, enabling it to evade the host immune system continuously. Similarly, viruses such as HIV mutate their epitopes rapidly, while some parasites enter a dormant or quiescent state to avoid immune recognition altogether (Schmid-Hempel, 2009).

In contrast, active evasion directly interferes with the host's immune response. Many pathogens produce or code for molecules that modulate or block immune functions. For example, bacterial adhesins and invasins facilitate pathogen entry into host cells. *Shigella* employs the Type III

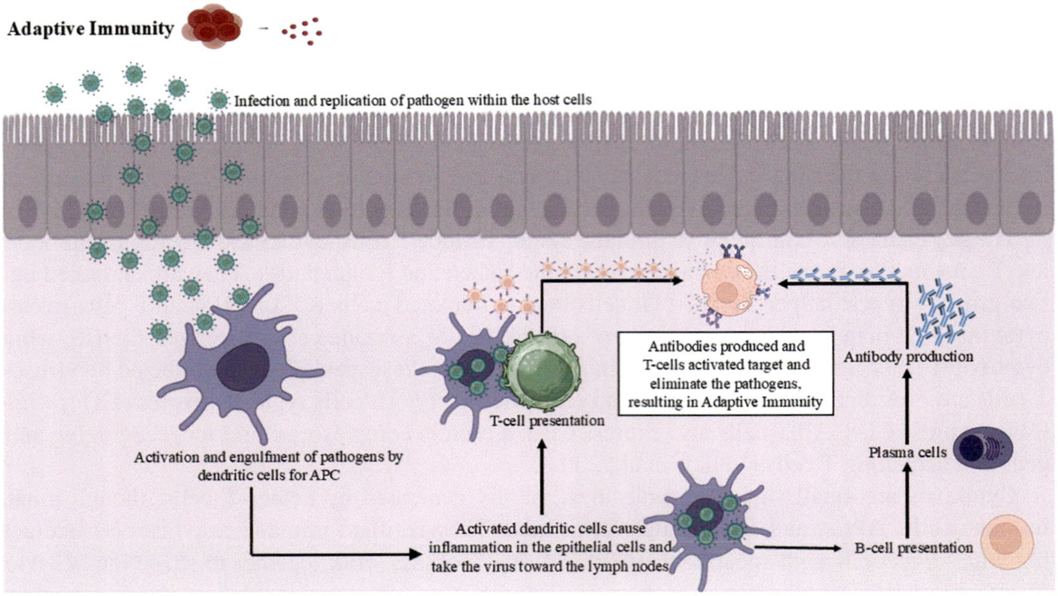

FIGURE 6.2 Adaptive immune response to pathogen invasion.

Secretion System to transfer proteins directly into host cells, disrupting crucial immune defense functions (Schmid-Hempel, 2009). Parasites such as schistosomes generate C-type lectins to inhibit host detection molecules (Loukas and Maizels, 2000), while viruses such as cytomegalovirus produce MHC decoy molecules to impair antigen presentation (Murphy, 1993). Additionally, *Plasmodium* and nematodes produce competing ligands that interfere with host recognition (Blaxter et al., 1992; Locksley, 1997).

Once the immune system recognizes the pathogen, evasion strategies often target key immune defense mechanisms such as the complement system and phagocytosis. For example, *Leishmania* degrades host proteins to inhibit the complement cascade (Nunes et al., 1997), while bacteria such as *Streptococcus* and *S. aureus* prevent complement binding to their surface. *S. aureus* produces the CHIPS protein to inhibit neutrophils to evade phagocytosis, while *Shigella* induces macrophage apoptosis. Other pathogens, such as *M. tuberculosis*, arrest phagosome development to escape destruction, whereas *Salmonella* alters vacuole maturation to avoid antimicrobial effects.

Parasites also deploy various mechanisms to neutralize immune effectors. *M. tuberculosis* breaks down reactive, toxic molecules for protection (Flynn and Chan, 2001), while *Pseudomonas* produces proteases and lipases to degrade immunoglobulins. These strategies exemplify convergent evolution across different pathogens, enabling them to overcome host defenses and establish persistent infections (Loh et al., 2023).

Like pathogens, tumor cells have developed multiple strategies to evade immune detection and destruction (Vinay et al., 2015). Immunosuppressive markers such as IDO, Siglec-9, and PD-L1 are upregulated in cancer cells, while MHC class I is downregulated, facilitating invasion, metastasis, and recurrence. The tumor microenvironment is infiltrated by immune cells, including neutrophils, fibroblasts, macrophages, regulatory T cells (Tregs), and myeloid-derived suppressor cells (MDSCs), contributing to immunosuppression and tumor progression. Additionally, cytokines and immunosuppressive molecules such as COX-2, TGF-β, PGE2, and IL-10 further promote immune evasion (Kuol et al., 2017).

NK cells play a crucial role in innate immunity by targeting tumor cells that lack MHC class I expression. However, tumor cells develop escape mechanisms that prevent their elimination. Soluble factors secreted by malignant cells, including prostaglandins, vascular endothelial growth factor, and immunosuppressive cytokines, inhibit immune responses and facilitate tumor growth. Additionally, malignant cells induce activation-induced cell death (AICD) to eliminate immune effector cells actively. Beyond producing inhibitory molecules, tumor cells also evade detection by modifying antigen presentation pathways. By altering the expression of key proteins required for antigen processing and presentation, they effectively conceal their pathogenic state from anti-tumor immune cells (Loose and Van de Wiele, 2009).

Thus, pathogens and tumor cells employ various sophisticated strategies to evade immune detection and suppression. While pathogens use passive and active immune evasion tactics to persist within the host, tumor cells exploit immunosuppressive pathways and modify antigen presentation to escape immune surveillance. Understanding these mechanisms is crucial for developing therapeutic interventions to enhance immune system's effectiveness against infections and cancer.

6.4 PATHOGENS AND HUMANS: THE EVOLUTIONARY CONFLICT

6.4.1 Antimicrobial Resistance: A Developing Problem

A pressing issue for global health today is AMR. Pathogens build resistance in several ways, including by producing enzymes that break down antibiotics, changing the targets of drugs, and altering the permeability of their membranes to block drug entry (Salam et al., 2023). Methicillin-resistant *S. aureus* (MRSA) and bacteria that produce beta-lactamases are some examples exhibiting resistance (GBD 2021 Antimicrobial Resistance Collaborator, 2024). Antibiotic abuse and overuse in agriculture and healthcare have sped up the emergence of resistant strains, making it more difficult or impossible to treat previously curable infections (Ventola, 2015).

6.4.2 Pathogens' Genetic Adaptability

Because of their extraordinary genetic flexibility, pathogens can quickly adjust to environmental stresses such as medication exposure (Munita and Arias, 2016). Horizontal gene transfer (HGT), mutations, and genetic recombination are essential processes that allow the formation of novel strains with increased virulence or treatment resistance (Emamalipour et al., 2020). Mutations that occur during replication are one important mechanism that can lead to drug resistance (Hughes and Andersson, 2015). For example, antibiotics can become ineffective due to changes in their target sites caused by single-nucleotide mutations in essential bacterial genes (Muteeb et al., 2023). Another adaptive mechanism that shields bacteria from antimicrobial drugs and makes illnesses more challenging to treat is the creation of biofilms (Sharma et al., 2023).

6.4.3 Human Behavior's Contribution to Resistance

Human activity significantly influences antibiotic resistance development and dissemination (Knobler et al., 2003). The development of resistance is fueled by the selection pressure created by the improper use of antibiotics, whether through self-medication or overprescription by medical professionals (Sachdev et al., 2022).

Noncompliance with recommended treatment plans further facilitates the survival and multiplication of partially resistant strains (Prestinaci et al., 2015). Beyond healthcare, more travel and globalization have allowed resistant infections to spread quickly across national boundaries, transforming local issues into global emergencies (Kumbhar et al., 2023). Furthermore, agricultural practices make the problem worse, especially the frequent use of antibiotics in animal husbandry to promote development and prevent disease, which breeds resistance in zoonotic bacteria that people can consume (Zhang et al., 2024).

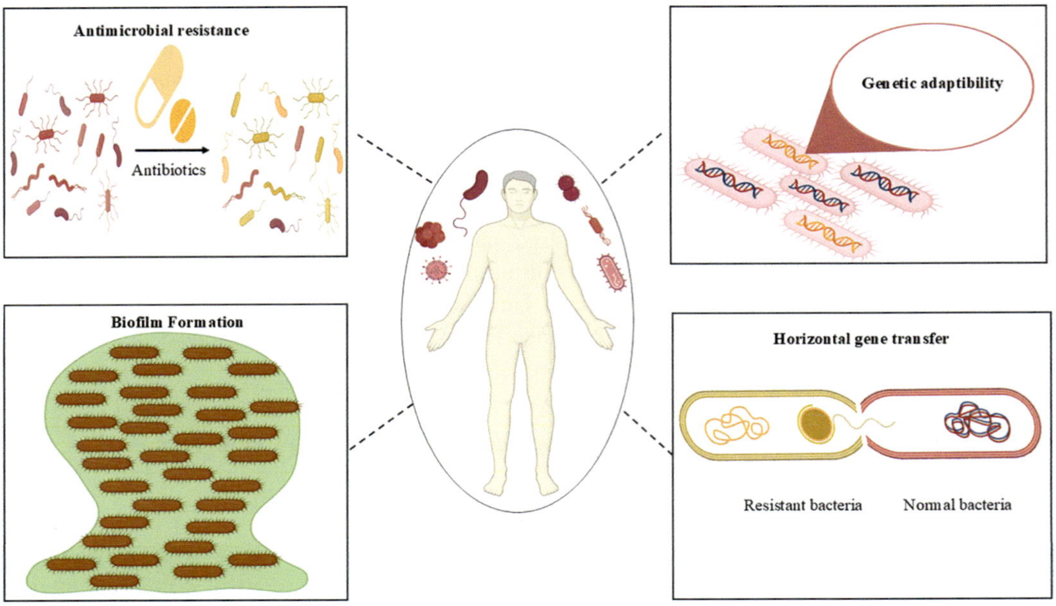

FIGURE 6.3 Dynamic host–pathogen interactions.

6.4.4 Fighting Resistance: Novel Approaches to Drug Development

Traditional antibiotics are losing effectiveness, prompting scientists to explore innovative therapies (Muteeb et al., 2023). A viable approach is the creation of novel antibiotics that target bacterial pathways that have not been explored before. Furthermore, employing viruses that infect and kill bacteria in bacteriophage therapy is a viable remedy for bacterial infections resistant to medication (Lin et al., 2017). Antimicrobial peptides (AMPs), which are naturally occurring compounds with broad-spectrum activity against infections, are another new strategy (Mba and Nweze, 2022). Additionally, CRISPR-based antimicrobial technologies are being studied by researchers because they allow for the precise targeting and eradication of resistant bacteria without endangering the host's regular microbiota (Mayorga-Ramos et al., 2023). The dynamic host–pathogen interactions are represented in **Figure 6.3**.

6.5 THE WORLDWIDE IMPACT OF INFECTIOUS DISEASES

The threat of infectious diseases to global well-being endures, continuing to significantly impact both mortality and morbidity despite advances in sanitation, vaccinations, and treatment. These diseases continue to be a foremost contributor to mortality, particularly in impoverished areas. In line with the WHO, diseases such as malaria, diarrheal infections, and respiratory illnesses account for millions of deaths annually. Beyond mortality, these diseases often lead to chronic illness, long-term disability, and a deterioration in the quality of life, imposing a significant strain on individuals, families, and healthcare systems. Diseases such as hepatitis, HIV/AIDS, and tuberculosis remain prevalent, especially in regions such as sub-Saharan Africa and parts of Asia. Moreover, new infectious diseases, such as COVID-19, have underscored how vulnerable populations are to novel pathogens, leading to a surge in global infectious disease prevalence (Greenwood, 2014).

In addition to their direct health consequences, pandemics and epidemics bring about significant socioeconomic disruptions that affect economies, livelihoods, and social structures. During outbreaks, healthcare systems often become overwhelmed, limiting access to medical treatment for infectious and non-infectious conditions. Economic disruptions ensue because supply chains are interrupted, healthcare costs soar, and workforce participation declines. The COVID-19 pandemic, for example, resulted in widespread job losses, business closures, and recessions across multiple countries, with low-income communities bearing the brunt of these economic shocks. Education systems are also heavily affected as schools close, while sectors such as travel and tourism face severe losses. Pandemics and epidemics often exacerbate pre-existing social inequalities, disproportionately affecting marginalized and vulnerable populations. The long-term socioeconomic impacts of such events can persist for years, with countries struggling to recover, rebuild their economies, and restore their healthcare systems (Alizadeh et al., 2023).

Infectious diseases disproportionately affect people with low incomes, chiefly in underprivileged and emerging economic countries, where they aggravate global health issues and disparities. These populations are particularly vulnerable due to poor nutrition, inadequate sanitation, and limited access to healthcare. Diseases that could be prevented with vaccines or basic hygiene practices continue to thrive in these regions. For example, HIV/AIDS, malaria, and tuberculosis remain widespread in sub-Saharan Africa, where healthcare infrastructure is often insufficient to provide timely treatments and interventions. Determinants of health within society, such as income, education, and living conditions, contribute to significant health disparities both within and between nations. While global health organizations have made some progress in addressing these inequities, infectious diseases continue to disproportionately impact the most vulnerable populations, perpetuating health disparities globally (Bhutta et al., 2014).

Climate change has become an increasingly important factor in the resurgence and spread of infectious diseases. Rising global temperatures, shifting rainfall patterns, and an escalation in the frequency of severe weather events create favorable conditions for many pathogens and their vectors, such as mosquitoes and ticks. Diseases such as malaria, dengue, and Zika are susceptible to environmental changes, with warmer temperatures expanding the geographic range of the insects that transmit these diseases. Climate change also affects food and water security, increasing the risk of waterborne diseases such as cholera and diarrheal infections. Extreme weather events, such as floods and droughts, can disrupt sanitation systems, raising the likelihood of outbreaks. Furthermore, the displacement caused by natural disasters leads to overcrowded living conditions, further facilitating the spread of infectious diseases. As climate change accelerates, the risk of new and re-emerging contagious diseases affecting vulnerable and developed regions poses a growing public health concern (Mojahed et al., 2022).

Effective management of infectious diseases requires strong healthcare systems and infrastructure. However, many countries face significant challenges, especially in low- and middle-income regions. Insufficient healthcare resources, including a lack of trained healthcare personnel, medical supplies, and infrastructure, hinder the timely diagnosis and treatment of infectious diseases. In rural and underserved areas, access to healthcare is limited, and patients may experience long delays in seeking care. Weak health systems cannot contain outbreaks, allowing diseases to spread rapidly and cause more severe consequences. Even in wealthier nations, the COVID-19 pandemic revealed weaknesses in healthcare systems, including overcrowded hospitals, shortages of critical medical supplies, and difficulties coordinating large-scale public health responses. Strengthening healthcare systems through investments in infrastructure, workforce development, and public health preparedness is essential for managing and preventing the spread of infectious diseases. This requires a global commitment to building resilient healthcare systems that effectively respond to emerging and re-emerging health threats (Kruk et al., 2018; Sucharitha et al.,2022).

6.6 PERSONALIZED MEDICINE IN INFECTIOUS DISEASE AND CANCER MANAGEMENT

As scientific advancements reshape therapeutic strategies for infections, the ongoing battle between microorganisms and human health continues to evolve. Emerging challenges such as antibiotic resistance, climate change, and increasing global interconnectivity necessitate innovative solutions for future infectious disease management. These solutions will be driven by cutting-edge technologies, international collaboration, and proactive strategies to anticipate new threats.

One such transformative technology is artificial intelligence (AI), which has shown immense promise in predicting and managing infectious disease outbreaks. While AI has been widely adopted in clinical medicine (Fong et al., 2021), its integration into public health has been slower (Budd et al., 2020). However, AI's proficiency in analyzing large datasets and identifying patterns that might elude human detection makes it a valuable resource for early disease detection and response. This is particularly significant in disease prevention, detection, and treatment, marking a shift toward more precise and proactive healthcare strategies.

The rapid growth of AI in clinical medicine has been driven by the availability of vast medical datasets facilitated by the digital transformation of medical reports and the sharing of de-identified health information (Colombo et al., 2020). This integration of AI in healthcare systems marks a new era of transformative advancements, particularly in machine learning, computational linguistics, and data analysis (Kasula, 2017). These innovations have enabled a more holistic approach to healthcare, improving early detection, personalized treatment strategies, and more efficient public health responses (Dey et al.,2023). This is especially crucial in managing infectious diseases, where swift and accurate interventions are essential.

In addition to AI, pioneering technologies such as single-cell sequencing and spatial gene profiling enhance the discovery of molecular markers for infectious diseases (Gomes et al., 2019; Ward et al., 2021). These innovations allow scientists to study individual cells in unprecedented detail, providing insights into specific molecular signatures linked to infections. The synergy between AI and advanced technologies has the potential to revolutionize how we detect and respond to infectious diseases.

AI's role in healthcare extends beyond diagnostics. Its advanced data analytics and pattern recognition capabilities enable the processing of vast datasets, including clinical records, laboratory results, and demographic information. This aids in the early detection of outbreaks and the identification of disease trends. Machine learning algorithms analyze historical and real-time data to support these efforts, incorporating climate and environmental conditions to predict disease spread and guide timely public health interventions. In personalized medicine, AI tailors treatment plans by analyzing patient-specific data, including genomic information, to optimize therapies and minimize adverse effects. AI-driven predictive models enhance outbreak forecasting by integrating travel trends, climate conditions, and healthcare system capabilities. Additionally, AI-powered diagnostic tools, such as image recognition and genetic analysis, accelerate pathogen identification and improve diagnostic accuracy (Isiaka et al., 2024).

Vaccines remain one of the most powerful tools for preventing infectious diseases, as they train the immune system to identify and respond to specific pathogens (Anilkumar et al.,2025). The conventional vaccine development process involves several stages, including pathogen identification, preclinical tests, clinical studies, and regulatory approval (Danasekaran, 2021;Dalsass et al., 2019). AI accelerates this process through predictive modeling and data analysis, where machine learning algorithms process large datasets on pathogen characteristics, host immune responses, and vaccine outcomes (Zohar, 2022). This helps identify promising vaccine candidates and enhances vaccine effectiveness. AI is also transforming drug and vaccine development in other ways. Companies such as BenevolentAI use AI to mine biomedical datasets for potential drug candidates (Bess et al., 2022), while Atomwise employs AI-powered virtual screening to discover new small-molecule drugs targeting infectious diseases (Batool et al., 2019).

In vaccine research, EpiVax utilizes AI-based algorithms to predict antigenic epitopes for vaccine development (Moise et al., 2015). Additionally, initiatives such as BenevolentAI's identification of baricitinib as a potential COVID-19 treatment highlight AI's groundbreaking role in drug repurposing. Integrating AI into infectious disease management, vaccine development, and personalized medicine, the healthcare landscape rapidly evolves, creating more efficient, targeted healthcare solutions and accelerating responses to emerging global health threats.

Despite significant advancements in molecular oncology, targeted therapeutic options for cancers with unknown carcinogenesis processes remain limited. While tumor cell biological traits are commonly used, clinical tumor features also serve as valuable biomarkers, guiding patient-specific and tumor-specific treatment approaches (Hoeben et al., 2021). Personalized medicine in oncology not only optimizes anticancer treatments but also enhances supportive care for cancer patients.

Proteomics has revolutionized cancer biomarker research by identifying differentially expressed proteins across various cancer types, providing new targets for precision treatment. Mapping human cancer proteomes helps address challenges such as chemotherapy resistance, leading to improved clinical outcomes through more precise prevention, diagnosis, and individualized treatment (Su et al., 2021). Next-generation sequencing (NGS) enables time- and cost-efficient tumor DNA sequencing, allowing targeted therapies for specific tumors and patient genotypes. Based on disease stage, such as in various cancers, NGS can categorize patients into distinct subpopulations and assess their response to therapy, including synthetic drugs and herbal formulations (Singh et al., 2024).

Cross-resistance to chemotherapy makes cancer cells resistant to multiple drugs. Nanoparticles offer a targeted approach to reduce toxicity and improve treatment. They can be designed for various applications, including antimicrobial therapy and tumor diagnosis, enhancing cancer management (Singh et al., 2024). Pharmacogenomics enhances personalized medicine by using genotyping to customize drug selection and dosage. Genetic variability influences drug efficacy, activation, adverse responses, and cancer treatment models. Pharmacogenes, regulated by coding and regulatory regions, play a crucial role in drug response and development (Anand et al., 2022). The steps involved in the generation of personalized medicine for both infectious diseases and cancer are depicted in **Figure 6.4**.

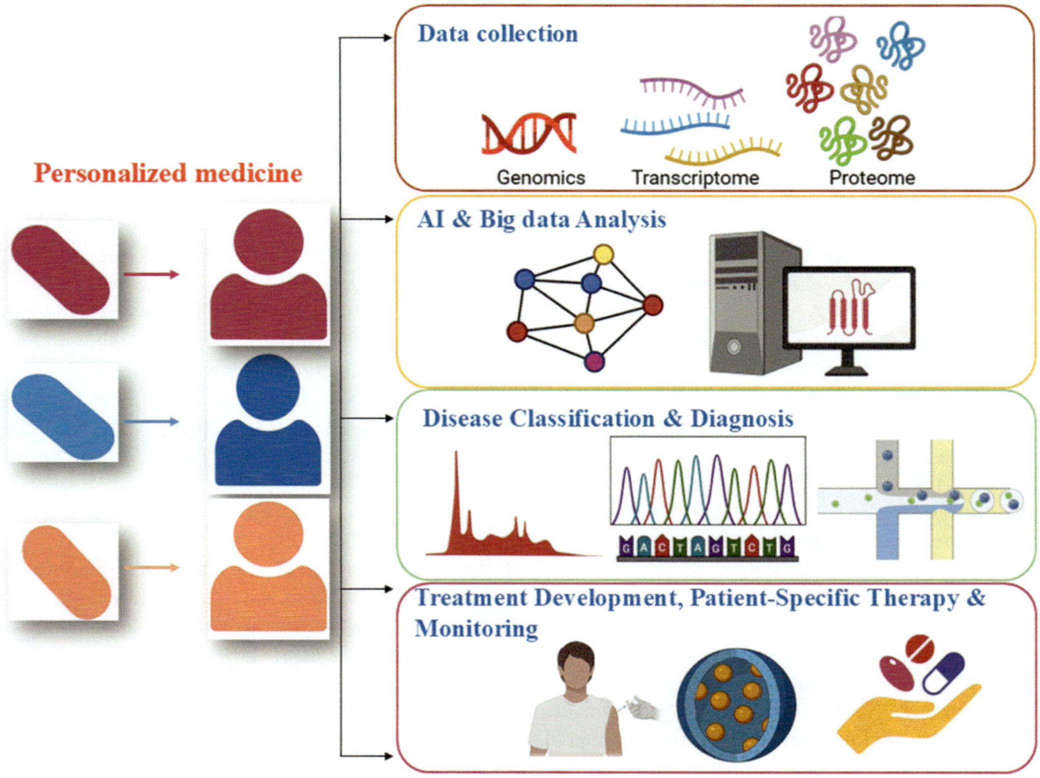

FIGURE 6.4 Steps in the generation of personalized medicine for both infectious diseases and cancer.

6.7 CONCLUSION

Infectious diseases and cancer pose interconnected challenges to human health, with infectious agents contributing to a significant proportion of cancers. Understanding the complex interactions between pathogens, the immune system, and host cells is crucial for effective disease management. Personalized medicine transforms the approach to infectious diseases and cancer by leveraging advanced technologies for tailored prevention, diagnosis, and treatment. AI-driven analytics enhance early disease detection and outbreak response, while proteomics and pharmacogenomics refine therapeutic strategies. NGS and nanoparticle-based drug delivery also improve targeted cancer therapies, addressing issues such as chemotherapy resistance. As global health threats evolve, integrating advancements in medicine, biotechnology, and public health is essential to combat the ongoing battle between infectious pathogens and cancer. Continued research and international collaboration will be key to optimizing precision medicine approaches, ultimately improving patient outcomes and reducing the burden of these diseases worldwide.

ACKNOWLEDGMENTS

The authors thank the Chettinad Academy of Research Education for their constant support and encouragement.

DECLARATION

Ethics approval and consent to participate: Not applicable
Consent for publication: Not applicable
Availability of data and materials: Not applicable
Competing interests: The authors declare no conflict of interest to report
Funding: Not applicable

REFERENCES

Abdulamir, A. S., Hafidh, R. R., & Abu Bakar, F. (2011). The association of Streptococcus bovis/gallolyticus with colorectal tumors: the nature and the underlying mechanisms of its etiological role. *Journal of experimental & clinical cancer research: CR*, *30*(1), 11. https://doi.org/10.1186/1756-9966-30-11

Alberts, B., Johnson, A., Lewis, J., Raff, M., Roberts, K., & Walter, P. (2002). Helper T cells and lymphocyte activation. In *Molecular biology of the cell*. 4th edition. Garland Science.

Alibek, K., Karatayeva, N., & Bekniyazov, I. (2012). The role of infectious agents in urogenital cancers. *Infectious agents and cancer*, *7*(1), 35. https://doi.org/10.1186/1750-9378-7-35

Alizadeh, H., Sharifi, A., Damanbagh, S., Nazarnia, H., & Nazarnia, M. (2023). Impacts of the COVID-19 pandemic on the social sphere and lessons for crisis management: a literature review. *Natural hazards*, *117*(3), 2139–2164.

Ameya, G., & Birri, D. J. (2023). The molecular mechanisms of virus-induced human cancers. *Microbial pathogenesis*, *183*, 106292. https://doi.org/10.1016/j.micpath.2023.106292

Anand, U., Dey, A., Chandel, A. K. S., Sanyal, R., Mishra, A., Pandey, D. K., De Falco, V., Upadhyay, A., Kandimalla, R., Chaudhary, A., Dhanjal, J. K., Dewanjee, S., Vallamkondu, J., & Pérez de la Lastra, J. M. (2022). Cancer chemotherapy and beyond: Current status, drug candidates, associated risks and progress in targeted therapeutics. *Genes & diseases*, *10*(4), 1367–1401. https://doi.org/10.1016/j.gendis.2022.02.007

Anilkumar, A. S., Thomas, S. M., & Veerabathiran, R. (2025). Next-generation cancer vaccines: targeting cryptic and non-canonical antigens for precision immunotherapy. *Exploration of targeted anti-tumor therapy*, *6*, 1002338. https://doi.org/10.37349/etat.2025.1002338

Balloux, F., & van Dorp, L. (2017). Q&A: What are pathogens, and what have they done to and for us?. *BMC biology*, *15*(1), 91. https://doi.org/10.1186/s12915-017-0433-z

Banerjee, S., Tian, T., Wei, Z., Shih, N., Feldman, M. D., Alwine, J. C., Coukos, G., & Robertson, E. S. (2017). The ovarian cancer oncobiome. *Oncotarget*, *8*(22), 36225–36245. https://doi.org/10.18632/oncotarget.16717

Bartlett, A., Padfield, D., Lear, L., Bendall, R., & Vos, M. (2022). A comprehensive list of bacterial pathogens infecting humans. *Microbiology (Reading, England)*, *168*(12). https://doi.org/10.1099/mic.0.001269

Batool, M., Ahmad, B., & Choi, S. (2019). A structure-based drug discovery paradigm. *International journal of molecular sciences*, *20*(11), 2783.

Bess, A., Berglind, F., Mukhopadhyay, S., Brylinski, M., Griggs, N., Cho, T., …, & Wasan, K. M. (2022). Artificial intelligence for the discovery of novel antimicrobial agents for emerging infectious diseases. *Drug discovery today*, *27*(4), 1099–1107.

Bhutta, Z. A., Sommerfeld, J., Lassi, Z. S., Salam, R. A., & Das, J. K. (2014). Global burden, distribution, and interventions for infectious diseases of poverty. *Infectious diseases of poverty*, *3*, 1–7.

Blaxter, M. L., Page, A. P., Rudin, W., & Maizels, R. M. (1992). Nematode surface coats: Actively evading immunity. *Parasitology today*, *8*(7), 243–247.

Bradley, J. E., & Jackson, J. A. (2008). Measuring immune system variation to help understand host-pathogen community dynamics. *Parasitology*, *135*(7), 807–823. https://doi.org/10.1017/S0031182008000322

Budd, J., Miller, B. S., Manning, E. M., Lampos, V., Zhuang, M., Edelstein, M., …, & McKendry, R. A. (2020). Digital technologies in the public-health response to COVID-19. *Nature medicine*, *26*(8), 1183–1192.

Chew, Q. H., Wei, K. C., Vasoo, S., Chua, H. C., & Sim, K. (2020). Narrative synthesis of psychological and coping responses towards emerging infectious disease outbreaks in the general population: Practical considerations for the COVID-19 pandemic. *Singapore medical journal*, *61*(7), 350–356. https://doi.org/10.11622/smedj.2020046

Ching-López, R., & Rodríguez Pavón, S. (2020). Talaromycosis in a lung cancer patient: A rare case. *Cureus*, *12*(9), e10615. https://doi.org/10.7759/cureus.10615

Chowdhury, M. A., Hossain, N., Kashem, M. A., Shahid, M. A., & Alam, A. (2020). Immune response in COVID-19: A review. *Journal of infection and public health*, *13*(11), 1619–1629.

Cockerill, K., Armstrong, M., Richter, J., & Okie, J. G. (2017). The human nature of infectious disease. In *Environmental realism: Challenging solutions* (pp. 45–65). https://doi.org/10.1007/978-3-319-52824-3_3

Coker, O. O., Nakatsu, G., Dai, R. Z., Wu, W. K. K., Wong, S. H., Ng, S. C., Chan, F. K. L., Sung, J. J. Y., & Yu, J. (2019). Enteric fungal microbiota dysbiosis and ecological alterations in colorectal cancer. *Gut*, *68*(4), 654–662. https://doi.org/10.1136/gutjnl-2018-317178

Colombo, F., Oderkirk, J., & Slawomirski, L. (2020). Health information systems, electronic medical records, and big data in global healthcare: Progress and challenges in OECD countries. In Haring, R., Kickbusch, I., Ganten, D., & Moeti, M. (Eds.), *Handbook of global health*. Springer. https://doi.org/10.1007/978-3-030-05325-3_71-1

Crowe, S. E. (2005). Helicobacter infection, chronic inflammation, and the development of malignancy. *Current opinion in gastroenterology*, *21*(1), 32–38.

Cummins, J., & Tangney, M. (2013). Bacteria and tumours: Causative agents or opportunistic inhabitants?. *Infectious agents and cancer*, *8*(1), 11. https://doi.org/10.1186/1750-9378-8-11

Dalsass, M., Brozzi, A., Medini, D., & Rappuoli, R. (2019). Comparison of open-source reverse vaccinology programs for bacterial vaccine antigen discovery. *Frontiers in immunology*, *10*, 113.

Danasekaran, R. (2021). Immunization among Healthcare Workers in India: A Need or a Want. *Journal of comprehensive health*, *9*(1), 50–51.

de Martel, C., & Franceschi, S. (2009). Infections and cancer: Established associations and new hypotheses. *Critical reviews in oncology/hematology*, *70*(3), 183–194. https://doi.org/10.1016/j.critrevonc.2008.07.021

Dey, A., Mitra, A., Pathak, S., Prasad, S., Zhang, A. S., Zhang, H., Sun, X. F., & Banerjee, A. (2023). Recent Advancements, Limitations, and Future Perspectives of the use of Personalized Medicine in Treatment of Colon Cancer. *Technology in cancer research & treatment*, *22*, 15330338231178403. https://doi.org/10.1177/15330338231178403

Dohlman, A. B., Klug, J., Mesko, M., Gao, I. H., Lipkin, S. M., Shen, X., & Iliev, I. D. (2022). A pan-cancer mycobiome analysis reveals fungal involvement in gastrointestinal and lung tumors. *Cell*, *185*(20), 3807–3822.e12. https://doi.org/10.1016/j.cell.2022.09.015

Efird, J. T., Davies, S. W., O'Neal, W. T., & Anderson, E. J. (2014). Animal viruses, bacteria, and cancer: A brief commentary. *Frontiers in public health*, *2*, 14. https://doi.org/10.3389/fpubh.2014.00014

Eisenreich, W., Rudel, T., Heesemann, J., & Goebel, W. (2019). How viral and intracellular bacterial pathogens reprogram the metabolism of host cells to allow their intracellular replication. *Frontiers in cellular and infection microbiology*, *9*, 42. https://doi.org/10.3389/fcimb.2019.00042

El-Gayar, E. K., & Mahmoud, M. M. (2014). Do protozoa play a role in carcinogenesis. *Parasitologists united journal*, *7*(2), 80.

Emamalipour, M., Seidi, K., Zununi Vahed, S., Jahanban-Esfahlan, A., Jaymand, M., Majdi, H., Amoozgar, Z., Chitkushev, L. T., Javaheri, T., Jahanban-Esfahlan, R., & Zare, P. (2020). Horizontal gene transfer: From evolutionary flexibility to disease progression. *Frontiers in cell and developmental biology*, *8*, 229. https://doi.org/10.3389/fcell.2020.00229

Engering, A., Hogerwerf, L., & Slingenbergh, J. (2013). Pathogen-host-environment interplay and disease emergence. *Emerging microbes & infections*, *2*(2), e5. https://doi.org/10.1038/emi.2013.5

Farber, D. L., Netea, M. G., Radbruch, A., Rajewsky, K., & Zinkernagel, R. M. (2016). Immunological memory: Lessons from the past and a look to the future. *Nature reviews immunology*, *16*(2), 124–128.

Ferrándiz-Pulido, C., Martin-Gomez, M. T., Repiso, T., Juárez-Dobjanschi, C., Ferrer, B., López-Lerma, I., Aparicio, G., González-Cruz, C., Moreso, F., Roman, A., & García-Patos, V. (2019). Cutaneous infections by dematiaceous opportunistic fungi: Diagnosis and management in 11 solid organ transplant recipients. *Mycoses*, *62*(2), 121–127. https://doi.org/10.1111/myc.12853

Ferreira, M. S., & Borges, A. S. (2002). Some aspects of protozoan infections in immunocompromised patients – A review. *Memorias do Instituto Oswaldo Cruz*, *97*(4), 443–457. https://doi.org/10.1590/s0074-02762002000400001

Flynn, J. L., & Chan, J. (2001). Immunology of tuberculosis. *Annual review of immunology*, *19*, 93–129. https://doi.org/10.1146/annurev.immunol.19.1.93

Fong, S. J., Dey, N., & Chaki, J. (2021). *Artificial intelligence for coronavirus outbreak*. Springer.

Garvey, M., Meade, E., & Rowan, N. J. (2022). Effectiveness of front line and emerging fungal disease prevention and control interventions and opportunities to address appropriate eco-sustainable solutions. *The science of the total environment*, *851*(Pt 2), 158284. https://doi.org/10.1016/j.scitotenv.2022.158284

GBD 2013 Mortality and Causes of Death Collaborators (2015). Global, regional, and national age-sex specific all-cause and cause-specific mortality for 240 causes of death, 1990-2013: A systematic analysis for the Global Burden of Disease Study 2013. *Lancet (London, England)*, *385*(9963), 117–171. https://doi.org/10.1016/S0140-6736(14)61682-2

GBD 2021 Antimicrobial Resistance Collaborators (2024). Global burden of bacterial antimicrobial resistance 1990-2021: A systematic analysis with forecasts to 2050. *Lancet (London, England)*, *404*(10459), 1199–1226. https://doi.org/10.1016/S0140-6736(24)01867-1

Gomes, T., Teichmann, S. A., & Talavera-López, C. (2019). Immunology driven by large-scale single-cell sequencing. *Trends in immunology*, *40*(11), 1011–1021.

Goncalves, P. H., Ziegelbauer, J., Uldrick, T. S., & Yarchoan, R. (2017). Kaposi sarcoma herpesvirus-associated cancers and related diseases. *Current opinion in HIV and AIDS*, *12*(1), 47–56. https://doi.org/10.1097/COH.0000000000000330

Greenwood, B. (2014). The contribution of vaccination to global health: Past, present and future. *Philosophical transactions of the Royal Society B: Biological sciences*, *369*(1645), 20130433.

Gros, P., Milder, F. J., & Janssen, B. J. (2008). Complement driven by conformational changes. *Nature reviews immunology*, *8*(1), 48–58.

Gulati, A., Kaur, D., Krishna Prasad, G. V. R., & Mukhopadhaya, A. (2018). PRR function of innate immune receptors in recognition of bacteria or bacterial ligands. *Advances in experimental medicine and biology*, *1112*, 255–280. https://doi.org/10.1007/978-981-13-3065-0_18

Han, J. J., Song, H. A., Pierson, S. L., Shen-Gunther, J., & Xia, Q. (2023). Emerging infectious diseases are virulent viruses – Are we prepared? An overview. *Microorganisms*, *11*(11), 2618. https://doi.org/10.3390/microorganisms11112618

Heesterbeek, H., Anderson, R. M., Andreasen, V., Bansal, S., De Angelis, D., Dye, C., Eames, K. T., Edmunds, W. J., Frost, S. D., Funk, S., Hollingsworth, T. D., House, T., Isham, V., Klepac, P., Lessler, J., Lloyd-Smith, J. O., Metcalf, C. J., Mollison, D., Pellis, L., Pulliam, J. R., …, & Isaac Newton Institute IDD Collaboration (2015). Modeling infectious disease dynamics in the complex landscape of global health. *Science (New York, N.Y.)*, *347*(6227), aaa4339. https://doi.org/10.1126/science.aaa4339

Hoeben, A., Joosten, E. A. J., & van den Beuken-van Everdingen, M. H. J. (2021). Personalized medicine: Recent progress in cancer therapy. *Cancers*, *13*(2), 242. https://doi.org/10.3390/cancers13020242

Holmes, K. K., Bertozzi, S., Bloom, B. R., & Jha, P. (Eds.). (2017). Major infectious diseases. *The international bank for reconstruction and development/the world bank*. 3rd edition. https://doi.org/10.1596/978-1-4648-0524-0

Hosseini, K., Ahangari, H., Chapeland-Leclerc, F., Ruprich-Robert, G., Tarhriz, V., & Dilmaghani, A. (2022). Role of fungal infections in carcinogenesis and cancer development: A literature review. *Advanced pharmaceutical bulletin*, *12*(4), 747–756. https://doi.org/10.34172/apb.2022.076

Hotchkiss, R. S., & Moldawer, L. L. (2014). Parallels between cancer and infectious disease. *The New England journal of medicine*, *371*(4), 380–383. https://doi.org/10.1056/NEJMcibr1404664

Hughes, D., & Andersson, D. I. (2015). Evolutionary consequences of drug resistance: Shared principles across diverse targets and organisms. *Nature reviews genetics*, *16*(8), 459–471.

Iannello, A., Debbeche, O., Martin, E., Attalah, L. H., Samarani, S., & Ahmad, A. (2006). Viral strategies for evading antiviral cellular immune responses of the host. *Journal of leukocyte biology*, *79*(1), 16–35.

Institute of Medicine (US) Forum on Emerging Infections, Knobler, S. L., Lemon, S. M., Najafi, M., & Burroughs, T. (Eds.). (2003). *The resistance phenomenon in microbes and infectious disease vectors: Implications for human health and strategies for containment*. National Academies Press.

Isiaka, A., Anakwenze, V., Ilodinso, C., Anaukwu, C., Ezeokoli, C. M. V., Noi, S. M., …, & Adonu, R. M. (2024). Harnessing artificial intelligence for early detection and management of infectious disease outbreaks. *International journal of innovative research and development*, *13*, 52–65.

Kasula, B. Y. (2017). Transformative applications of artificial intelligence in healthcare: A comprehensive review. *International journal of statistical computation and simulation*, *9*(1).

Keselowsky, B. G., Acharya, A., & Lewis, J. S. (2020). Innate and adaptive immunity: The immune response to foreign materials. In *Biomaterials science* (pp. 747–775). Academic Press.

Khabbaz, R., Bell, B. P., Schuchat, A., Ostroff, S. M., Moseley, R., Levitt, A., & Hughes, J. M. (2015). Emerging and reemerging infectious disease threats. *Mandell, Douglas, and Bennett's principles and practice of infectious diseases*, 158–177.e6. https://doi.org/10.1016/B978-1-4557-4801-3.00014-X

Koo, S., Kejariwal, D., Al-Shehri, T., Dhar, A., & Lilic, D. (2017). Oesophageal candidiasis and squamous cell cancer in patients with gain-of-function STAT1 gene mutation. *United European gastroenterology journal*, *5*(5), 625–631. https://doi.org/10.1177/2050640616684404

Kruk, M. E., Gage, A. D., Arsenault, C., Jordan, K., Leslie, H. H., Roder-DeWan, S., & Pate, M. (2018). High-quality health systems in the sustainable development goals era: Time for a revolution. *The lancet global health*, *6*(11), e1196–e1252.

Kumbhar, U. T., Ashok, W. V., Nashte, A., Limkar, S., Patil, V. C., & Chaudhari, K. (2023). Globalization and public health: An examination of cross-border health issues. *South Eastern European journal of public health*, *XXI*, 171–180.

Kuol, N., Stojanovska, L., Nurgali, K., & Apostolopoulos, V. (2017). The mechanisms tumor cells utilize to evade the host's immune system. *Maturitas*, *105*, 8–15. https://doi.org/10.1016/j.maturitas.2017.04.014

Langefeld, T. W., Muehling, J., Engel, J., Harbach, H., & Chakraborty, T. (2009). Part 2: The acquired immune system. *Anasthesiologie & intensivmedizin*, *50*, 29–35.

Lin, D. M., Koskella, B., & Lin, H. C. (2017). Phage therapy: An alternative to antibiotics in the age of multi-drug resistance. *World journal of gastrointestinal pharmacology and therapeutics*, *8*(3), 162–173. https://doi.org/10.4292/wjgpt.v8.i3.162

Lindahl, J. F., & Grace, D. (2015). The consequences of human actions on risks for infectious diseases: A review. *Infection ecology & epidemiology*, *5*, 30048. https://doi.org/10.3402/iee.v5.30048

Liongue, C., John, L. B., & Ward, A. (2011). Origins of adaptive immunity. *Critical reviews™ in immunology*, *31*(1).

Liu, C., Hong, Q., Chang, R. Y. K., Kwok, P. C. L., & Chan, H. K. (2022). Phage-antibiotic therapy as a promising strategy to combat multidrug-resistant infections and to enhance antimicrobial efficiency. *Antibiotics (Basel, Switzerland)*, *11*(5), 570. https://doi.org/10.3390/antibiotics11050570

Locksley, R. M. (1997). Exploitation of immune and other defence mechanisms by parasites: An overview. *Parasitology*, *115*(7), 5–7.

Loh, J. M., Aghababa, H., & Proft, T. (2023). Eluding the immune system's frontline defense: Secreted complement evasion factors of pathogenic Gram-positive Cocci. *Microbiological research*, *277*, 127512. https://doi.org/10.1016/j.micres.2023.127512

Loose, D., & Van de Wiele, C. (2009). The immune system and cancer. *Cancer biotherapy & radiopharmaceuticals*, *24*(3), 369–376. https://doi.org/10.1089/cbr.2008.0593

Loukas, A., & Maizels, R. M. (2000). Helminth C-type lectins and host–parasite interactions. *Parasitology today*, *16*(8), 333–339.

Mager, D. L. (2006). Bacteria and cancer: Cause, coincidence or cure? A review. *Journal of translational medicine*, *4*, 14. https://doi.org/10.1186/1479-5876-4-14

Masrour-Roudsari, J., & Ebrahimpour, S. (2017). Causal role of infectious agents in cancer: An overview. *Caspian journal of internal medicine*, *8*(3), 153–158. https://doi.org/10.22088/cjim.8.3.153

Mayorga-Ramos, A., Zúñiga-Miranda, J., Carrera-Pacheco, S. E., Barba-Ostria, C., & Guamán, L. P. (2023). CRISPR-Cas-based antimicrobials: Design, challenges, and bacterial mechanisms of resistance. *ACS infectious diseases*, *9*(7), 1283–1302. https://doi.org/10.1021/acsinfecdis.2c00649

Mba, I. E., & Nweze, E. I. (2022). Antimicrobial peptides therapy: An emerging alternative for treating drug-resistant bacteria. *The Yale journal of biology and medicine*, *95*(4), 445–463.

McArthur, D. B. (2019). Emerging infectious diseases. *The nursing clinics of North America*, *54*(2), 297–311. https://doi.org/10.1016/j.cnur.2019.02.006

Merlo, L. M., & Mandik-Nayak, L. (2013). Adaptive immunity: B cells and antibodies. In *Cancer immunotherapy* (pp. 25–40). Academic Press.

Miranda, M. N., Pingarilho, M., Pimentel, V., Torneri, A., Seabra, S. G., Libin, P. J., & Abecasis, A. B. (2022). A tale of three recent pandemics: Influenza, HIV and SARS-CoV-2. *Frontiers in microbiology*, *13*, 889643.

Mogensen, T. H. (2009). Pathogen recognition and inflammatory signaling in innate immune defenses. *Clinical microbiology reviews*, *22*(2), 240–273.

Moise, L., Gutierrez, A., Kibria, F., Martin, R., Tassone, R., Liu, R., …, & De Groot, A. S. (2015). iVAX: An integrated toolkit for the selection and optimization of antigens and the design of epitope-driven vaccines. *Human vaccines & immunotherapeutics*, *11*(9), 2312–2321.

Mojahed, N., Mohammadkhani, M. A., & Mohamadkhani, A. (2022). Climate crises and developing vector-borne diseases: A narrative review. *Iranian journal of public health*, *51*(12), 2664.

Moradi, S., Tadris Hasani, M., Darvish, L., & Roozbeh, N. (2017). Evaluating cervicovaginal infections and cervical cancer in women with low socioeconomic levels. *Iranian journal of public health*, *46*(6), 867–868.

Munita, J. M., & Arias, C. A. (2016). Mechanisms of antibiotic resistance. *Microbiology spectrum*, *4*(2). https://doi.org/10.1128/microbiolspec.VMBF-0016-2015

Murphy, P. M. (1993). Molecular mimicry and the generation of host defense protein diversity. *Cell*, *72*(6), 823–826.

Murray, K. A., Preston, N., Allen, T., Zambrana-Torrelio, C., Hosseini, P. R., & Daszak, P. (2015). Global biogeography of human infectious diseases. *Proceedings of the National Academy of Sciences of the United States of America*, *112*(41), 12746–12751. https://doi.org/10.1073/pnas.1507442112

Muteeb, G., Rehman, M. T., Shahwan, M., & Aatif, M. (2023). Origin of antibiotics and antibiotic resistance, and their impacts on drug development: A narrative review. *Pharmaceuticals (Basel, Switzerland)*, *16*(11), 1615. https://doi.org/10.3390/ph16111615

Narunsky-Haziza, L., Sepich-Poore, G. D., Livyatan, I., Asraf, O., Martino, C., Nejman, D., Gavert, N., Stajich, J. E., Amit, G., González, A., Wandro, S., Perry, G., Ariel, R., Meltser, A., Shaffer, J. P., Zhu, Q., Balint-Lahat, N., Barshack, I., Dadiani, M., Gal-Yam, E. N., …, & Straussman, R. (2022). Pan-cancer analyses reveal cancer-type-specific fungal ecologies and bacteriome interactions. *Cell*, *185*(20), 3789–3806.e17. https://doi.org/10.1016/j.cell.2022.09.005

Nii-Trebi, N. I. (2017). Emerging and neglected infectious diseases: Insights, advances, and challenges. *BioMed research international*, *2017*, 5245021. https://doi.org/10.1155/2017/5245021

Nucci, M., & Anaissie, E. (2001). Revisiting the source of candidemia: Skin or gut? *Clinical infectious diseases: An official publication of the Infectious Diseases Society of America*, *33*(12), 1959–1967. https://doi.org/10.1086/323759

Nunes, A. C., Almeida-Campos, F. R., Horta, M. F., & Ramalho-Pinto, F. J. (1997). *Leishmania amazonensis* promastigotes evade complement killing by interfering with the late steps of the cascade. *Parasitology*, *115*(6), 601–609.

Ofoezie, E. F., Ogbonna, C. A., Olisakwe, S. C., Anunobi, C. J., George, E. T., Babarinde, S., Chukwuemeka, C. G., Ogbonna, U. E., Amafili, C. C., Alisigwe, C. V., & Omaba, O. J. (2025, Mar 31). Role of infectious agents in cancer pathogenesis and therapy. *Microbe (Netherlands)*, *6*, 100284.

Oluwasola, A. O., & Adeoye, A. O. (2005). Infectious agents and cancer. *Annals of Ibadan postgraduate medicine*, *3*(1), 74–81.

Pagano, J. S., Blaser, M., Buendia, M. A., Damania, B., Khalili, K., Raab-Traub, N., & Roizman, B. (2004). Infectious agents and cancer: Criteria for a causal relation. *Seminars in cancer biology*, *14*(6), 453–471. https://doi.org/10.1016/j.semcancer.2004.06.009

Pallavi, P., Harini, K., Elboughdiri, N., Gowtham, P., Girigoswami, K., & Girigoswami, A. (2023). Infections associated with SARS-CoV-2 exploited via nanoformulated photodynamic therapy. *ADMET & DMPK*, *11*(4), 513–531. https://doi.org/10.5599/admet.1883

Premachandra, N. M., & Jayaweera, J. A. A. S. (2022). *Chlamydia pneumoniae* infections and development of lung cancer: systematic review. *Infectious agents and cancer*, *17*(1), 11. https://doi.org/10.1186/s13027-022-00425-3

Prestinaci, F., Pezzotti, P., & Pantosti, A. (2015). Antimicrobial resistance: A global multifaceted phenomenon. *Pathogens and global health*, *109*(7), 309–318. https://doi.org/10.1179/2047773215Y.0000000030

Rahman, M. T., Sobur, M. A., Islam, M. S., Ievy, S., Hossain, M. J., El Zowalaty, M. E., Rahman, A. T., & Ashour, H. M. (2020). Zoonotic diseases: Etiology, impact, and control. *Microorganisms*, *8*(9), 1405. https://doi.org/10.3390/microorganisms8091405

Roberts, M., Dobson, A., Restif, O., & Wells, K. (2021). Challenges in modelling the dynamics of infectious diseases at the wildlife–human interface. *Epidemics*, *37*, 100523. https://doi.org/10.1016/j.epidem.2021.100523

Ruddle, N. H., & Akirav, E. M. (2009). Secondary lymphoid organs: Responding to genetic and environmental cues in ontogeny and the immune response. *The journal of immunology*, *183*(4), 2205–2212.

Sachdev, C., Anjankar, A., & Agrawal, J. (2022). Self-medication with antibiotics: An element increasing resistance. *Cureus*, *14*(10), e30844. https://doi.org/10.7759/cureus.30844

Salam, M. A., Al-Amin, M. Y., Salam, M. T., Pawar, J. S., Akhter, N., Rabaan, A. A., & Alqumber, M. A. A. (2023). Antimicrobial resistance: A growing serious threat for global public health. *Healthcare (Basel, Switzerland)*, *11*(13), 1946. https://doi.org/10.3390/healthcare11131946

Schiller, J. T., & Lowy, D. R. (2021). An introduction to virus infections and human cancer. In *Recent results in cancer research. Fortschritte der Krebsforschung. Progres dans les recherches sur le cancer* (Vol. 217, pp. 1–11). https://doi.org/10.1007/978-3-030-57362-1_1

Schmid-Hempel, P. (2009). Immune defence, parasite evasion strategies and their relevance for 'macroscopic phenomena' such as virulence. *Philosophical transactions of the Royal Society B: Biological sciences*, *364*(1513), 85–98.

Schmidt, C. Q., Lambris, J. D., & Ricklin, D. (2016). Protection of host cells by complement regulators. *Immunological reviews*, *274*(1), 152–171.

Shanker, A. (2010). Adaptive control of innate immunity. *Immunology letters*, *131*(2), 107–112.

Sharan, M., Vijay, D., Yadav, J. P., Bedi, J. S., & Dhaka, P. (2023). Surveillance and response strategies for zoonotic diseases: A comprehensive review. *Science in one health*, *2*, 100050. https://doi.org/10.1016/j.soh.2023.100050

Sharma, S., Mohler, J., Mahajan, S. D., Schwartz, S. A., Bruggemann, L., & Aalinkeel, R. (2023). Microbial biofilm: A review on formation, infection, antibiotic resistance, control measures, and innovative treatment. *Microorganisms*, *11*(6), 1614. https://doi.org/10.3390/microorganisms11061614

Shen, C., Jiang, X., Li, M., & Luo, Y. (2023). Hepatitis virus and hepatocellular carcinoma: Recent advances. *Cancers*, *15*(2), 533. https://doi.org/10.3390/cancers15020533

Singh, D., Dhiman, V. K., Pandey, M., Dhiman, V. K., Sharma, A., Pandey, H., Verma, S. K., & Pandey, R. (2024). Personalized medicine: An alternative for cancer treatment. *Cancer treatment and research communications*, *42*, 100860. https://doi.org/10.1016/j.ctarc.2024.100860

Solares, S., León, J., & García-Gutiérrez, L. (2024). The functional interaction between Epstein-Barr virus and MYC in the pathogenesis of Burkitt lymphoma. *Cancers*, *16*(24), 4212. https://doi.org/10.3390/cancers16244212

Strathdee, S. A., Hatfull, G. F., Mutalik, V. K., & Schooley, R. T. (2023). Phage therapy: From biological mechanisms to future directions. *Cell*, *186*(1), 17–31. https://doi.org/10.1016/j.cell.2022.11.017

Su, M., Zhang, Z., Zhou, L., Han, C., Huang, C., & Nice, E. C. (2021). Proteomics, personalized medicine and cancer. *Cancers*, *13*(11), 2512. https://doi.org/10.3390/cancers13112512

Sucharitha, S. T., Manoharan, A., Vasudevan, J., & Fernando, A. (2022). Contextual narratives associated with immunization services during COVID-19 disease outbreak in Chennai, Tamil Nadu. *Natl J Community Med*, *13*, 352–8.https://doi.org/10.55489/njcm.130620221711

Sutrave, S., & Richter, M. H. (2021). The Truman Show for protozoan parasites: A review of in vitro cultivation platforms. *PLoS neglected tropical diseases*, *15*(8), e0009668. https://doi.org/10.1371/journal.pntd.0009668

Thomas, S.M., Veerabathiran, R. Influence of COVID-19 on pediatric immunocompromised children: mechanism and implications for pathogenesis. *VirusDis*. **36**, 263–274 (2025). https://doi.org/10.1007/s13337-025-00923-z

Trinchieri, G. (2015). Cancer immunity: Lessons from infectious diseases. *The journal of infectious diseases*, *212*(Suppl 1), S67–S73. https://doi.org/10.1093/infdis/jiv070

Turvey, S. E., & Broide, D. H. (2010). Innate immunity. *Journal of allergy and clinical immunology*, *125*(2), S24–S32.

Uthaisangsook, S., Day, N. K., Bahna, S. L., Good, R. A., & Haraguchi, S. (2002). Innate immunity and its role against infections. *Annals of allergy, asthma & immunology*, *88*(3), 253–265.

Vaishnavi, C., Kochhar, R., Singh, G., Kumar, S., Singh, S., & Singh, K. (2005). Epidemiology of typhoid carriers among blood donors and patients with biliary, gastrointestinal and other related diseases. *Microbiology and immunology*, *49*(2), 107–112. https://doi.org/10.1111/j.1348-0421.2005.tb03709.x

Vallejo, A. N., Davila, E., Weyand, C. M., & Goronzy, J. J. (2004). Biology of T lymphocytes. *Rheumatic disease clinics*, *30*(1), 135–157.

van Duin, D., & Paterson, D. L. (2016). Multidrug-resistant bacteria in the community: Trends and lessons learned. *Infectious disease clinics of North America*, *30*(2), 377–390. https://doi.org/10.1016/j.idc.2016.02.004

Ventola, C. L. (2015). The antibiotic resistance crisis: Part 1: Causes and threats. *P & T: A peer-reviewed journal for formulary management*, *40*(4), 277–283.

Vinay, D. S., Ryan, E. P., Pawelec, G., Talib, W. H., Stagg, J., Elkord, E., Lichtor, T., Decker, W. K., Whelan, R. L., Kumara, H. M. C. S., Signori, E., Honoki, K., Georgakilas, A. G., Amin, A., Helferich, W. G., Boosani, C. S., Guha, G., Ciriolo, M. R., Chen, S., Mohammed, S. I., …, & Kwon, B. S. (2015). Immune evasion in cancer: Mechanistic basis and therapeutic strategies. *Seminars in cancer biology*, *35*(Suppl), S185–S198. https://doi.org/10.1016/j.semcancer.2015.03.004

Wahab, A., Sanborn, D., Vergidis, P., Razonazole, R., Yadav, H., & Pennington, K. M. (2024). Diagnosis and prevention of invasive fungal infections in the immunocompromised host. *Chest*, *167*(2), 374–386. https://doi.org/10.1016/j.chest.2024.08.046

Wahab, B. A. A., Merah, M. H. M., Latif, A. D., & Gharban, H. A. J. (2024). Alternative therapeutic approach of ovine subclinical mastitis using the ethanolic roots extract of *Capparis spinosa*. *Open veterinary journal*, *14*(3), 814–821. https://doi.org/10.5455/OVJ.2024.v14.i3.8

Wang, W. H., Thitithanyanont, A., Urbina, A. N., & Wang, S. F. (2021). Emerging and re-emerging diseases. *Pathogens (Basel, Switzerland)*, *10*(7), 827. https://doi.org/10.3390/pathogens10070827

Ward, R. A., Aghaeepour, N., Bhattacharyya, R. P., Clish, C. B., Gaudillière, B., Hacohen, N., …, & Vyas, J. M. (2021, November). Harnessing the potential of multiomics studies for precision medicine in infectious disease. In *Open forum infectious diseases* (Vol. 8, No. 11, p. ofab483). Oxford University Press.

Yi, M., Li, T., Niu, M., Zhang, H., Wu, Y., Wu, K., & Dai, Z. (2024). Targeting cytokine and chemokine signaling pathways for cancer therapy. *Signal transduction and targeted therapy*, *9*(1), 176.

Yusuf, K., Sampath, V., & Umar, S. (2023). Bacterial infections and cancer: Exploring this association and its implications for cancer patients. *International journal of molecular sciences*, *24*(4), 3110. https://doi.org/10.3390/ijms24043110

Zipfel, P. F. (2009). Complement and immune defense: from innate immunity to human diseases. *Immunology letters*, *126*(1–2), 1–7.

Zohar, T. (2022). *Methods, Models, and Machine Learning Approaches for Understanding Pathogen-Specific Humoral Immunity* (Doctoral dissertation, Massachusetts Institute of Technology).

Zhang, G., Qiu, Y., Boireau, P., Zhang, Y., Ma, X., Jiang, H., Xin, T., Zhang, M., Tadesse, Z., Wani, N. A., Song, J., & Ding, J. (2024). Modern agriculture and One Health. *Infectious diseases of poverty*, *13*(1), 74. https://doi.org/10.1186/s40249-024-01240-1

Zong, Z., Zhou, F., & Zhang, L. (2023). The fungal mycobiome: a new hallmark of cancer revealed by pan-cancer analyses. *Signal transduction and targeted therapy*, *8*(1), 50. https://doi.org/10.1038/s41392-023-01334-6

7 Artificial Intelligence-Integrated Precision Oncology of Colorectal Cancer

Maduravani Ramasundaram and Thirumurthy Madhavan
School of Bioengineering, SRM Institute of Science and Technology, Kattankulathur, Tamil Nadu, India

7.1 INTRODUCTION

Colorectal cancer (CRC) ranks as the third most prevalent cancer and is the second most lethal malignancy for both males and females combined (Gabralla et al. 2023). The root cause of the disease is believed to entail a mutation in the adenomatous polyposis coli tumor suppressor gene, leading to the development of benign carcinomas that may progress to malignant stages within a decade after polyp growth (Sung et al. 2021). Chromosomal instability, microsatellite instability, and the CpG island methylator phenotype are primary molecular processes of CRC, linked to loss of heterozygosity, impaired DNA repair mechanisms, and gene silence (Mármol et al. 2017). The primary treatment modalities for localized CRC were surgery and endoscopic resection. Chemotherapy-oriented fluoropyrimidines have enhanced prognosis in malignant patients (Andrei et al. 2022). Latest research has clarified the molecular underpinnings, broadening the treatment strategies for CRC, including immunotherapy and personalized therapy (Gore 2020; MacEachern and Forkert 2021). In the epoch of personalized therapy, the tailored choice of therapeutic methods is crucial for delivering optimal care for patients. This presents a challenge for physicians: forecasting surgical results, thereby determining suitable treatment options (Lin and Semrad 2018). Furthermore, precise prognostic predictions for CRC patients might offer guidance in the selection of therapy methods. Unlike conventional biomarkers for therapeutic outcomes and prognosis prediction, individualized cancer treatment prediction can enter a new age with advancements in computer technology (Swiderska et al. 2014).

The advent of artificial intelligence (AI) in pathological diagnostics plays a crucial part in the quick detection of disease, allowing a more precise and successful strategy for cancer treatment. AI is a contemporary concept that incorporates a range of techniques and neural networks (NNs) which improve available tools/methods or provide a fresh perspective in the anticipation, prognosis, and treatment of disease. AI, equipped with adequate data, can categorize patients to determine individualized treatment approaches (Kantarjian and Yu 2015). Machine learning (ML) employs algorithms to analyze and derive insights from data, subsequently making choices and predictions regarding real-world entities. The independent and extensive learning capacity of AI, together with its capability to extract progressively intricate characteristics from photos or videos beyond individual intervention, underscores its influence in the distinctive field. The velocity and precision were augmented in comparison to mortal intercession (Yamashita et al. 2021). Widely utilized ML techniques like support vector machines (SVMs) were engaged in the medical sector to serve numerous purposes, including disease prediction and categorization (Mitsala et al. 2021). Deep learning (DL)

DOI: 10.1201/9781003644309-7

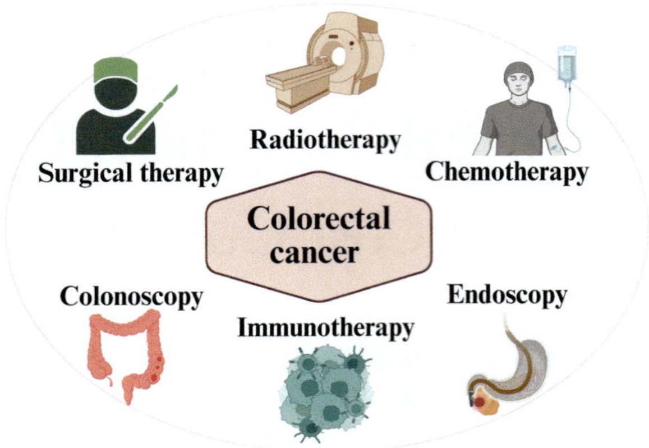

FIGURE 7.1 An illustration of the main diagnostic and therapeutic modalities used in the management of colorectal cancer. They are: surgical therapy, radiotherapy, chemotherapy, endoscopy, immunotherapy, and colonoscopy. These methods collectively depict the multidisciplinary approach used for the diagnosis, staging, and treatment of colorectal cancer. (Created in https://BioRender.com.)

is an innovative approach to education that leverages ML and uses multi-layered NN algorithms to perform the function (Tran et al. 2021). ML exhibited expertise in identifying complex structures within high-dimensional data. DL has surpassed classical ML, which is constrained in its ability to analyze raw data, in domains such as recognition of images, gene expression forecasting, and disease impact (Corti et al. 2022). Multimodal data, including virtual pathology, molecular data, radiographic images, and digital health records, are accessible for cancer patients. Convolutional NNs (CNNs) exemplify a DL technique capable of analyzing complex data faster on an individual level to facilitate precision prognosis resolution-manufacturing (Yang and Yu 2021). The recent advancement of multimodal perspectives has facilitated the consolidated analysis of this data (Lobato-Delgado et al. 2022). Due to its enhanced predictive and classificatory powers, AI is currently employed in the management of CRC. This chronological review will address the application of AI in therapeutic strategies, biomarker identification, and prognostic evaluation for CRC patients. We analyze the role of AI technologies in chemotherapy, toxicity prognostics, endoscopic precision, and surgical oversight. We present an overview of the efficacy of NNs in CRC concerning precision oncology. **Figure 7.1** depicts diverse treatment options for CRC.

7.2 AI-IMPACT ON BIOMARKER DISCOVERY

Epigenomic biomarker discovery was accomplished due to the remarkable potential of AI. Different ML algorithms like SVM, LR, and XGB have been utilized for the identification of nine gene expression stemness biomarkers from 1048 patient samples. The two-clustered statistical analysis expressed a p-value of 0.01 in the validation set obtained from TCGA and GEO cohort (Liu et al. 2022a). Discovery of around 43 long non-coding RNAs and IRLS signature from 816 patient samples achieved AUC in a time-dependent manner with a validation dataset. LASSO, SVM, and RSF were used with 232 test sets from publicly available datasets, TCGA, and GEO. The AUC for first, third, and fifth years were 0.840, 0.776, and 0.818 with a C-index of 0.765 (Liu et al. 2022b). The growing popularity of ML has facilitated a significant advancement in the prediction of molecular instabilities. A diagnostic investigation utilizing the DL model MSINet was conducted with complete-slide pictures of a hundred stained H&E from an affected person with CRC resection. The educational tool surpassed seasoned gastrointestinal physicians in forecasting microsatellite instability, with negative result in the diagnosis of 93.7% (Yamashita et al. 2021). An EPLA-based DL model was developed using multi-instance learning using the slide images and the patch-level

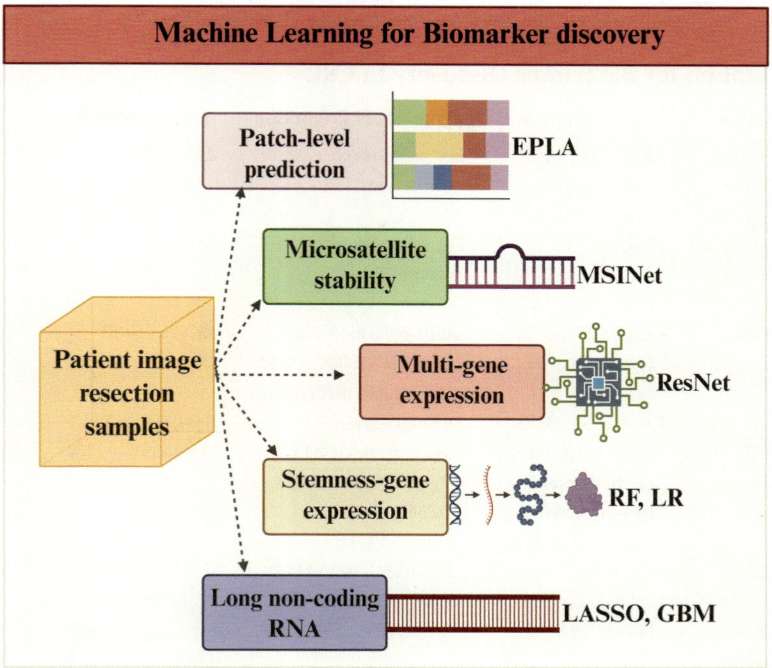

FIGURE 7.2 Illustration titled "Machine learning for Biomarker discovery" highlights the integration of histological data with various machine learning models to derive predictive molecular features for CRC biomarker discovery. (1) "Patch-level prediction" utilizing the EPLA model, (2) "Microsatellite stability" using MSINet, (3) "Multi-gene expression" processed via ResNet, (4) "Stemness-gene expression" analyzed by Random Forest (RF) and Linear Regression (LR), and (5) "Long non-coding RNA" modeled through LASSO and Gradient Boosting Machine (GBM). (Created in https://BioRender.com.)

likelihood of patients. The model achieved an AUC of around 0.88, which was better than MSINet (Cao et al. 2020). Bilal and his team developed algorithms using ResNet34 and ResNet18 for predicting BRAF, TP53, and CpG methylation on patient samples with CRC. The results were compared with the prediction of Cao et al. (2020). ResNet method accomplished greater prediction, whose an AUC of 0.90, obtained from the ROC curve (Bilal et al. 2021). **Figure 7.2** represents different prediction approaches for biomarker discovery. The implementation of AI for biomarker discovery using specific ML algorithms is stated in **Table 7.1**.

Tumor adipose features (TAF) have been utilized for patients in CRC prognosis by implementing DL methods, a remarkable study in CRC pathology (Wulczyn et al. 2021). Limperio and his group reproduced TAF as an independent histopathologic biomarker in a test study for CRC pathology (Limperio et al. 2023). Jiang and his group conducted a prognostic study to highlight the crucial role of tumor-infiltrated fat for poor prognosis (Jiang et al. 2024). DL methods were implemented on initial CRC hematoxylin and eosin slides, which facilitated the findings of inflammatory fatty tissue as an element of danger for lymphoid tissue metastases (Brockmoeller et al. 2022). SARIFA (Stroma A Reactive Invasion Front Areas) was a unique histopathological entity exclusively on H&E staining, which is a biomarker in CRC, characterized by uninterrupted contact via tumor tissues and adipocytes at the intervention point. This may associate SARIFA with the unique tumor medicine marked by enhanced fatty metabolism and immunological deterioration (Grosser et al. 2022; Reitsam et al. 2024b, 2024c). SARIFA, as a manhood-declared biomarker, and TAF, as a feature produced using DL, exhibit notable parallels with some significant variances. This unique architecture was expected to impact treatment response and may possibly be targeted therapeutically through immunotherapeutic strategies or innovative drugs (Pelka et al. 2021).

TABLE 7.1
AI Implementation for Biomarker Discovery in CRC

Dataset Information	ML Methods	Biomarkers Prediction	Evaluation Results	References
100 whole slide images from CRC resection patients	EPLA, TCGA-COAD cohort	For patch-level prediction	AUC = 0.884, AUC = 0.845	Cao et al. (2020)
100 whole slide images from CRC resection patients	MSINet	For microsatellite instability	ACC = 93.7%	Yamashita et al. (2021)
499 patient samples	ResNet18 and ResNet34	Multi-gene expression with BRAF, TP53, and CpG island methylation	AUC = 0.900	Bilal et al. (2021)
1048 (616 train /72 test) from TCGA, GEO, and FAHZ institution	LR, RF, SVM, and XGB for stemness prediction and two-clustered statistical analysis	*Stemness-gene expression*: GFPT1, PTMAP9, MOGAT3, DPM3, S100A12, PGM5, FUT6, SEMA3C, ADAM33	P = 0.01 for two clusters	Liu et al. (2022a)
816 (584 train/ 232 test) from TCGA, GEO, and public datasets	LASSO, Ridge, GBM, SVM, and RSF	*43 long non-coding RNAs*: IRLS Signature	AUC-time dependent First year = 0.840 Third year = 0.776 Fifth year = 0.818 C-index = 0.765	Liu et al. (2022b)

Abbreviations: ACC, accuracy; AUC, area under the ROC curve; EPLA, ensembled patch likelihood aggregation; FAHZ, First Affiliated Hospital Zhengzhou; GBM, gradient boosting machine; GEO, Gene Expression Omnibus; IRLS, immune-related lncRNA signature; LASSO, least absolute shrinkage and selection operator; LR, linear regression; RF, random forest; RSF, random survival forest; SVM, support vector machine; TCGA, The Cancer Genome Atlas Program; XGB, extreme gradient boosting.

7.3 NEURAL NETWORKS FOR CRC PROGNOSIS

Precision oncology in CRC necessitates a comprehensive investigation of the genetic biomarkers implicated in the progression of the disease. As colonoscopy is the primary diagnostic tool for CRC, strategies must be developed to integrate it with AI. Visual representation of intricate connections with DNA methylation was carried out using ANN models. Novel variables, MLH1 hypermethylation, and right colon disposition were detected using ANN connections. This led to the environmental factor understanding for the identified molecular CRC subtypes (Coppedè et al. 2015). Diagnosis of CRC was implemented in the selection of miRNA biomarkers. A three-layered MATLAB-based perceptron was built using an ANN model comprising four miRNAs. The highest score sample was utilized as the training set. Furthermore, miRNAs were included depending on the scores. This was continued in iterations till the maximum performance of the ANN model. The ROC curve and confusion matrix demonstrated outstanding results in prediction (Afshar et al. 2019). The CP-ANN model was developed for the detection of between BRAF V600E and wild-type mutants. The samples used were around 104 in total, embedded with paraffin. The model attained 100% sensitivity, 87.5% specificity, and 93.8% accuracy. This method was rapid and more efficient compared to traditional methods like PCR and NIR detection (Zhang et al. 2019).

Choi and his team developed a DL method with three baseline models, Inception-v3, ResNet-50, and DenseNet-161, using 3000 CRC images. The developed models were compared with different endoscopists of diverse expertise. This CNN model achieved good accuracy and sensitivity (Choi et al. 2020). Wu and team utilized region proposal networks (RPN) to develop a faster CNN using 183 patient samples from retrospective analysis. Training of the model was done by RPN, while validation was carried out using CNN. Autonomic feature combination led to an efficient and unbiased approach. The MRI image identification achieved 100% accuracy and demonstrated excellent performance in AUC analysis. It enables AI to enhance productivity and promote progress inside a new field, augmenting the impact of computational technology (Wu et al. 2021). **Table 7.2** depicts the list of AI-based NNs for CRC diagnosis. A total of 12 colon data and 10 esophagogastric data were utilized for training the three-dimensional CNN. This model achieved a better AUC score than SVM and MLP by 0.04. The 3DCNN exhibited substantially superior performance compared to the existing models, excluding training on the integrated data (Collins et al. 2021). Hamabe and his colleagues analyzed 201 patient images and 103 resected specimens using the U-net DNN. This technique accomplished the accurate estimation of the tumor area, rectum, and mesorectum. The model showed enhanced performance with SN, SP, and ACC of 77.3%, 76.8%, and 77.1%, at the T-stage (Hamabe et al. 2022). Investigations into integrated Fourier transform infrared (FTIR) hyperspectral imaging have garnered attention for its capacity to depict various disease conditions in biopsy slides. FTIR-HSI exhibited remarkable pattern recognition skills, effectively differentiating between malignant, healthy, and inflammatory tissues, achieving up to 99% accuracy in the majority of studied folds (Muniz et al. 2023).

TABLE 7.2
Neural Networks in CRC Prognosis and Treatment

Dataset Information	Neural Network Implemented	Evaluation Results	References
83 patient samples	An ANN with auto contractive map analysis	MLH1 hypermethylation	Coppedè et al. (2015)
miRNAs of 200 patients from GEO dataset	An ANN model implemented which provided four best miRNA scores. Confusion matrix analysis was performed.	AUC = 1	Afshar et al. (2019)
312 tissue samples: 104 paraffin-embedded CRC samples	CP-ANN model on BRAF V600E mutant	ACC = 93.8% SN = 100% SP = 87.5%	Zhang et al. (2019)
3000 colonoscopic images into four divisions	CNN model with ResNet-50, Inception-v3, and DenseNet-161	ACC = 92.48%	Choi et al. (2020)
183 retrospective patient samples	Faster R-CNN with ROC curve analysis	ACC = 100%	Wu et al. (2021)
22 patients: 12 (colon), 10 (esophagogastric data)	3D-CNN	Dice score = 0.41	Collins et al. (2021)
201 patient MRI images and 103 resected specimens	U-Net DNN	ACC = 77.1% SN = 77.3% SP = 76.8%	Hamabe et al. (2022)
55 patient's hyperspectral data	FCNN	ACC = 99%	Muniz et al. (2023)

Abbreviations: 3D-CNN, 3-Dimensional convolutional neural networks; ACC, accuracy; ANN, artificial neural network; AUC, area under the ROC curve; BRAF, v-raf murine sarcoma viral oncogene homolog B1; CNN, convolutional neural networks; CP-ANN, counter-propagation artificial neural networks; DNN, deep neural network; GEO, Gene Expression Omnibus; MLH1, MutL Homolog 1; R-CNN, region-based convolutional neural networks; ROC, receiver operating characteristic; SN, sensitivity; SP, specificity.

7.4 AI TOOLS FOR CRC-PRECISION ONCOLOGY

AI might be integrated into clinical practice as an innovative instrument that may surpass healthcare professionals in predicting cardiotoxicity. Huang and team demonstrated logistic regression as the most effective method due to its high sensitivity of 0.911, making it suitable as a diagnostic toolkit for truncated antecedent abscission syndrome (Huang et al. 2023). AImmunoscore was a metric derived from several immunohistopathological pictures of diverse subdivisions of immunological cells. The findings indicated that AImmunoscore serves as an unrestrained precision indicator for CRC and can forecast therapeutic retaliation to perioperative therapy.

In professional therapy, AImmunoscore can furnish doctors with another justification for administering perioperative chemotherapy. The AImmunoscore may serve as a decision-making instrument for physicians to enhance precision medicine (Li et al. 2022). Colonoscopy or stool testing serves as the fundamental method for CRC prevention. Recent technological advancements in colonoscopy, like virtual chromoendoscopy, have enhanced the detection of concerning injury (Roelandt et al. 2019). The excision of adenomatous cysts during colonoscopy is essential in minimizing deaths related to CRC. The adenoma detection rate (ADR), a crucial caliber parameter for assessing endoscopy operations, and research indicates that a higher ADR correlates with a decrease in post-colonoscopy or interval CRC. Regrettably, the ADR is markedly affected and exhibits substantial variability, ranging from 7.0% to 53% (Barret et al. 2014). Numerous impending intermixed studies have shown that AI-oriented computer-assisted detection (CADe) improved the ADR analyzed compared to a standard group that did not utilize CADe.

AI techniques could immediately deduce some molecular characteristics, including mutational status, MMR/MSI position, and CMS subdivision, from H&E slides, requiring minimal or no additional molecular experimental identification. Furthermore, AI methods have the potential to evaluate clinically significant outcomes directly from histological slides, including survival and recurrent infections, therapeutic response, and metastatic potential, such as lymph node metastases. Immediate clinical applications are possible for all these diverse uses (Reitsam et al. 2024a). **Figure 7.3** depicts the overview of AI-assisted tools in different domains for CRC therapy.

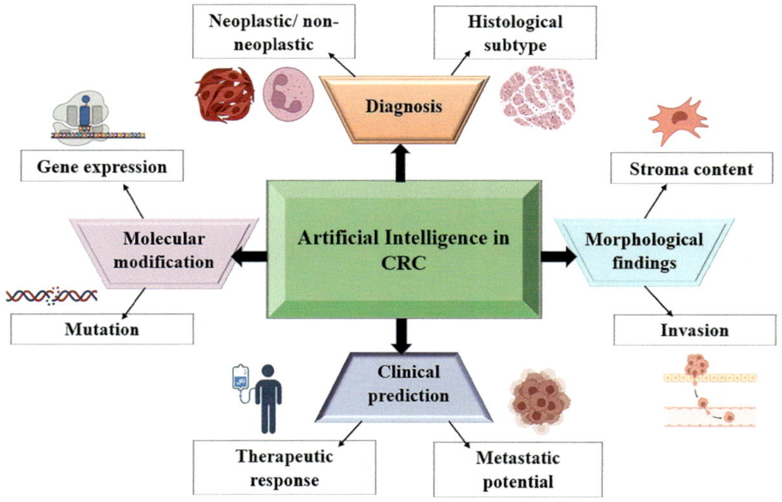

FIGURE 7.3 Illustration titled "Artificial Intelligence in CRC" depicts the applications of AI-assisted tools across four main domains: (1) "Diagnosis," which includes determining neoplastic vs. non-neoplastic status and histological subtype; (2) "Molecular modification," comprising mutation analysis and gene expression profiling; (3) "Morphological findings," involving assessment of stroma content and invasion; and (4) "Clinical prediction," which encompasses evaluating therapeutic response and metastatic potential. Each domain highlights the integrative role of AI in advancing precision oncology for CRC. (Created in https://BioRender.com.)

7.5 DISCUSSION

Since its emergence in CRC, AI has been a fundamental force, providing multiple benefits and improvements in the prognostic perspective to CRC. The extensive AI accomplishment, ranging from complex genetic interpretation to effective association with equipment such as the endoscope, highlights the feasibility and positive results seen in the preliminary assessment. Although the existing study mostly encompasses a restricted sample size, it is essential to emphasize the need for diversification of affected individual data. This diversity is not only a schematic need but a crucial measure for enhancing cohort discrimination, vital for creating cognitive models with increased sensitivity and specificity. Besides aiding in precise diagnosis, AI may also significantly contribute to prognosis prediction and patient therapy. Imaging of affected individuals can be utilized to forecast the viability, assess characteristics, and ascertain the required amount of intervention to get optimum endurance. The forecasting of habituation, disease progression, therapeutic means, and surgical responses can be utilized to develop an effective treatment approach for each of the affected individuals (Preuss et al. 2022). Nonetheless, ANN-based multimodal strategies offer improved translation for increased-computative data, such as omics information (Lobato-Delgado et al. 2022). This partially illustrates the advantages of employing NNs for personalized cancer treatment prognosis. Moreover, due to its enhanced characteristics, DL-based NNs can outperform ML in the processing and interpretation of medical imaging data.

7.6 FUTURE POSSIBILITIES

AI is seen as a valuable tool for transforming precision oncology and healthcare. Surgeons and medical personnel may find AI-based Clinical Decision Support Systems beneficial for making judgments regarding CRC therapy in clinical environments in the future. The regular improvement of extensive clinical data will facilitate the rapid advancement of AI in medicine. The early detection rate and diagnosis of CRC necessitate the prompt and thorough assessment of patients. AI, utilizing diverse algorithms in conjunction with extensive medical imaging datasets, enhances performance. Furthermore, it augments the efficacy of adjuvant therapies, including NCRT and targeted treatments, therefore reinforcing the monitoring of patient prognosis. Future research will be essential to provide adequate privacy and security measures for the management and protection of medical data. With ongoing improvement and advancement, AI will significantly enhance the detection and treatment of CRC in the precision medicine paradigm.

REFERENCES

Afshar, Saeid, Sepideh Afshar, Emily Warden, Hamed Manochehri, and Massoud Saidijam. 2019. "Application of Artificial Neural Network in miRNA Biomarker Selection and Precise Diagnosis of Colorectal Cancer." *Iranian Biomedical Journal* 23 (3): 175–83. https://doi.org/10.29252/ibj.23.3.175

Andrei, Pietro, Paolo Battuello, Gaia Grasso, Emanuele Rovera, Nicolò Tesio, and Alberto Bardelli. 2022. "Integrated Approaches for Precision Oncology in Colorectal Cancer: The More You Know, the Better." *Seminars in Cancer Biology* 84: 199–213. https://doi.org/10.1016/j.semcancer.2021.04.007

Barret, Maximilien, Stanislas Chaussade, and Romain Coriat. 2014. "Adenoma Detection Rate and Risk of Colorectal Cancer and Death." *The New England Journal of Medicine* 370 (26): 2540–41. https://doi.org/10.1056/NEJMc1405329#SA2

Bilal, Mohsin, Shan E. Ahmed Raza, Ayesha Azam, Simon Graham, Mohammad Ilyas, Ian A. Cree, David Snead, Fayyaz Minhas, and Nasir M. Rajpoot. 2021. "Development and Validation of a Weakly Supervised Deep Learning Framework to Predict the Status of Molecular Pathways and Key Mutations in Colorectal Cancer from Routine Histology Images: A Retrospective Study." *The Lancet. Digital Health* 3 (12): e763–72. https://doi.org/10.1016/S2589-7500(21)00180-1

Brockmoeller, Scarlet, Amelie Echle, Narmin Ghaffari Laleh, Susanne Eiholm, Marie Louise Malmstrøm, Tine Plato Kuhlmann, Katarina Levic, et al. 2022. "Deep Learning Identifies Inflamed Fat as a Risk Factor for Lymph Node Metastasis in Early Colorectal Cancer." *The Journal of Pathology* 256 (3): 269–81. https://doi.org/10.1002/path.5831

Cao, Rui, Fan Yang, Si-Cong Ma, Li Liu, Yu Zhao, Yan Li, De-Hua Wu, et al. 2020. "Development and Interpretation of a Pathomics-Based Model for the Prediction of Microsatellite Instability in Colorectal Cancer." *Theranostics* 10 (24): 11080–91. https://doi.org/10.7150/thno.49864

Choi, Kihwan, Seong Ji Choi, and Eun Sun Kim. 2020. "Computer-Aided Diagonosis for Colorectal Cancer Using Deep Learning with Visual Explanations." *Annual International Conference of the IEEE Engineering in Medicine and Biology Society. IEEE Engineering in Medicine and Biology Society. Annual International Conference 2020*: 1156–59. https://doi.org/10.1109/EMBC44109.2020.9176653

Collins, Toby, Marianne Maktabi, Manuel Barberio, Valentin Bencteux, Boris Jansen-Winkeln, Claire Chalopin, Jacques Marescaux, Alexandre Hostettler, Michele Diana, and Ines Gockel. 2021. "Automatic Recognition of Colon and Esophagogastric Cancer with Machine Learning and Hyperspectral Imaging." *Diagnostics (Basel, Switzerland)* 11 (10): 1810. https://doi.org/10.3390/diagnostics11101810

Coppedè, Fabio, Enzo Grossi, Angela Lopomo, Roberto Spisni, Massimo Buscema, and Lucia Migliore. 2015. "Application of Artificial Neural Networks to Link Genetic and Environmental Factors to DNA Methylation in Colorectal Cancer." *Epigenomics* 7 (2): 175–86. https://doi.org/10.2217/epi.14.77

Corti, Chiara, Marisa Cobanaj, Federica Marian, Edward C. Dee, Maxwell R. Lloyd, Sara Marcu, Andra Dombrovschi, et al. 2022. "Artificial Intelligence for Prediction of Treatment Outcomes in Breast Cancer: Systematic Review of Design, Reporting Standards, and Bias." *Cancer Treatment Reviews* 108 (102410): 102410. https://doi.org/10.1016/j.ctrv.2022.102410

Gabralla, Lubna Abdelkareim, Ali Mohamed Hussien, Abdulaziz AlMohimeed, Hager Saleh, Deema Mohammed Alsekait, Shaker El-Sappagh, Abdelmgeid A. Ali, and Moatamad Refaat Hassan. 2023. "Automated Diagnosis for Colon Cancer Diseases Using Stacking Transformer Models and Explainable Artificial Intelligence." *Diagnostics (Basel, Switzerland)* 13 (18). https://doi.org/10.3390/diagnostics13182939

Gore, John C. 2020. "Artificial Intelligence in Medical Imaging." *Magnetic Resonance Imaging* 68: A1–4. https://doi.org/10.1016/j.mri.2019.12.006

Grosser, Bianca, Marie-Isabelle Glückstein, Christine Dhillon, Stefan Schiele, Sebastian Dintner, Alison VanSchoiack, David Kroeppler, et al. 2022. "Stroma AReactive Invasion Front Areas (SARIFA) – A New Prognostic Biomarker in Gastric Cancer Related to Tumor-Promoting Adipocytes." *The Journal of Pathology* 256 (1): 71–82. https://doi.org/10.1002/path.5810

Hamabe, Atsushi, Masayuki Ishii, Rena Kamoda, Saeko Sasuga, Koichi Okuya, Kenji Okita, Emi Akizuki, et al. 2022. "Artificial Intelligence-Based Technology for Semi-Automated Segmentation of Rectal Cancer Using High-Resolution MRI." *PLoS One* 17 (6): e0269931. https://doi.org/10.1371/journal.pone.0269931

Huang Ming Jun, Lin Ye, Ke Xin Yu, Jing Liu, Ka Li, et al. 2023. "Development of Prediction Model of Low Anterior Resection Syndrome for Colorectal Cancer Patients after Surgery Based on Machine learning Technique." *Cancer Medicine* 12: 1501–19. https://doi.org/10.1002/cam4.5041

Jiang, Xiaofeng, Michael Hoffmeister, Hermann Brenner, Hannah Sophie Muti, Tanwei Yuan, Sebastian Foersch, Nicholas P. West, et al. 2024. "End-to-End Prognostication in Colorectal Cancer by Deep Learning: A Retrospective, Multicentre Study." *The Lancet. Digital Health* 6 (1): e33–43. https://doi.org/10.1016/S2589-7500(23)00208-X

Kantarjian, Hagop, and Peter Paul Yu. 2015. "Artificial Intelligence, Big Data, and Cancer." *JAMA Oncology* 1 (5): 573–74. https://doi.org/10.1001/jamaoncol.2015.1203

Li, Moying, Qiyun Xiao, Nachiyappan Venkatachalam, Ralf-Dieter Hofheinz, Marlon R. Veldwijk, Carsten Herskind, Matthias P. Ebert, and Tianzuo Zhan. 2022. "Predicting Response to Neoadjuvant Chemoradiotherapy in Rectal Cancer: From Biomarkers to Tumor Models." *Therapeutic Advances in Medical Oncology* 14: 17588359221077972. https://doi.org/10.1177/17588359221077972

Limperio, Vincenzo, Ellery Wulczyn, Markus Plass, Heimo Muller, Nicolo Tamini, and Luca Gianotti, et al. 2023. "Pathologist Validation of a Machine Learning-Derived Feature for Colon Cancer Risk Stratification." *JAMA Netw Open* 6 (3).

Lin, Patrick S., and Thomas J. Semrad. 2018. "Molecular Testing for the Treatment of Advanced Colorectal Cancer: An Overview." *Methods in Molecular Biology (Clifton, N.J.)* 1765: 281–97. https://doi.org/10.1007/978-1-4939-7765-9_18

Liu, Zaoqu, Long Liu, Siyuan Weng, Chunguang Guo, Qin Dang, Hui Xu, Libo Wang, et al. 2022a. "Machine Learning-Based Integration Develops an Immune-Derived lncRNA Signature for Improving Outcomes in Colorectal Cancer." *Nature Communications* 13 (1): 816. https://doi.org/10.1038/s41467-022-28421-6

Liu, Zaoqu, Hui Xu, Siyuan Weng, Yuqing Ren, and Xinwei Han. 2022b. "Stemness Refines the Classification of Colorectal Cancer with Stratified Prognosis, Multi-Omics Landscape, Potential Mechanisms, and Treatment Options." *Frontiers in Immunology* 13: 828330. https://doi.org/10.3389/fimmu.2022.828330

Lobato-Delgado, Barbara, Blanca Priego-Torres, and Daniel Sanchez-Morillo. 2022. "Combining Molecular, Imaging, and Clinical Data Analysis for Predicting Cancer Prognosis." *Cancers* 14 (13): 3215. https://doi.org/10.3390/cancers14133215

MacEachern, Sarah J., and Nils D. Forkert. 2021. "Machine Learning for Precision Medicine." *Genome* 64 (4): 416–25. https://doi.org/10.1139/gen-2020-0131

Mármol, Inés, Cristina Sánchez-de-Diego, Alberto Pradilla Dieste, Elena Cerrada, and María Jesús Rodriguez Yoldi. 2017. "Colorectal Carcinoma: A General Overview and Future Perspectives in Colorectal Cancer." *International Journal of Molecular Sciences* 18 (1): 197. https://doi.org/10.3390/ijms18010197

Mitsala, Athanasia, Christos Tsalikidis, Michail Pitiakoudis, Constantinos Simopoulos, and Alexandra K. Tsaroucha. 2021. "Artificial Intelligence in Colorectal Cancer Screening, Diagnosis and Treatment. A New Era." *Current Oncology (Toronto, Ont.)* 28 (3): 1581–607. https://doi.org/10.3390/curroncol28030149

Muniz, Frederico Barbosa, Matheus de Freitas Oliveira Baffa, Sergio Britto Garcia, Luciano Bachmann, and Joaquim Cezar Felipe. 2023. "Histopathological Diagnosis of Colon Cancer Using Micro-FTIR Hyperspectral Imaging and Deep Learning." *Computer Methods and Programs in Biomedicine* 231: 107388. https://doi.org/10.1016/j.cmpb.2023.107388

Pelka, Karin, Matan Hofree, Jonathan H. Chen, Siranush Sarkizova, Joshua D. Pirl, Vjola Jorgji, Alborz Bejnood, et al. 2021. "Spatially Organized Multicellular Immune Hubs in Human Colorectal Cancer." *Cell* 184 (18): 4734–52.e20. https://doi.org/10.1016/j.cell.2021.08.003

Preuss, Kiersten, Nate Thach, Xiaoying Liang, Michael Baine, Justin Chen, Chi Zhang, Huijing Du, et al. 2022. "Using Quantitative Imaging for Personalized Medicine in Pancreatic Cancer: A Review of Radiomics and Deep Learning Applications." *Cancers* 14 (7): 1654. https://doi.org/10.3390/cancers14071654

Reitsam Nic Gabriel, Grosser, Bianca, Enke, Johanna Sophie, Mueller, Wolfram, Westwood, Alice, West, Nicholas Paul, Quirke, Philip, Märkl, Bruno, and Grabsch, Heike Irmgard. 2024a. "Stroma AReactive Invasion Front Areas (SARIFA): A Novel Histopathologic Biomarker in Colorectal Cancer Patients and Its Association with the Luminal Tumour Proportion." *Translational Oncology* 44: 101913. https://doi.org/10.1016/j.tranon.2024.101913

Reitsam, Nic G., Veselin Grozdanov, Chiara M. L. Löffler, Hannah S. Muti, Bianca Grosser, Jakob N. Kather, and Bruno Märkl. 2024b. "Novel Biomarker SARIFA in Colorectal Cancer: Highly Prognostic, Not Genetically Driven and Histologic Indicator of a Distinct Tumor Biology." *Cancer Gene Therapy* 31 (2): 207–16. https://doi.org/10.1038/s41417-023-00695-y

Reitsam, Nic Gabriel, Johanna Sophie Enke, Kien Vu Trung, Bruno Märkl, and Jakob Nikolas Kather. 2024c. "Artificial Intelligence in Colorectal Cancer: From Patient Screening over Tailoring Treatment Decisions to Identification of Novel Biomarkers." *Digestion* 105 (5): 331–44. https://doi.org/10.1159/000539678

Roelandt, Philip, Ingrid Demedts, Hilde Willekens, Talat Bessissow, Lieve Braeye, Georges Coremans, Pieter-Jan Cuyle, et al. 2019. "Impact of Endoscopy System, High Definition, and Virtual Chromoendoscopy in Daily Routine Colonoscopy: A Randomized Trial." *Endoscopy* 51 (03): 237–43. https://doi.org/10.1055/a-0755-7471

Sung, Hyuna, Jacques Ferlay, Rebecca L. Siegel, Mathieu Laversanne, Isabelle Soerjomataram, Ahmedin Jemal, and Freddie Bray. 2021. "Global Cancer Statistics 2020: GLOBOCAN Estimates of Incidence and Mortality Worldwide for 36 Cancers in 185 Countries." *CA: A Cancer Journal for Clinicians* 71 (3): 209–49. https://doi.org/10.3322/caac.21660

Swiderska, Magdalena, Barbara Choromańska, Ewelina Dąbrowska, Emilia Konarzewska-Duchnowska, Katarzyna Choromańska, Grzegorz Szczurko, Piotr Myśliwiec, Jacek Dadan, Jerzy Robert Ladny, and Krzysztof Zwierz. 2014. "The Diagnostics of Colorectal Cancer." *Contemporary Oncology (Poznan, Poland)* 18 (1): 1–6. https://doi.org/10.5114/wo.2013.39995

Tran, Khoa A., Olga Kondrashova, Andrew Bradley, Elizabeth D. Williams, John V. Pearson, and Nicola Waddell. 2021. "Deep Learning in Cancer Diagnosis, Prognosis and Treatment Selection." *Genome Medicine* 13 (1). https://doi.org/10.1186/s13073-021-00968-x

Wu, Qing-Yao, Shang-Long Liu, Pin Sun, Ying Li, Guang-Wei Liu, Shi-Song Liu, Ji-Lin Hu, Tian-Ye Niu, and Yun Lu. 2021. "Establishment and Clinical Application Value of an Automatic Diagnosis Platform for Rectal Cancer T-Staging Based on a Deep Neural Network." *Chinese Medical Journal* 134 (7): 821–28. https://doi.org/10.1097/CM9.0000000000001401

Wulczyn, Ellery, David F. Steiner, Melissa Moran, Markus Plass, Robert Reihs, Fraser Tan, Isabelle Flament-Auvigne, et al. 2021. "Interpretable Survival Prediction for Colorectal Cancer Using Deep Learning." *npj Digital Medicine* 4 (1): 71. https://doi.org/10.1038/s41746-021-00427-2

Yamashita, Rikiya, Jin Long, Teri Longacre, Lan Peng, Gerald Berry, Brock Martin, John Higgins, Daniel L. Rubin, and Jeanne Shen. 2021. "Deep Learning Model for the Prediction of Microsatellite Instability in Colorectal Cancer: A Diagnostic Study." *The Lancet Oncology* 22 (1): 132–41. https://doi.org/10.1016/S1470-2045(20)30535-0

Yang, Ruixin, and Yingyan Yu. 2021. "Artificial Convolutional Neural Network in Object Detection and Semantic Segmentation for Medical Imaging Analysis." *Frontiers in Oncology* 11. https://doi.org/10.3389/fonc.2021.638182

Zhang, Xue, Yang Yang, Yalan Wang, and Qi Fan. 2019. "Detection of the BRAF V600E Mutation in Colorectal Cancer by NIR Spectroscopy in Conjunction with Counter Propagation Artificial Neural Network." *Molecules (Basel, Switzerland)* 24 (12): 2238. https://doi.org/10.3390/molecules24122238

8 Precision Medicine in Breast Cancer

An Immuno-Oncology Approach

Juvin Ann Thomas and Suboj Babykutty
Mar Ivanios College, Thiruvananthapuram, Kerala, India

8.1 INTRODUCTION

Breast cancer (BC) ranks as the second most frequently diagnosed cancer in women and is the primary reason for cancer-related deaths among women globally (1). The evolution of BC diagnostics and treatments over the decades contributed to early diagnostics and a reduction in mortality rate. The decline in mortality rate can be attributed to better screening methods, together with modernized treatment options, including surgery, chemotherapy, targeted therapy, and radiotherapy (2). Conventionally, oncology trials are drug centered, focusing on identifying common attributes in patients to fit all participants in one treatment plan (3). This led to different survival outcomes, despite receiving similar therapies. The variability has driven the development of precision medicine, where patient care is given based on individual prognosis and disease progression (4). Precision medicine offers tailored treatments for patients with specific diseases by considering their genotypic, phenotypic, and psychological characteristics, thereby significantly improving patient care. In addition to offering customized care, it can also serve to precisely identify a disease condition in a patient (5). The higher mortality rate in BC is largely due to its high metastasis rate and heterogeneity (6). The disease has multiple molecular subtypes. The most accepted classification is based on hormone receptor (HR) and human epidermal growth factor 2 (HER2) status – luminal A, luminal B, HER2-positive ($HER2^+$), and triple-negative (7). The emergence of precision medicine marks a breakthrough in the field of BC (8). BC is diverse, featuring different subtypes influenced by unique genetic mutations. Understanding this diversity is essential for customized treatment approaches that aim at particular vulnerabilities in each tumor. Genetic testing, especially for mutations in BRCA genes linked to DNA repair, aids in evaluating hereditary risks and affects treatment choices. Molecular subtyping directs individualized therapies. For example, HR-positive (HR^+) cancers generally respond favorably to hormonal therapies, whereas $HER2^+$ cancers gain advantages from HER2-targeted therapies. In contrast, triple-negative breast cancers (TNBCs) do not have these receptors and often need alternative methods, like chemotherapy (9). Molecular subtypes of BC were initially suggested by Perou et al. to clarify the variations in treatment responses and clinical results that go beyond what tumor nuclear grade and size could explain by themselves (10). Recently, the integration of immuno-oncology in precision medicine has expanded the possibilities of personalized therapeutic strategies (11). Cancer immunotherapy was voted "breakthrough of the year" by the journal *Science* in 2013 and has revolutionized the field of oncology. It aims to utilize the specificity and cytotoxic functions of the immune system to identify and eliminate cancerous cells (12). The immune system plays an unavoidable role in TME, both by escalating disease

DOI: 10.1201/9781003644309-8

progression and portraying anti-tumor effects (13). In BC, tumors show higher levels of immune cell infiltration when compared to normal tissues. Different subtypes show variations, with increased levels found in triple-negative and $HER2^+$ tumors associated with improved survival. In comparison, ER^+ tumors show reduced immune infiltration, linked to worse results. Additionally, metastatic locations often display a more immunosuppressive microenvironment. Thus, targeting the tumor immune microenvironment (TIME) in BC is promising and achieving encouraging outcomes. This chapter discusses the role of immune system in shaping TME, the necessity of prioritizing them, and various immunotherapy approaches in diagnosing and treating the disease.

8.2 CONVENTIONAL THERAPIES IN BC – ARE THEY SUFFICIENT?

The four conventional cancer treatment therapies in BC are surgery, hormonal therapy, radiation therapy, and chemotherapy. Surgery succeeded by radiotherapy and chemotherapy is the standard therapeutic approach for BC management (14). Surgery is a well-established and essential method for diagnosing and treating solid tumors. In diagnostics, tumor tissue biopsy serves as the ideal choice for cancer subtyping and grading; however, limited sample size and frequent agonizing observation hinder its effectiveness (15). The post-operative introduction of immunosuppressants to promote wound healing helps tumor cells avoid detection by the immune system. This leads to diminished natural killer (NK) cytotoxicity and impaired macrophage activity associated with enhanced tumor growth after surgery. Surgical procedures may also decrease the levels of circulating dendritic cells (DC), essential for immune monitoring after tumor excision (16). Among all, the surgical procedures also entail possible complications, such as infections, reduced quality of life, and difficulties during post-operative recovery. Cancer patients with solid tumors might gain additional protection against recurring disease through the administration of perioperative immunotherapy alongside standard surgical care (17).

Radiotherapy is a worthwhile cancer therapy that employs high-energy particles like X-rays, gamma rays, and protons to eliminate cancer cells by harming their DNA. Since the advent of X-rays, they have been employed in the treatment of cancers from different origins. Current studies aim to create sophisticated radiation delivery methods that reduce harm to adjacent healthy tissues, including FLASH radiotherapy and brachytherapy (internal radiotherapy) to inoperable tumors by directly placing the radiation source within or close to the tumor location (18,19). However, certain cancer cells continue to resist radiotherapy, and the chances of relapses remain elevated (18). Moreover, ionizing radiation exposure leads to hydrolysis and the formation of reactive oxygen species (ROS), particularly hydroxyl radicals (•OH), resulting in DNA lesion (19). The influence of oxygen levels, genetic factors, and metabolites on the response to radiotherapy encompasses intricate mechanisms that affect DNA damage and the expression of hypoxia-inducible factor-1α (HIF-1α), consequently impacting treatment outcomes (20).

Chemotherapy is among the most commonly utilized standard methods for treating cancer. It focuses on crucial phases of the cell cycle to trigger cell death. The major chemotherapeutic agents employed in BC are anthracyclines (e.g., Doxorubicin, Epirubicin), taxanes (e.g., Paclitaxel, Docetaxel), alkylating agents (e.g., Cyclophosphamide), and antimetabolites (e.g., 5'Fluorouracil, Capecitabine, Methotrexate) (21–24). Chemoresistance is the main hindrance for effective chemotherapy. Chemoresistance can be either acquired, developing during treatment, or intrinsic, being present before therapy due to genetic changes, tumor diversity, and additional factors such as poor drug absorption or metabolism. Tumor heterogeneity is the major cause behind chemoresistance. Initial tumors are small and more uniform; therefore, they can be treated with various therapies. As the size increases and there is extended exposure to a particular chemotherapeutic agent, chemoresistance develops, prompting a re-evaluation of the treatment given.

In the case of hormonal therapy, early diagnosis is crucial for improved results. As 60–70% of BCs exhibit estrogen receptors, treatments that manage estrogen levels have been shown to be effective. The efficacy of these therapies frequently varies between patients, affected by genetic variations, tumor diversity, and the changing characteristics of cancer. This underscores the necessity for precision medicine and improved biomarkers to inform treatment choices.

8.3 THE SIGNIFICANCE OF IMMUNOTHERAPY

BC has conventionally been viewed as an immunologically "cold" tumor (cancers that do not trigger a strong immune response or respond well to immunotherapy (25)), unreactive to immunotherapy. Nonetheless, recent clinical trials have revealed immunotherapy to be an effective treatment choice for certain patients (26). The clinical development of immunotherapy in BC started more than 20 years ago, but it was only with the introduction of immune checkpoint inhibitors (ICIs) that the quantity of clinical trials assessing immunotherapeutic strategies increased. In January 2022, there were 745 clinical trials related to immunotherapy that involved individuals with solid tumors, including BC, as listed on clinicaltrials.gov, with 450 (60.4%) exclusively concentrating on BC. There have been a growing number of clinical trials in both advanced and early BC. Significantly, in 2018, neoadjuvant trials surpassed adjuvant trials, indicating a notable change in research focus. Furthermore, there is a distinct advancement from phase 1 to phase 2 and 3 trials, indicating the evolution of the discipline. Although major phase 3 trials are primarily funded by the industry, the rise in phase 2 studies initiated by investigators underscores a worldwide academic initiative to investigate new immunotherapy methods (27). The past two decades marked the unavoidable role of immunotherapy in BC (28). Cancer cells modify their TIME, establishing an immunosuppressive setting via several mechanisms, including alterations in signaling, limitation of antigen recognition, and triggering of T cell exhaustion (29). Cancer cells employ strategic methods to evade detection and destruction. One approach to achieve this is by strengthening the interaction between programmed death-ligand 1 (PD-L1) and Programmed death receptor-1 (PD-1), which ultimately prevents immune T cells from eliminating tumor cells. ICIs allow immune T cells to recognize and destroy tumor cells by blocking the interaction between PD-L1 and PD-1. These medications enhance the full potential of immune cells by removing the barriers that hinder their anti-tumor activities, allowing the immune system to recognize and destroy cancer cells that were previously ignored or tolerated (30). In this chapter we are reviewing the new successes as well as new approaches of immunotherapy in BC.

8.4 LIQUID BIOPSY IN THE ERA OF IMMUNOTHERAPY

The traditional screening methods for BC include mammography, ultrasound, MRI, biopsy, and histopathology. Mammography, as the main screening technique, has assisted many in identifying breast tumors and is linked to a notable decrease in BC mortality (31). Ultrasound, and MRI on the other hand, increases the sensitivity of screening along with mammography (32). Taking into consideration the critical role of immune system in TME, immunological markers have a promising potential in diagnosing BC in both neoadjuvant and adjuvant settings. Here we are discussing some of the major prognostic and predictive immunological biomarkers in BC, which could personalize the treatment, analyze the patient's response to specific therapies, and improve outcomes by avoiding ineffective treatment strategies.

8.4.1 Circulating Immune Cells

Peripheral blood monitoring represents a practical alternative to repeated biopsies (33). Blood-based biomarkers such as circulating tumor cells (CTCs), cell-free tumor-derived DNA, mRNA and miRNA, proteins, autoantibodies, and metabolites are being explored recently. Numerous research suggests that they are potential candidates for BC detection, diagnosis, or monitoring (34). However, monitoring peripheral immune cells is another frontier approach in liquid biopsy, considering the critical influence of immune system in tumor growth (35,36). Thus, identifying specific circulating immune cells would be a great tool in early BC diagnosis as well as to analyze the response of cancer patients toward therapies (34,37). It has been proven that tumor cells chemotactically recruit immune-inflammatory cells to their microenvironment, serving their function to promote immunosuppression, angiogenesis, cancer cell survival, growth, invasion, and metastasis (38–41). The immune system exhibits paradoxical behavior during the development of cancer; while some immune cells can help activate immune escape mechanisms, other cells can identify tumor cells and defend the host (immunosurveillance) (42). The peripheral immunological alterations that are influenced by or facilitate metastasis still need clarification. A prior study using mass spectrometry proteomics revealed phenotypic resemblances between PBMCs and the TME of corresponding BC tissues, where the expression patterns of IL-17, PI3K-Akt, and elements of HIF-1 signaling pathways were observed to be maintained in both circulating and tumor-infiltrating immune cells (43,44). Another study reported that an elevated proportion of immunosuppressive cells, including granulocytic MDSCs, intermediate $CD14^{+}$+$CD16^{+}$ monocytes, and CD127negCD25highFoxP3^{+} Treg cells, was noted in patients diagnosed with BC, particularly those with stage 3 and 4 disease, irrespective of ER status (45).

8.4.1.1 MDSCs

MDSCs are immature myeloid cells that suppress T cells by altering the local T cell extracellular environment and through direct cell interactions (46). Their involvement in cancer has been elucidated, demonstrating in various studies that elevated levels of MDSCs serve as a negative prognostic indicator, including responses to immunotherapies (47–49). MDSCs are identifiable in the peripheral blood of cancer patients, particularly during advanced stages. Nonetheless, the inherent diversity of these cells has made analytical characterization difficult. At present, MDSCs are usually identified by the expression of $CD45^{+}CD3^{-}CD19^{-}CD20^{-}CD56^{-}CD16^{-}HLADR^{-}CD33+$ $CD11b^{+}$ through flow cytometry, with the $CD14^{+}$ subset categorized as monocytic and the $CD15^{+}$ subset as granulocytic MDSCs, respectively (50). According to a study, MDSCs can forecast both survival and reaction to ICIs, and it was noted that a reduction in MDSCs was linked to an improved prognosis (51). A connection has been established between increased circulating MDSCs and prognosis, associating with advanced cancer stages, heightened tumor burden, decreased progression-free survival (PFS), and overall survival (OS) rates, while also affecting cancer treatment responses by reducing the effectiveness of chemotherapy, radiotherapy, immunotherapy, or other targeted therapies (49–55).

8.4.1.2 Neutrophils

Neutrophils are the most prevalent myeloid cells found in the blood and play a significant immunological role in the tumor microenvironment (56). Nonetheless, their functional significance has frequently been overlooked, as they have consistently been viewed as a one-dimensional group of terminally differentiated, short-lived cells. In the past ten years, the application of advanced, single-cell technologies has transformed the traditional perspective of these cells, revealing their phenotypic and functional diversity. They are significant immune elements in tumors, exhibiting either anti-tumor (N1) or pro-tumor functions (N2) (57). Mirroring the polarization of TANs, circulating neutrophils can also be divided into two subpopulations – high-density neutrophils (HDN) and low-density neutrophils (LDN); LDN are uncommon in non-disease situations, but common in cancer, showing a pro-tumor characteristic (58–60). LDN are perceived as a blend of both mature and immature neutrophils, exhibiting modified functions and immunosuppressive characteristics, like the activation of regulatory T cells (Tregs), the secretion of ROS, nitric oxide, and arginase, which will obstruct activity of effector $CD8^{+}$ T lymphocytes (61,62). A study demonstrated that LDN are not present in the bloodstream of healthy people and that patients with metastatic BC exhibit a greater proportion of LDN compared to those without metastases, supporting the notion that LDN play a role in metastasis and accumulate steadily as cancer advances (61,63,64). Furthermore, they noted that non-metastatic BC patients who did not respond to neoadjuvant chemotherapy (NACT) exhibited a notably greater percentage of LDN prior to initiating the treatment, in contrast to patients who responded to NACT. While a significant presence of neutrophils in the low-density fraction has been noted in cancer patients, such as those with breast and lung cancers, the majority of participants in earlier studies had advanced illness, and no link between treatment response and LDN propagation was found (60,60).

8.4.1.3 Monocytes

The TME attracts circulating monocytes, which are then stimulated to develop into macrophages, which are essential for the TME. These cells are also directly linked to CTCs in advanced BC patients' peripheral blood, particularly in TNBC patients (65). Additionally, the presence and subtype of M2-polarized macrophages, especially M2c induced by IL-10, are linked to increased tumor invasiveness, advanced disease stages, and worse prognosis, especially in ER^- patients (66). The presence, signaling behavior, and differentiation status of peripheral immune cells reflect the interactions between tumor and immune cells as well as the patient's reaction to immunotherapy. A study indicated alterations in blood leukocytes linked to primary BC, surgical excision, and supplementary radiotherapy. Specifically, it identified increased levels of $CD117^+$ granulocytes, memory, and regulatory $CD4^+$ T cells as potential biomarkers of BC and radiotherapy, respectively (34). Another study by the same group has shown that metastatic BC patients have elevated frequencies of $TIE2^+CD11b^+$ and $CD117^+CD11b^+$ leukocytes circulating in the blood, and that circulating $CD11b^+$ cells express higher mRNA levels of the M2 polarization markers CD163, ARG1, and IL-10 (67).

8.4.1.4 Monocyte–lymphocyte Ratio (MLR) and Neutrophil–Lymphocyte Ratio (NLR)

In terms of the examination of tumor development and prognosis in BC patients, it is worth noting that the ratio of immune cellular counts (e.g., monocyte–lymphocyte ratio (MLR), neutrophil–lymphocyte ratio (NLR)) may play a pivotal role. The availability and non-invasive nature of these indices signify that they can serve as significant and affordable biological markers. The most commonly used inflammatory index is NLR. The NLR index's prognostic significance in BC has been investigated. Numerous research have indicated that an increased NLR correlates with poor survival outcomes, impacting both disease-free survival (DFS) and OS, as well as most advanced and aggressive BC (68–73). According to a systematic review of 15 studies that examined 8,563 patients, patients with BC who have a high NLR are more likely to have poor OS, and DFS, particularly those with TNBC and $HER2^+$ BC than those who have HR^+ BC (70,74). A study carried out in Spain indicated that the likelihood of BC increased with elevated neutrophil percentages and NLR in luminal A and HER2-negative ($HER2^-$) BCs, affecting both pre- and postmenopausal women, although it was notably more pronounced in postmenopausal women. A study carried out in South Korea showed that LMR has the strong potential to predict DFS and OS in BC (75). Elevated monocyte levels indicate a significant tumor burden in cancer patients. In this mechanism, LMR is thought to indicate the immune condition of the host and the extent of tumor advancement. Since both a low lymphocyte count and high monocyte count indicate inadequate anti-tumor immunity and an increased tumor load, a low LMR is consequently linked to a worse prognosis (76). Also, an elevated lymphocyte-to-monocyte ratio (LMR) has emerged as a significant independent prognostic marker for poor OS in advanced BC, particularly in triple-negative subtypes, and its variation during treatment correlates with outcomes. Weijuan et al. also found that a reduced LMR was significantly linked to a worse prognosis for the TNBC subtype in their study involving 1,570 patients (77).

8.4.2 Cytokine Profiles

Cytokines are small proteins of up to 70 kDa, classified in distinct superfamilies, including interferons (INFs), interleukins (ILs), tumor necrosis factors (TNFs), transforming growth factors (TGFs), chemotactic cytokines (chemokines), and colony-stimulating factors (CSFs) (78,79). They generally notify infections and tissue damage to immune cells, but repeated production of cytokine from a particular body site stimulates immune cells to release more cytokines, causing chronic inflammatory state that promotes tumor growth (80). Bidirectional signaling mediated by cytokines between tumor and stromal cells is crucial for the development and progression of solid tumors, such as BC (82). Serum cytokine levels may correlate with their expression in tumors, rendering them significant prognostic markers for cancer patients. For instance, the serum concentrations of IL-8, macrophage inflammatory protein (MIP)-1α, and MIP-1β were notably elevated in patients with BC (83). A team of researchers examined 45 distinct cytokines in the serum samples from patients with metastatic breast cancer (MBC) through ProcartaPlex Immunoassays and discovered that the cytokines HGF, IL-8, FGF2, VEGF, IL-18, MCP-1, MIP-1β, IFN-γ, IP-10, and NGF-β had a significant correlation with mortality in MBC (81). Similarly, solid-phase antibody array and ELISA assay were used for screening 274 biomarkers in serum from BC patients. There was a significant increase in levels of IL-8, MIP-1 alpha, MIP-1 beta, MMP-8, resistin, FLRG, and BCAM, but LAP and TSH-b levels were lower, suggesting that these cytokines might serve as novel inflammatory markers in BC patients (82). BC and non-cancer groups can be distinguished by profiling GCSF, IL-6, and IL-17, also IL-6 contributing to recurrence and metastasis in BC. Wang *et al.* reported that serum IL-6, IL-8, IL-10, SCC-Ag, and CYFRA 21-1 may serve as potential markers for predicting metastasis and prognosis of BC (83). Vilsmaier *et al.* reported that IL-1α is a candidate marker for the release of tumor cells, and IL-1β, IL-12, sFlt1, and PlGF appear to be related to CTC release in patients with BC (83,84). The interaction of serum IL-17 levels with an increased level of both bFGF and G-CSF has been shown to correlate with poor DFS among BC patients (85). Blood based biomarkers and functions are portrayed in **Figure 8.1**.

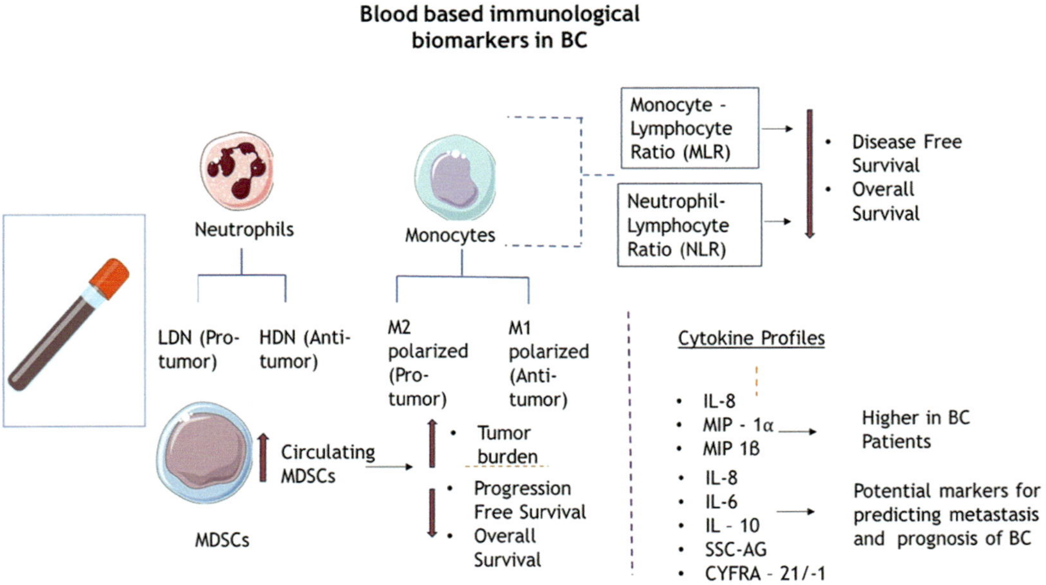

FIGURE 8.1 Blood based immunological biomarkers: The circulating neutrophils having both pro- and anti-tumor phenotypes, LDN (Low Density Neutrophil) and HDN (High Density Neutrophil) respectively. LDN exhibits immunosuppressive characteristics. Monocytes also have pro- and anti-tumor circulating phenotypes. Both NLR and MLR are significant prognostic markers for poor overall survival and disease-free survival. In the case of MDSCs, an elevated range shows reduced progression free survival as well as overall survival. Serum cytokine levels also serve as valuable biomarkers for BC.

8.4.3 Immune Score/Immune Gene Signatures

The revolution in high-throughput genomic and transcriptomic technologies enabled researchers to delve deep into the TIME; immune gene signatures (IGIs) are one of them. IGIs are a set of genes, whose expression could make us know the type, presence, and activity of immune cells in the TME, emerging as a novel prognostic tool for numerous cancer types. Immune score is quantitative index derived from the expression of immune-related genes, used to measure immune cell infiltration and activity within a tumor (86). The expression signatures of the primary tumor are prognostic and predict a patient's outcome, since the genetic and epigenetic characteristics of a primary tumor determine its fate and potential for metastasis (87). Various gene signature assays have been developed and proven in numerous clinical trials over the last 20 years to categorize patients into various risk groups. Commonly used genomic tests, such as MammaPrint,4 Oncotype DX,5, and PAM50 Prosigna Assay, predict the recurrence risk of patients with ER^+HER2-subtype BC (88–90). Oncological professional communities advise the use of these gene expression signatures and help physicians in clinical practice. But the genes identified by these assays only exhibit activity related to the biology of tumor cells, which includes invasion, metastasis, angiogenesis, apoptosis, and proliferation (87). Immune cell markers are not used in any commonly used multi-gene expression assay (91). Nevertheless, numerous studies have been carried out to develop predictive as well as prognostic immune signatures in BC. Some of the most common tools used to analyze IGSs in BC include CIBERSORT/CIBERSORTx, ESTIMATE, xCell, Immucell AI, MCP-Counter, and TISIDB (92–96). Scientists often attempt to figure out the cellular makeup of the TME in order to investigate immune signatures and their prognostic significance. This indicates that specific lymphocyte subsets may be important for the development of tumors. IRS, or immune-related score, is a quantitative value used as a method of assessing the immune system's role in cancer and its potential for treatment response, particularly immunotherapy. A shorter OS is linked to a higher IRS score. Patients with low IRS have significantly higher levels of B lymphocyte and $CD8^+$ T cell infiltration. Macrophage Marker Genes (MMGs) are another immune-related signature scientists have been developing. For instance, one group performed bioinformatics analysis of BC scRNA-seq profiles and found out MMGs in the BC tissue. MMGS demonstrated superior ability to discriminate between high- and low-risk groups in the HR^+ and HER2– subgroup ($HR^+/HER2^-$). Macrophages are thought to be crucial in BC, particularly in luminal subtypes (91). Tan, Wen, et al. analyzed the OS, time-dependent receiver operating characteristic (ROC), and protein–protein interaction (PPI) network, and all of them were linked to a good prognosis in BC, particularly CD226 and KLRC4-KLRK1, and low immune score groups were linked to a better prognosis. They have been screened and validated in both TCGA and GEO (Gene Expression Omnibus) database (97). Immune signatures are significant in the context of therapeutic options based on ICIs. They have shown that PD-L1-positive expression in immune cells was linked with a longer PFS; similarly, PD-L1 overexpression in tumor cells also showed a favorable prognostic association trend (98). Anti-PD-1 and anti-PD-L1 have been tested in patients with TNBC who express PD-L1 in two early clinical trials that were presented at the San Antonio Breast Cancer Symposium. This inclusion criterion was primarily founded on the finding that a greater percentage of TNBC exhibits elevated TIL, particularly if they express PD-L1 (99,100).

8.5 TUMOR-INFILTRATING LYMPHOCYTES

Tumor-infiltrating lymphocytes (TILs) are immune cells within the TME that contribute to anti-tumor immunity (101). They reflect the patient's immune response against cancer and have shown robust prognostic value in BC, particularly in $HER2^+$ and TNBC subtypes. TILs in BC are primarily composed of $CD8^+$ cells, $CD4^+$ cells, $FOXP3^+$ cells, and $CD19^+$ cells, with $CD56^+$ NK cells being less common. Majority of these TILs are found in the stroma, with fewer intratumoral. Their capacity to predict treatment outcomes makes them worthy biomarker in guiding immunotherapies and personalized treatment strategies (102). They can be a predictive factor in both neoadjuvant as well as adjuvant setting (103). For example, an elevated level of $CD8^+$ T cells before the treatment and after preoperative therapy is associated with a higher incidence of pathologic complete response (pCR) (104). On the other hand, a higher number of $FOXP3^+$ is associated with shorter OS (105). One study revealed that the anti-tumor activity of anti-PDL-1 agents should be performed on patients with low TIL scores and higher tumor PD-L1 expression levels (106). Loi et al. demonstrated a clear association between the presence of TILs at diagnosis and significantly better clinical outcomes for TNBC patients. The study highlighted that an increase in its levels reduced the risk of relapse and death regardless of the type of chemotherapy scheme (anthracyclines vs doxorubicin plus docetaxel). In $HER2^+$ BC population, TILs were also associated with improved outcomes in accordance with anthracycline-based treatment (107). A study conducted in a tertiary care cancer center in South India underscores the fact that TILs are strongly associated with tumor regression since tumors with higher TILs have better response to NACT (108). TNBCs with higher TILs had a greater amount of $CD56^+$, $CD57^+$, $GNLY^+$, and $GZMB^+$ TILs not only in absolute number but also in proportion relative to $CD4^+$ or $CD8^+$ TILs. High TIL and its subset ($CD4^+$, $CD8^+$, $CD56^+$, $CD57^+$, $GNLY^+$, and $GZMB^+$ TIL) infiltration correlated with favorable clinicopathological features of tumor. The same team also explored the spatial arrangement of TILs in triple-negative BC, discovering that consistently high TIL infiltration correlated with improved DFS, while cases with varied infiltration exhibited no survival difference relative to the former (109). When it comes to its identification or analysis, it can be done using hematoxylin and eosin-stained slides of BC samples using light microscopy that could be performed easily by pathologists (110). Thus, evaluating TILs as the biomarkers for prognostic and treatment could be routinely performed, especially in aggressive subtypes of BC such as TNBC and ER^+.

8.6 IMMUNE THERAPEUTICS FOR BC

Cancer immunotherapy has emerged as one of the most important breakthroughs in oncology in recent years. It has shown remarkable anti-tumor effects and a lasting clinical advantage in various cancers, with recent achievements in TNBC. Traditionally regarded as having low immunogenicity, BC was not thoroughly explored for its potential response to immunotherapy. Nonetheless, recent advancements with ICIs in various malignancies along with growing evidence of the immune system's impact on cancer behavior have prompted the initiation of clinical trials assessing various immune therapeutic approaches for BC patients. Here we are attempting to update major immune therapeutics in BC.

8.6.1 Immune Checkpoint Inhibitors

ICIs is a revolutionary approach in cancer treatment for the past ten years (111). Patients who respond to ICIs generally show a "hot" (immune-inflamed) phenotype, which is characterized by immune cell infiltration, whereas non-responders may show a "cold" (immune-desert/immune-excluded) phenotype, which is characterized by a lower or absent infiltration of immune cells in the tumor (112).

8.6.1.1 PD-1/PDL-1 Inhibitors

PD-1 is a suppressive transmembrane protein found on T cells, B cells, and NK cells. They possess two ligands, specifically PD-L1, referred to as B7-H1, and PD-L2, identified as B7-H2 (115). Various cell types, such as tumor and hematopoietic cells, display PD-L1 on their surfaces, whereas PD-L2 is mainly found on hematopoietic cells. PD-1's interaction with its specific ligands directly leads to the inhibition of tumor cell apoptosis, encourages peripheral T effector cell fatigue, and facilitates the transformation of T effector cells into immunosuppressive T regulatory (Treg) cells.

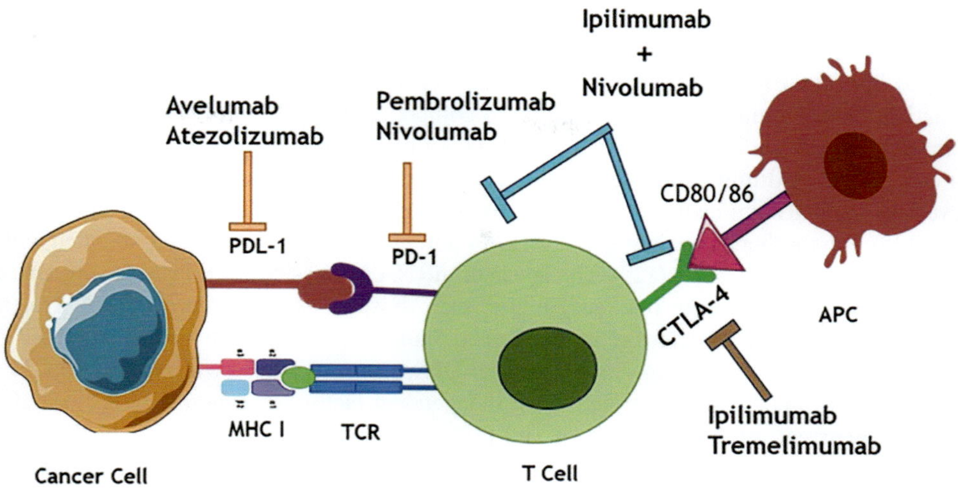

FIGURE 8.2 In BC, PDL-1 from tumor cells binds with PD-1 on T effector cells, making them exhausted. Antibodies targeting PDL-1 like Avelumab and Atezolizumab blocks it from binding to its receptor on T cells. Similarly, antibodies such as Pembrolizumab and Nivolumab hinders the binding of PD-1 on T cells to their cognate ligands from tumor cells. On the other hand, CTLA-4 another antigen helping immune escape of cancer cells also being blocked by antibodies targeting it such as Ipilimumab and Tremelimumab. The bi-specific antibodies targeting both PD-1 and CTLA-4 has also encourages effectiveness and survival advantages.

ICIs work by releasing this inhibitory control, allowing the immune system to target cancer cells (113) **(Figure 8.2)**. Generally, PD-1 and PD-L1/L2 are upregulated in correlation with pro-effector cytokines (such as IFN-gamma) secreted by $CD8^+$ TILs, emphasizing their role as immune checkpoints (114). Approximately 20% of BCs express PD-L1 with TNBC and $HER2^+$ BCs showing higher levels of expression than ER-positive BCs (114). The prognostic impact of PD-1/PD-L1 antibodies on human cancers and their clinical significance have been validated by several studies in recent years (115,116). However, there is a lack of clarity and variation in the relationship between this biomarker and its clinical significance across various human cancer types (117). At the same time, both PD-1 and PDL-1 blockade in PD-L1-positive cancers show greater response in patients. Anti-PD-1 and anti-PD-L1 antibodies are in clinical use for treating various tumors, with ongoing trials evaluating their efficacy (118). It is encouraging to know that certain PD-1/PD-L1 antibodies can successfully block either PD-1 or PD-L1 in BC. PD-1/PD-L1 inhibitors might be effective in treating metastatic TNBC (mTNBC) as well. Pembrolizumab was the first ICI to be approved as a first-line treatment and the first PD-1-targeted therapy to be approved after melanoma trials. It has significant anti-tumor activity and safety in patients with PD-L1-positive mTNBC (114). Furthermore, anti-PD-L1 antibody, atezolizumab, sustains PFS in patients with mTNBC. Atezolizumab is a high-affinity, engineered, fully human IgG1 monoclonal antibody that inhibits the interaction of PD-L1 with PD-1 and B7.1 (CD80), both of which are negative regulators of T-lymphocyte activation (119). Avelumab is another human anti-PD-L1 IgG1 monoclonal antibody (mAb) that inhibits the interaction between PD-1 and PD-L1. MBC patients with higher PD-L1 expression levels showed a favorable response when treated with avelumab (anti-PD-L1). Those who had immune cells positive for PD-L1 had a significantly higher objective response rate (ORR), indicating that PD-L1 is linked to higher response rates to avelumab in MBC patients. Not only that, avelumab demonstrated cytotoxic effects on TNBC patients via NK cells. Immune responses have also increased by improving NK cell cytotoxicity and tumor recognition (118). Another PD-1 inhibitor, nivolumab though not FDA approved yet, demonstrated anti-tumor activity in inflammatory BC with high pCR rate (120).

8.6.1.2 CTLA-4 Inhibitors

It was initially found that cytotoxic T-lymphocyte-associated protein 4 (CTLA-4) delivers an inhibitory signal important for terminating immune responses (121,122). CTLA-4 negatively regulates T cell activation in a number of ways, including by competing with CD28 for binding to their shared ligands B7.1 and B7.2 (123). Theoretically, the CTLA4 produced by tumor cells is expected to aid tumor cell escape by diminishing the immune surveillance from surrounding immune cells (124). However, the clinical significance of CTLA4 in forecasting the prognosis of different cancers is still unclear (125). Researchers have found that CTLA4 polymorphisms are notably associated with the risk of BC in Asian populations (129). The levels of mRNA expression for CTLA4 in unstimulated PBMCs from BC patients were markedly higher than those in healthy controls (130). Treatment targeting CTLA4 has proven effective in the clinical management of BC. In luminal B $HER2^-$ BC, patients with $CTLA4^+$ tumors experienced shorter DFS, similar to those with interstitial $CTLA4^+$ tumors. $CTLA4^+$ tumors were identified as an independent factor associated with decreased DFS (133). The concurrent inhibition of PD-L1 and CTLA-4, targeting distinct stages of the immune response, has progressed to first-line therapy for various cancers, and recent results could suggest its application in BC, particularly with elevated PD-L1 levels (134). In HR^+ BC, the ICON trial aimed to assess ipilimumab (anti-CTLA-4) and nivolumab (anti-PD-1) alongside chemotherapy in patients with HR^+ metastatic disease. This trial did not achieve its main objectives but indicated a possible advantage for patients undergoing sequential dual blockade instead of combined with chemotherapy. In the randomized phase 2 KEYNOTE-046 trial, a bispecific protein targeting anti-PD-L1/CTLA-4 was employed alongside nab-paclitaxel. The findings indicated encouraging effectiveness and survival advantages, particularly in individuals with PD-L1-positive advanced TNBC (126). Ipilimumab, a fully human immunoglobulin (Ig)G1 monoclonal antibody targeting CTLA-4, activates T cells by sterically blocking the interaction of CTLA-4 – CD80 and CD86 on antigen-presenting cells (APCs) or T cells, preventing the inhibitory effect of CTLA-4, so allowing CD28 to bind to CD80/CD86 **(Figure 8.2).** Tremelimumab is another human IgG2 monoclonal antibody directed against CTLA-4. It has a similar mechanism of action to ipilimumab, hindering the interaction between CTLA-4 and CD28, thus preventing CTLA-4-mediated immune-cell inactivation. Ipilimumab and tremelimumab have demonstrated great clinical benefits in many different malignancies, including melanoma, lung carcinoma, and renal cell carcinoma, but not in BC. In a clinical phase 2 trial, NCT02527434, patients with multiple advanced solid tumors (TNBC, pancreatic ductal adenocarcinoma, and uroepithelial bladder cancer) were evaluated for tremelimumab's safety and effectiveness. This study shows that treating TNBC with tremelimumab is feasible. In addition, ipilimumab's safety in patients with early-stage mammary gland cancer is presently being assessed by the clinical phase 1 trial NCT01502592 (26).

8.6.1.3 LAG-3

LAG-3 is significantly expressed by activated human T and NK cells, along with TILs, in different tumors (127). LAG-3 restricts T cell growth and sustains T cell exhaustion through its interaction with major histocompatibility complex class II (128). Relatlimab, a monoclonal antibody targeting LAG-3, is the inaugural LAG-3 inhibitor authorized by the FDA in conjunction with nivolumab for treating previously untreated unresectable or metastatic melanoma, following the findings of the RELATIVITY-047 trial (129). Results from the I-SPY 2 arm presented at the San Antonio Breast Cancer Symposium 2022, investigating the co-inhibition of PD-L1 and LAG-3, revealed an impressive pCR rate of 60% in $HR^-/HER2^-$ BC and 37% in $HR^+/HER2^-$ BC (130,131).

8.6.1.4 TIGIT

TIGIT is a novel immunomodulatory receptor found on the surface of NK and T cells. Tiragolumab (anti-TIGIT) received breakthrough therapy designation from the U.S. Food and Drug Administration for its combined use with atezolizumab in treating non–small cell lung cancer, supported by findings from the phase 2 CITYSCAPE trial. In a large clinicopathologic series involving 1,222 invasive BCs, TIGIT expression was significantly elevated when compared to matching normal tissue (132). The ongoing ICI therapies were listed in **Table 8.1**. Furthermore, patients exhibiting higher TIGIT

TABLE 8.1
Trial Number, Agent, Phase of Clinical Trial and Outcome of Ongoing Immune Checkpoint Inhibitor Therapies

Trial (NCT Identifier)	Agent/Target	Phase	Outcome
KEYNOTE-5222 (133) (NCT03036488)	Pembrolizumab (anti-PD-1)	Phase 3, randomized trial for high-risk early-stage triple-negative breast cancer (TNBC)	• *5-Year OS*: Enhanced to 86.6% with pembrolizumab plus chemo compared to 81.7% with chemo only • *Event-Free Survival*: Markedly improved with pembrolizumab in various subgroups • *Pathologic Complete Response (pCR)*: Increased rates observed with pembrolizumab combined with chemotherapy
KEYNOTE-355 (134) (NCT02819518)	Pembrolizumab (anti-PD-1)	Phase 3 trial of patients with advanced TNBC with PD-L1 Combined Positive Score ≥10	• Pembrolizumab–chemotherapy resulted in significantly longer overall survival than chemotherapy alone among patients with advanced triple-negative breast cancer whose tumors expressed PD-L1 with a Combined Positive Score of 10 or more
ICON (NCT03409198) (126)	Ipilimumab (anti-CTLA-4) + nivolumab (anti-PD-1) + anthracycline	Phase 2b trial	• Combination of chemotherapy with ipilimumab and nivolumab led to a high rate of (immune-related adverse effect) irAEs • Administering ipilimumab/nivolumab alone post-chemotherapy showed clinical advantages with an improved safety profile
(NCT03872791) (135)	Anti-PD-L1/CTLA-4 bispecific (KN046) + nab-paclitaxel	Multicenter phase 2 trial	• Positive effectiveness and survival advantages with manageable toxicity in the first-line therapy of metastatic TNBC, particularly in PD-L1-positive cases
I-SPY 210 (136) (NCT01042379)	Co-inhibition with cemiplimab (anti-PD-1) + REGN3767 (anti-LAG-3)	Multicenter open-label adaptively randomized phase 2 trial	• Elevated anticipated pCR rate in both $HR^-/HER2^-$ and $HR^+/HER2^-$ • Patients with immune-positive HR^+ BC exhibited a PCR rate of 91%
(NCT02460224) (137)	Co-inhibition with ieramilimab (anti-LAG-3) with spartalizumab (anti-PD-1)	Phase 2, multicenter, open-label study	• The primary endpoint was objective response rate (ORR) TNBC

expression showed a correlation with extended progression-free intervals and improved OS. In preclinical research, blocking TIGIT alongside PD-L1 inhibition has shown the ability to diminish the metastatic potential of BC tumors, likely by boosting NK cell surveillance and also enhancing T cell anti-tumor effects in ex vivo models (128).

8.7 ADOPTIVE CELL THERAPIES

In general, adoptive cell therapy (ACT) artificially generates lymphocytes that have a strong affinity for identifying and attacking target tumor cells in vivo. ACT provides an expanding set of tools to address antigenic variability and the extensive range of immune evasion strategies present in advanced BC. To maximize the benefits of these tailored treatments, there is a need to tackle both approach-specific obstacles and overarching issues (138). We are briefly describing the advancements of CAR-T, CAR-NK, and TILs in breast carcinoma.

8.7.1 Chimeric Antigen Receptor T Cell (CAR-T Cell) Therapy

Chimeric antigen receptor (CAR) T cells, or genetically modified T cells, have become a viable treatment option for a number of cancers. The purpose of CAR-T cells is to target cancer-related antigens specifically (139). CAR-T therapy is an immunotherapy technique that modifies T cells to identify cancer cells and more effectively target and eliminate them. To target tumors, patients are given human T cells after they have been extracted and genetically altered. Usually, CAR or chimeric antigen receptors are used to engineer T cells. Since they are a single receptor that combines the abilities of T cell activation and antigen binding, receptors are chimeric. The treatment of luminal A subtype with CAR-T therapy is still being researched. For instance, a significant percentage of patients with the luminal A subtype express diganglioside GD2, a tumor-associated antigen. Seitz et al. found that while the GD2-targeted CAR-T cells exhibited good cytolytic activity against the GD2-positive luminal A cell line MCF-7, they did not show any anti-tumor activity against the luminal A cell line T-47D (140). Nevertheless, CAR-T treatment for luminal B tumors is less explored. Thus, it demands more investigations of CAR-T cells for treating luminal A and luminal B subtypes. On the other hand, targeting $HER2^+$ cancers, HER2-CAR-T cells showed a significant reduction in tumor growth and a regression in brain tumor metastases in preclinical studies (141,142). Also, in trastuzumab-resistant JIMT-1 cell line–derived xenograft mouse models, HER2-CAR-T cells penetrated into the tumor matrix and eradicated the established solid tumor, which subsequently resulted in an improved long-term survival (143). These findings imply that CAR-T cell therapy for BC may target HER2.

In the case of TNBC, it is noteworthy that the exploration of mesothelin-specific CAR-T therapy for treatment has been the subject of extensive preclinical and clinical studies. A recent phase 1 clinical trial focused on evaluating the safety and efficacy of this treatment, although the current status of this trial is yet to be disclosed (NCT02580747) (144). Another phase 1 study was conducted by the University of Pennsylvania, demonstrating that there was no evidence of drug-related side effects and that the immunotherapy had been well tolerated by patients, causing an inflammatory response within TNBC tumors. Assessing the effectiveness of autologous MUC-specific CAR-T cells in TNBC patients was the most explored cell therapy [NCT02587689]. NKG2D ligand and ROR1 are two additional target antigens undergoing clinical trials. A phase 1 trial [NCT04107142] is being conducted to assess the safety and effectiveness of allogeneic gamma delta ($\gamma\delta$) T cells transduced with CARs that target NKG2D ligands on TNBC cells. To further investigate the effectiveness of ROR1-specific CAR-T cells, TNBC patients are also being enrolled. Altogether, the increasing number of clinical trials being carried out on various CAR-T antigens indicates that these initiatives will result in a revolutionary era of immunotherapy (139,145,146).

8.7.2 CAR-NK Cell Therapy

CAR-NK cells are NK cells that have been genetically modified to display CARs. These CARs connect antigen-recognizing domains (like antibodies or receptors aimed at cancer or virus-infected cells) with activating signaling components. This alteration improves NK cell specificity and cytotoxicity by bypassing inhibitory signals and encouraging focused immune responses (147). Contrary to CAR-T therapy, CAR-NK therapy offers distinct benefits and features stemming from the switch of carrier cells from T cells to NK cells. NK cells exhibit cytotoxic activity and operate in a manner akin to $CD8^+$ T cells. In $HER2^+$ BC, research indicates that HER2 CAR-NK cells – modified from NK cells of healthy donors or patients – demonstrate strong anti-tumor effects against $HER2^-$ expressing cancer cells, irrespective of MHC class I expression. In comparison to matched HER2 CAR-T cells, CAR-NK cells show greater cytotoxicity. Crucially, they maintain strong cytotoxicity even in immunosuppressive tumor settings, emphasizing their effectiveness and safety for immunotherapy targeting solid tumors (148). In the context of TNBC, Liu et al. showed that therapy using EGFR-CAR-NK cells (second-generation CAR) could represent a promising option for patients with TNBC. Standard cancer treatments and conventional immunotherapy are ineffective for patients with TNBC. CAR-NK cells targeting EGFR specifically trigger the elimination of TNBC cells in vitro. Alternatively, it could be used for managing TNBC patients who show heightened levels of EGFR expression (149).

8.7.3 TIL Therapy

This therapy centers on the ex vivo expansion of TILs obtained from cancer patients and their subsequent reinfusion into the same patients (150). Successful TIL expansion has been documented in various cancer types, such as melanoma, colorectal carcinoma, renal cell carcinoma, and pancreatic carcinoma. Concerning BC, several reports have detailed initial TIL cultures; however, the sample sizes in these investigations were limited (<20), and the responsiveness of TILs to autologous tumors along with the ratio exhibiting memory T cell phenotype, essential factors for forecasting therapeutic effectiveness, were not outlined, complicating the assessment of ACT's utility (151). NCT01174121 is a phase 2 study assessing the effectiveness and safety of TILs alongside pembrolizumab in metastatic cancer instances. Pembrolizumab was given before TIL infusion to prevent the inhibition of activated cells. A patient with HR^+ MBC involved in this clinical trial, who was treated with TILs aimed at four mutated proteins, had a regression of her MBC that lasted over 22 months (160). Additional clinical trials are available on clinicaltrials.gov, such as NCT04111510, a phase 1 study evaluating TILs in patients with triple-negative MBC who have progressed after three prior systemic treatments. TIL therapy has constraints such as the necessity to acquire enough tissue, producing a sufficient number of T cells that respond to tumor-specific mutations, and often requires a hospital stay of several weeks for lymphodepletion (152).

8.8 CHALLENGES IN IMMUNOTHERAPY

While cancer immunotherapy has become a focal point in conventional oncology, leading to complete and enduring tumor regression, only a fraction of patients treated demonstrate a response, with some experiencing relapse after an initial positive outcome. Various tumor types have varying responses, and even among cancer types that do respond (hot tumors), unresponsive tumors (cold tumors) can still be observed, indicating resistance exists (153). Tumors referred to as "hot" are those that exhibit signs of inflammation, indicating that T cells have already invaded the tumor to combat the cancerous cells. On the other hand, nonimmunogenic "cold" tumors have not been penetrated by T cells, indicating that the immune response is ineffective for some reason. The absence of T cells hinders the ability to initiate an immune response using immunotherapy medications. These tumors are primarily managed with conventional cancer treatments (154).

Additionally, it was reported that a patient who received the checkpoint inhibitor nivolumab had suddenly developed type 1 diabetes, which occurs when the body destroys cells in the pancreas that make insulin. Hopefully, checkpoint inhibitor developing pharmaceutical companies have collected blood, biopsies, and clinical data from trial participants, which may reveal why some patients develop immune-related adverse events. UCSF immunologist Jeffrey Bluestone, CEO of the Parker Institute, is seeking anonymized samples to identify genetic or biomarker-based predictors of these toxicities (155).

8.9 COMBINATION THERAPIES

A major challenge in BC is the molecular diversity that restricts the effectiveness of numerous treatment strategies. Clinical trials have demonstrated positive clinical results with immunotherapeutic options in certain subtypes of BC. Nevertheless, ICI monotherapy might not be adequate for every BC patient, highlighting the necessity for combination strategies. Current studies aim to elucidate the interactions of ICI with both traditional and new cancer treatment strategies in preclinical BC models (156). Chemoimmunotherapy is a new treatment approach for cancer that merges conventional chemotherapy with immunotherapy. This method seeks to enhance the effectiveness of cancer treatment by concurrently attacking cancer cells with chemotherapy while also strengthening the immune system's capacity to combat cancer using immunotherapy (157). For instance, TNBC has the poorest BC prognosis but shows high PD-L1 expression and TILs, making it responsive to ICIs. In PD-L1$^+$ cases (CPS u10), pembrolizumab plus chemotherapy reduced progression/death risk by 35%, earning FDA approval. In early TNBC, it improved outcomes with neoadjuvant chemo (151). The IMpassion130 phase 3 study assessed atezolizumab combined with nab-paclitaxel in 902 individuals with advanced TNBC, demonstrating a notable OS improvement from 15.5 to 25 months in PD-L1$^+$ patients, resulting in FDA approval in 2019. Follow-up studies IMpassion131 and IMpassion132 are evaluating atezolizumab alongside different chemotherapies in several TNBC scenarios (156). When it comes to combining targeted therapy and immunotherapy, a phase 1 dose-escalation trial is exploring the use of utomilumab in combination with either trastuzumab or T-DM1 for the treatment of patients with advanced HER2$^+$ BC (NCT03364348). The impact of utomilumab combined with avelumab is currently being examined in a phase 2 trial (AVIATOR, NCT03414658). The preclinical results indicated that utomilumab, when paired with an mAb directed at the PD-1/PD-L1 pathway, can enhance a robust immune reaction (158). Although single agent immunotherapies, particularly ICIs, have exhibited promising results and disease prognoses, their benefits are also limited (159). In fact, some studies have stated the adverse effect of ICIs due to supra-stimulation of immunity (155). It may be possible to determine which patients will respond to monotherapy by using predictive biomarkers. Additionally, combining immunological agents may increase response rates and lengthen the duration of response by promoting an anti-tumor immunological memory (160). Numerous Phase 1 trials have reported encouraging results from combinations with PD1 and PD-L1 inhibitors, such as CTLA4 blockers, cytotoxic chemotherapy, radiation therapy, or small-molecule inhibitors like the vascular endothelial growth factor receptor (VEGFR) tyrosine kinase inhibitors sunitinib (Sutent; Pfizer) or pazopanib (Votrient; Novartis) (159). Immunotherapy in conjunction with a second immunotherapy modality, as well as chemotherapy or radiation, are used in recent preclinical research and clinical trials of combination therapies (159,161). There is also potential for improving therapeutic results for TNBC by combining CAR-T therapy with other forms of treatment. Targeting elements of the tumor microenvironment, such as extracellular matrix (ECM) or cancer-associated fibroblasts (CAF), can increase the tumoricidal effects of CAR-T cells. Furthermore, anti-angiogenic medications or substances that target macrophages and monocytes can be used to enhance the anti-tumor activity of CAR-T therapy in solid tumors (139). Overall, it is indeed beneficial to combine different therapeutic strategies for better outcome and DFS. Another phase 1 clinical trial conducted by Criscitiello et al. found out that combined targeted chemotherapy (PI3K/AKT/mTOR inhibitor) with immunotherapy (PD1/PD-L1 inhibitor) in 151 patients with metastatic BC, which included 70 with HR+, 18 with HER2, and 63 with TNBC. But it was shown that patients with TNBC experience poor outcomes (162).

8.10 CONCLUSION

Precision medicine is a milestone in the field of oncology, marking a shift from all-size-fits-all treatments to tailored treatments where patient care is given based on individual prognosis and disease progression. Precision medicine starts from identifying precise biomarker to personalized treatment strategies, avoiding ineffective therapies. BC, being the second most cancer in mortality rate in women and heterogenous in subtypes, demands more accurate or personalized care. Targeting the whole TME despite simply targeting the tumor has proved better outcomes in several studies. Thus, precision medicine approaches in immune-oncology regimen also need peculiar attention. Immune oncology markers such as circulating immune cells, TILs, cytokine profile, and IGIs are promising approaches in BC diagnostics for neoadjuvant and adjuvant settings. Immunotherapy, proven strategy in preclinical as well as clinical trials in BC, include ICIs, adoptive cell therapies, and combination therapies. Given the immune system's significant variability between individuals, research must examine the varying tolerance to these combination therapies across different patient groups. The personalization of precise immunotherapies aided by predictive biomarkers is anticipated to improve the clinical effectiveness and reaction to treatment in patients, making this a significant and compelling field for additional research.

REFERENCES

1. Zhang Y, Ji Y, Liu S, Li J, Wu J, Jin Q, et al. Global burden of female breast cancer: New estimates in 2022, temporal trend and future projections up to 2050 based on the latest release from GLOBOCAN. J Natl Cancer Cent [Internet] 2025 Feb 13 [cited 2025 May 26]; Available from: https://www.sciencedirect.com/science/article/pii/S2667005425000225
2. Vetter M, Kurzeder C. Breast cancer treatment in the era of precision medicine. Heal TIMES Oncol Hematol. 2020 Oct 11;5(3):26–37.
3. Tsimberidou AM, Fountzilas E, Nikanjam M, Kurzrock R. Review of precision cancer medicine: Evolution of the treatment paradigm. Cancer Treat Rev. 2020 Jun 1;86:102019.
4. Rassy E, Mosele MF, Meglio AD, Pistilli B, Andre F. Precision oncology in patients with breast cancer: Towards a 'screen and characterize' approach. ESMO Open [Internet]. 2024 Oct 1 [cited 2025 Apr 22];9(10). Available from: https://www.esmoopen.com/article/S2059-7029(24)01486-8/fulltext
5. Yadav P, Sreelakshmi M, Chauhan V, Mishra R. Precision medicine: Unveiling progress amidst challenges. Int J Pharm Investig. 2025 Apr 21;14(4):1010–8.
6. Subhan MA, Parveen F, Shah H, Yalamarty SSK, Ataide JA, Torchilin VP. Recent advances with precision medicine treatment for breast cancer including triple-negative sub-type. Cancers. 2023 Apr 8;15(8):2204.
7. Johnson KS, Conant EF, Soo MS. Molecular subtypes of breast cancer: A review for breast radiologists. J Breast Imaging. 2021 Jan 1;3(1):12–24.
8. Sarhangi N, Hajjari S, Heydari SF, Ganjizadeh M, Rouhollah F, Hasanzad M. Breast cancer in the era of precision medicine. Mol Biol Rep. 2022 Oct;49(10):10023–37.
9. Papalexis P, Georgakopoulou VE, Drossos PV, Thymara E, Nonni A, Lazaris AC, et al. Precision medicine in breast cancer (review). Mol Clin Oncol. 2024 Nov;21(5):78.
10. Perou CM, Sørlie T, Eisen MB, van de Rijn M, Jeffrey SS, Rees CA, et al. Molecular portraits of human breast tumours. Nature. 2000 Aug;406(6797):747–52.
11. Azmal M, Miah MM, Prima FS, Paul JK, Haque ASNB, Ghosh A. Advances and challenges in cancer immunotherapy: Strategies for personalized treatment. Semin Oncol. 2025 Jun 1;52(3):152345.
12. Sahu M, Suryawanshi H. Immunotherapy: The future of cancer treatment. J Oral Maxillofac Pathol. 2021;25(2):371.
13. Moura T, Laranjeira P, Caramelo O, Gil AM, Paiva A. Breast cancer and tumor microenvironment: The crucial role of immune cells. Curr Oncol. 2025 Mar;32(3):143.

14. Moo TA, Sanford R, Dang C, Morrow M. Overview of breast cancer therapy. PET Clin. 2018 Jul;13(3):339–54.
15. Zafar A, Khatoon S, Khan MJ, Abu J, Naeem A. Advancements and limitations in traditional anticancer therapies: A comprehensive review of surgery, chemotherapy, radiation therapy, and hormonal therapy. Discov Oncol. 2025 Apr 24;16(1):607.
16. Tohme S, Simmons RL, Tsung A. Surgery for cancer: A trigger for metastases. Cancer Res. 2017 Apr 1;77(7):1548–52.
17. Bakos O, Lawson C, Rouleau S, Tai LH. Combining surgery and immunotherapy: Turning an immunosuppressive effect into a therapeutic opportunity J Immunother Cancer. 2018 Sep 3;6:86.
18. Jaber T, Waguespack SG, Cabanillas ME, Elbanan M, Vu T, Dadu R, et al. Targeted therapy in advanced thyroid cancer to resensitize tumors to radioactive iodine. J Clin Endocrinol Metab. 2018 Oct 1;103(10):3698–705.
19. Richardson RB, Harper ME. Mitochondrial stress controls the radiosensitivity of the oxygen effect: Implications for radiotherapy. Oncotarget. 2016 Apr 19;7(16):21469–83.
20. Mulder SL, Heukelom J, McDonald BA, Van Dijk L, Wahid KA, Sanders K, et al. MR-guided adaptive radiotherapy for OAR sparing in head and neck cancers. Cancers. 2022 Apr 10;14(8):1909.
21. Morris PG, Hudis CA, Dang CT. Anthracyclines are a critical component of adjuvant chemotherapy. 2011 Feb 18 [cited 2025 May 28];25. Available from: https://www.cancernetwork.com/view/anthracyclines-are-critical-component-adjuvant-chemotherapy
22. von Minckwitz G. Docetaxel/anthracycline combinations for breast cancer treatment. Expert Opin Pharmacother. 2007 Mar;8(4):485–95.
23. Germiniani R, Pipino G, Lavorato F, Bressani Doldi S. [Combination of antimetabolites and alkylating agents in the treatment of advanced breast cancer]. Minerva Med. 1977 Mar 17;68(13):831–4.
24. Park JH, Im SA, Byun JM, Kim KH, Kim JS, Choi IS, et al. Cyclophosphamide, methotrexate, and 5-fluorouracil as palliative treatment for heavily pretreated patients with metastatic breast cancer: A multicenter retrospective analysis. J Breast Cancer. 2017 Dec 1;20(4):347–55.
25. Wang M, Wang S, Desai J, Trapani JA, Neeson PJ. Therapeutic strategies to remodel immunologically cold tumors. Clin Transl Immunol. 2020 Dec 8;9(12):e1226.
26. Zhang H, Mi J, Xin Q, Cao W, Song C, Zhang N, et al. Recent research and clinical progress of CTLA-4-based immunotherapy for breast cancer. Front Oncol. 2023 Oct 4;13:1256360.
27. Debien V, De Caluwé A, Wang X, Piccart-Gebhart M, Tuohy VK, Romano E, et al. Immunotherapy in breast cancer: An overview of current strategies and perspectives. npj Breast Cancer. 2023 Feb 13;9:7.
28. Heater NK, Warrior S, Lu J. Current and future immunotherapy for breast cancer. J Hematol Oncol. 2024 Dec 25;17(1):131.
29. Kim SK, Cho SW. The evasion mechanisms of cancer immunity and drug intervention in the tumor microenvironment. Front Pharmacol. 2022;13:868695.
30. Dvir K, Giordano S, Leone JP. Immunotherapy in breast cancer. Int J Mol Sci. 2024 Jul 9;25(14):7517.
31. Gegios AR, Peterson MS, Fowler AM. Breast cancer screening and diagnosis: Recent advances in imaging and current limitations. PET Clin. 2023 Oct 1;18(4):459–71.
32. Sardanelli F, Magni V, Rossini G, Kilburn-Toppin F, Healy NA, Gilbert FJ. The paradox of MRI for breast cancer screening: High-risk and dense breasts—Available evidence and current practice. Insights Imaging. 2024 Mar 27;15(1):96.
33. Ocampo AA, Sun X, Balko JM. Peripheral blood biomarkers in monitoring treatment response in breast cancer patients. Expert Rev Mol Diagn. 2025 Apr 3;25(4):87–90.
34. Cattin S, Fellay B, Calderoni A, Christinat A, Negretti L, Biggiogero M, et al. Circulating immune cell populations related to primary breast cancer, surgical removal, and radiotherapy revealed by flow cytometry analysis. Breast Cancer Res. 2021;23:64.
35. Kotsifaki A, Alevizopoulos N, Dimopoulou V, Armakolas A. Unveiling the immune microenvironment's role in breast cancer: A glimpse into promising frontiers. Int J Mol Sci. 2023 Oct 18;24(20):15332.
36. Qian Y, Tao J, Li X, Chen H, Lu Q, Yang J, et al. Peripheral inflammation/immune indicators of chemosensitivity and prognosis in breast cancer patients treated with neoadjuvant chemotherapy. Onco Targets Ther. 2018;11:1423–32.
37. Griffiths JI, Wallet P, Pflieger LT, Stenehjem D, Liu X, Cosgrove PA, et al. Circulating immune cell phenotype dynamics reflect the strength of tumor–immune cell interactions in patients during immunotherapy. Proc Natl Acad Sci. 2020 Jul 7;117(27):16072–82.
38. Hanahan D, Weinberg RA. Hallmarks of cancer: The next generation. Cell. 2011 Mar 4;144(5):646–74.
39. Nagarajan D, McArdle SEB. Immune landscape of breast cancers. Biomedicines. 2018 Feb 11;6(1):20.

40. Labani-Motlagh A, Ashja-Mahdavi M, Loskog A. The tumor microenvironment: A milieu hindering and obstructing antitumor immune responses. Front Immunol [Internet]. 2020 May 15 [cited 2024 Jul 30];11. Available from: https://www.frontiersin.org/journals/immunology/articles/10.3389/fimmu.2020.00940/full
41. Tie Y, Tang F, Wei Y-Q, Wei X-W. Immunosuppressive cells in cancer: Mechanisms and potential therapeutic targets. J Hematol Oncol. 2022 May 18;15(1):61.
42. de Visser KE, Eichten A, Coussens LM. Paradoxical roles of the immune system during cancer development. Nat Rev Cancer. [cited 2025 May 6]. 2006 Jan;6(1):24–37. Available from: https://www.nature.com/articles/nrc1782
43. Moradpoor R, Gharebaghian A, Shahi F, Mousavi A, Salari S, Akbari ME, et al. Identification and validation of stage-associated PBMC biomarkers in breast cancer using MS-based proteomics. Front Oncol. 2020;10:1101.
44. Mangiola S, Brown R, Zhan C, Berthelet J, Guleria S, Liyanage C, et al. Circulating immune cells exhibit distinct traits linked to metastatic burden in breast cancer. Breast Cancer Res. 2025 May 8;27(1):73.
45. Foulds GA, Vadakekolathu J, Abdel-Fatah TMA, Nagarajan D, Reeder S, Johnson C, et al. Immune-phenotyping and transcriptomic profiling of peripheral blood mononuclear cells from patients with breast cancer: Identification of a 3 gene signature which predicts relapse of triple negative breast cancer. Front Immunol. 2018;9:2028.
46. Payne KK, Zoon CK, Wan W, Marlar K, Keim RC, Kenari MN, et al. Peripheral blood mononuclear cells of patients with breast cancer can be reprogrammed to enhance anti-HER-2/neu reactivity and overcome myeloid-derived suppressor cells. Breast Cancer Res Treat. 2013 Nov;142(1):45–57.
47. Tesi RJ. MDSC; the most important cell you have never heard of. Trends Pharmacol Sci. 2019 Jan;40(1):4–7.
48. Markowitz J, Wesolowski R, Papenfuss T, Brooks TR, Carson WE. Myeloid-derived suppressor cells in breast cancer. Breast Cancer Res Treat. 2013 Jul;140(1):13–21.
49. Diaz-Montero CM, Salem ML, Nishimura MI, Garrett-Mayer E, Cole DJ, Montero AJ. Increased circulating myeloid-derived suppressor cells correlate with clinical cancer stage, metastatic tumor burden, and doxorubicin-cyclophosphamide chemotherapy. Cancer Immunol Immunother. 2009 Jan;58(1):49–59.
50. Ma P, Beatty PL, McKolanis J, Brand R, Schoen RE, Finn OJ. Circulating myeloid derived suppressor cells (MDSC) that accumulate in premalignancy share phenotypic and functional characteristics with MDSC in cancer. Front Immunol. 2019;10:1401.
51. Yu J, Du W, Yan F, Wang Y, Li H, Cao S, et al. Myeloid-derived suppressor cells suppress antitumor immune responses through IDO expression and correlate with lymph node metastasis in patients with breast cancer. J Immunol. 1950. 2013 Apr 1;190(7):3783–97.
52. Yang G, Shen W, Zhang Y, Liu M, Zhang L, Liu Q, et al. Accumulation of myeloid-derived suppressor cells (MDSCs) induced by low levels of IL-6 correlates with poor prognosis in bladder cancer. Oncotarget. 2017 Jun 13;8(24):38378–88.
53. Jordan KR, Amaria RN, Ramirez O, Callihan EB, Gao D, Borakove M, et al. Myeloid-derived suppressor cells are associated with disease progression and decreased overall survival in advanced-stage melanoma patients. Cancer Immunol Immunother. 2013 Nov;62(11):1711–22.
54. Kawano M, Mabuchi S, Matsumoto Y, Sasano T, Takahashi R, Kuroda H, et al. The significance of G-CSF expression and myeloid-derived suppressor cells in the chemoresistance of uterine cervical cancer. Sci Rep. 2015 Dec 15;5:18217.
55. Weber J, Gibney G, Kudchadkar R, Yu B, Cheng P, Martinez AJ, et al. Phase I/II study of metastatic melanoma patients treated with nivolumab who had progressed after ipilimumab. Cancer Immunol Res. 2016 Apr;4(4):345–53.
56. Nolan E, Malanchi I. Connecting the dots: Neutrophils at the interface of tissue regeneration and cancer. Semin Immunol. 2021 Oct 1;57:101598.
57. Saraiva DP, Correia BF, Salvador R, de Sousa N, Braga S, Cabral MG. Circulating low density neutrophils of breast cancer patients are associated with their worse prognosis due to the impairment of T cell responses.
58. Cloke T, Munder M, Taylor G, Müller I, Kropf P. Characterization of a novel population of low-density granulocytes associated with disease severity in HIV-1 infection. PLoS One. 2012;7(11):e48939.
59. Fu J, Tobin MC, Thomas LL. Neutrophil-like low-density granulocytes are elevated in patients with moderate to severe persistent asthma. Ann Allergy Asthma Immunol. 2014 Dec;113(6):635–40.e2.
60. Liu Y, Hu Y, Gu F, Liang J, Zeng Y, Hong X, et al. Phenotypic and clinical characterization of low density neutrophils in patients with advanced lung adenocarcinoma. Oncotarget. 2017 Oct 31;8(53):90969–78.

61. Sagiv JY, Michaeli J, Assi S, Mishalian I, Kisos H, Levy L, et al. Phenotypic diversity and plasticity in circulating neutrophil subpopulations in cancer. Cell Rep. 2015 Feb 3;10(4):562–73.
62. Michaeli J, Shaul ME, Mishalian I, Hovav AH, Levy L, Zolotriov L, et al. Tumor-associated neutrophils induce apoptosis of non-activated CD8 T-cells in a TNFα and NO-dependent mechanism, promoting a tumor-supportive environment. Oncoimmunology. 2017;6(11):e1356965.
63. Tabariès S, Ouellet V, Hsu BE, Annis MG, Rose AAN, Meunier L, et al. Granulocytic immune infiltrates are essential for the efficient formation of breast cancer liver metastases. Breast Cancer Res. 2015 Mar 27;17(1):45.
64. Coffelt SB, Wellenstein MD, de Visser KE. Neutrophils in cancer: Neutral no more. Nat Rev Cancer. 2016 Jul;16(7):431–46.
65. De Giorgi U, Mego M, Scarpi E, Giordano A, Giuliano M, Valero V, et al. Association between circulating tumor cells and peripheral blood monocytes in metastatic breast cancer. Ther Adv Med Oncol. 2019 Aug 14;11:1758835919866065. doi:10.1177/1758835919866065
66. Gianni C, Palleschi M, Schepisi G, Casadei C, Bleve S, Merloni F, et al. Circulating inflammatory cells in patients with metastatic breast cancer: Implications for treatment. Front Oncol [Internet]. 2022 Aug 8 [cited 2025 May 6];12. doi: 10.3389/fonc.2022.882896
67. Cattin S, Fellay B, Pradervand S, Trojan A, Ruhstaller T, Rüegg C, et al. Bevacizumab specifically decreases elevated levels of circulating KIT+CD11b+ cells and IL-10 in metastatic breast cancer patients. Oncotarget. 2016 Mar 8;7(10):11137–50.
68. Azab B, Bhatt VR, Phookan J, Murukutla S, Kohn N, Terjanian T, et al. Usefulness of the neutrophil-to-lymphocyte ratio in predicting short- and long-term mortality in breast cancer patients. Ann Surg Oncol. 2012 Jan;19(1):217–24.
69. Proctor MJ, McMillan DC, Morrison DS, Fletcher CD, Horgan PG, Clarke SJ. A derived neutrophil to lymphocyte ratio predicts survival in patients with cancer. Br J Cancer. 2012 Aug 7;107(4):695–9.
70. Ethier JL, Desautels D, Templeton A, Shah PS, Amir E. Prognostic role of neutrophil-to-lymphocyte ratio in breast cancer: A systematic review and meta-analysis. Breast Cancer Res. 2017 Jan 5;19(1):2.
71. Ozyalvacli G, Yesil C, Kargi E, Kizildag B, Kilitci A, Yilmaz F. Diagnostic and prognostic importance of the neutrophil lymphocyte ratio in breast cancer. Asian Pac J Cancer Prev. 2014;15(23):10363–6.
72. Guthrie GJK, Charles KA, Roxburgh CSD, Horgan PG, McMillan DC, Clarke SJ. The systemic inflammation-based neutrophil-lymphocyte ratio: Experience in patients with cancer. Crit Rev Oncol Hematol. 2013 Oct;88(1):218–30.
73. Koh CH, Bhoo-Pathy N, Ng KL, Jabir RS, Tan GH, See MH, et al. Utility of pre-treatment neutrophil-lymphocyte ratio and platelet-lymphocyte ratio as prognostic factors in breast cancer. Br J Cancer. 2015 Jun 30;113(1):150–8.
74. Wei B, Yao M, Xing C, Wang W, Yao J, Hong Y, et al. The neutrophil lymphocyte ratio is associated with breast cancer prognosis: An updated systematic review and meta-analysis. Onco Targets Ther. 2016 Sep 8;9:5567–75.
75. Lee KH, Kim EY, Yun JS, Park YL, Do SI, Chae SW, et al. The prognostic and predictive value of tumor-infiltrating lymphocytes and hematologic parameters in patients with breast cancer. BMC Cancer. 2018 Oct 1;18(1):938.
76. Goto W, Kashiwagi S, Asano Y, Takada K, Takahashi K, Hatano T, et al. Predictive value of lymphocyte-to-monocyte ratio in the preoperative setting for progression of patients with breast cancer. BMC Cancer. 2018 Nov 19;18(1):1137.
77. Jia W, Wu J, Jia H, Yang Y, Zhang X, Chen K, Su F. The peripheral blood neutrophil-to-lymphocyte ratio is superior to the lymphocyte-to-monocyte ratio for predicting the long-term survival of triple-negative breast cancer patients. PLoS One [Internet]. [cited 2025 Jun 2]. 2015 Nov 18;10(11):e0143061. Available from: https://journals.plos.org/plosone/article?id=10.1371/journal.pone.0143061
78. Stenken JA, Poschenrieder AJ. Bioanalytical chemistry of cytokines – A review. Anal Chim Acta. 2015 Jan 1;853:95–115.
79. Miller MD, Krangel MS. Biology and biochemistry of the chemokines: A family of chemotactic and inflammatory cytokines. Crit Rev Immunol. 1992 Jan 1;12(1–2):17–46.
80. Greten FR, Grivennikov SI. Inflammation and cancer: Triggers, mechanisms, and consequences. Immunity. 2019 Jul 16;51(1):27–41.
81. Huang H, Zhang Y, Li S, Zhao J, Wang X, Zhou X, et al. Multiplexed immunoassay-based serum cytokine profiling for potential prognosis predictors in patients with metastatic breast cancer. Transl Cancer Res [Internet]. 2018 Dec [cited 2025 May 8];7(6). Available from: https://tcr.amegroups.org/article/view/25669

82. Li L, Chen L, Zhang W, Liao Y, Chen J, Shi Y, et al. Serum cytokine profile in patients with breast cancer. Cytokine. 2017 Jan;89:173–8.
83. Vilsmaier T, Rack B, Janni W, Jeschke U, Weissenbacher T. Angiogenic cytokines and their influence on circulating tumour cells in sera of patients with the primary diagnosis of breast cancer before treatment. PubMed [Internet]. [cited 2025 May 8]. 2016 Jul 27;16:547. Available from: https://pubmed.ncbi.nlm.nih.gov/27464822/
84. Vilsmaier T, Rack B, König A, Friese K, Janni W, Jeschke U, et al. Influence of circulating tumour cells on production of IL-1α, IL-1β and IL-12 in sera of patients with primary diagnosis of breast cancer before treatment. Anticancer Res. 2016 Oct;36(10):5227–36.
85. Kawaguchi K, Sakurai M, Yamamoto Y, Suzuki E, Tsuda M, Kataoka TR, et al. Alteration of specific cytokine expression patterns in patients with breast cancer. Sci Rep. 2019 Feb 27;9(1):2924.
86. Yoshihara K, Shahmoradgoli M, Martínez E, Vegesna R, Kim H, Torres-Garcia W, et al. Inferring tumour purity and stromal and immune cell admixture from expression data. Nat Commun. 2013 Oct 11;4(1):2612.
87. Yang B, Chou J, Tao Y, Wu D, Wu X, Li X, et al. An assessment of prognostic immunity markers in breast cancer. npj Breast Cancer. 2018 Oct 29;4(1):1–9.
88. van de Vijver MJ, He YD, van't Veer LJ, Dai H, Hart AAM, Voskuil DW, et al. A gene-expression signature as a predictor of survival in breast cancer. N Engl J Med. 2002 Dec 19;347(25):1999–2009.
89. Kaklamani V. A genetic signature can predict prognosis and response to therapy in breast cancer: Oncotype DX. Expert Rev Mol Diagn. 2006 Nov;6(6):803–9.
90. Boccia RV. Translating research into practice: The Prosigna® (PAM50) gene signature assay. Clin Adv Hematol Oncol. 2015 Jun;13(6 Suppl 6):3–13.
91. Li Y, Zhao X, Liu Q, Liu Y. Bioinformatics reveal macrophages marker genes signature in breast cancer to predict prognosis. Ann Med. 2021 Dec;53(1):1019–31.
92. Aran D, Hu Z, Butte AJ. xCell: Digitally portraying the tissue cellular heterogeneity landscape. Genome Biol. 2017 Nov 15;18(1):220.
93. Newman AM, Liu CL, Green MR, Gentles AJ, Feng W, Xu Y, et al. Robust enumeration of cell subsets from tissue expression profiles. Nat Methods. 2015 May;12(5):453–7.
94. Miao YR, Zhang Q, Lei Q, Luo M, Xie GY, Wang H, et al. ImmuCellAI: A unique method for comprehensive T-Cell subsets abundance prediction and its application in cancer immunotherapy. Adv Sci. 2020;7(7):1902880.
95. Becht E, Giraldo NA, Lacroix L, Buttard B, Elarouci N, Petitprez F, et al. Estimating the population abundance of tissue-infiltrating immune and stromal cell populations using gene expression. Genome Biol. 2016 Oct 20;17(1):218.
96. Ru B, Wong CN, Tong Y, Zhong JY, Zhong SSW, Wu WC, et al. TISIDB: An integrated repository portal for tumor–immune system interactions. Bioinformatics. 2019 Oct 15;35(20):4200–2.
97. Tan W, Liu M, Wang L, Guo Y, Wei C, Zhang S, et al. Novel immune-related genes in the tumor microenvironment with prognostic value in breast cancer. BMC Cancer. 2021 Feb 6;21(1):126.
98. Choi JE, Lee JS, Jin MS, Nikas IP, Kim K, Yang S, et al. The prognostic value of a combined immune score in tumor and immune cells assessed by immunohistochemistry in triple-negative breast cancer. Breast Cancer Res. 2023;25:134.
99. Nanda R, Chow LQ, Dees EC, Berger R, Gupta S, Geva R, Pusztai L, Pathiraja K, Aktan G, Cheng JD, Karantza V, Buisseret L. Abstract PD1-6: Inhibition of PD-L1 by MPDL3280A leads to clinical activity in patients with metastatic triple-negative breast cancer. Cancer Research. American Association for Cancer Research [Internet]. 2016 Jul 20;34(21):2460–7. Available from: https://aacrjournals.org/cancerres/article/75/9_Supplement/PD1-6/607658/Abstract-PD1-6-Inhibition-of-PD-L1-by-MPDL3280A
100. Nanda R, Chow LQM, Dees EC, Berger R, Gupta S, Geva R, et al. Pembrolizumab in patients with advanced triple-negative breast cancer: Phase Ib KEYNOTE-012 study. J Clin Oncol. 2016 Jul 20;34(21):2460–7.
101. Valenza C, Taurelli Salimbeni B, Santoro C, Trapani D, Antonarelli G, Curigliano G. Tumor infiltrating lymphocytes across breast cancer subtypes: Current issues for biomarker assessment. Cancers. 2023 Jan 26;15(3):767.
102. Ciarka A, Piątek M, Pęksa R, Kunc M, Senkus E. Tumor-infiltrating lymphocytes (TILs) in breast cancer: Prognostic and predictive significance across molecular subtypes. Biomedicines. 2024 Apr;12(4):763.
103. Ravelli A, Roviello G, Cretella D, Cavazzoni A, Biondi A, Cappelletti MR, et al. Tumor-infiltrating lymphocytes and breast cancer: Beyond the prognostic and predictive utility. Tumor Biol. 2017 Apr 1;39(4):1010428317695023.

104. Ladoire S, Arnould L, Apetoh L, Coudert B, Martin F, Chauffert B, et al. Pathologic complete response to neoadjuvant chemotherapy of breast carcinoma is associated with the disappearance of tumor-infiltrating foxp3+ regulatory T cells. Clin Cancer Res. 2008 Apr 15;14(8):2413–20.
105. Shou J, Zhang Z, Lai Y, Chen Z, Huang J. Worse outcome in breast cancer with higher tumor-infiltrating FOXP3+ Tregs : A systematic review and meta-analysis. BMC Cancer. 2016 Aug 26;16(1):687.
106. Andre F, Dieci MV, Dubsky P, Sotiriou C, Curigliano G, Denkert C, Loi S. Molecular pathways: Involvement of immune pathways in the therapeutic response and outcome in breast cancer. Clinical Cancer Research. American Association for Cancer Research [Internet]. 2013 Jan 1; 19(1):28–33. Available from: https://aacrjournals.org/clincancerres/article/19/1/28/78002/Molecular-Pathways-Involvement-of-Immune-Pathways
107. Loi S, Sirtaine N, Piette F, Salgado R, Viale G, Van Eenoo F, Rouas G, Francis P, Crown JP, Hitre E, de Azambuja E, Quinaux E, Di Leo A, Michiels S, Piccart MJ, Sotiriou C. Prognostic and predictive value of tumor-infiltrating lymphocytes in a phase III randomized adjuvant breast cancer trial in node-positive breast cancer comparing the addition of docetaxel to doxorubicin with doxorubicin-based chemotherapy: BIG 02-98. J Clin Oncol [Internet]. 2013 Mar 1; 31(7):860–7. Available from: https://ascopubs.org/doi/full/10.1200/JCO.2011.41.0902
108. Mishra B, Kodandapani S, Challa S, Dash S. Significance of tumor-infiltrating lymphocytes in tumor regression in breast cancer: A study in a tertiary care cancer center in South India. J Cancer Res Ther. 2023 Dec;19(7):1837.
109. Han E, Choi HY, Kwon HJ, Chung YR, Shin HC, Kim EK, et al. Characterization of tumor-infiltrating lymphocytes and their spatial distribution in triple-negative breast cancer. Breast Cancer Res. 2024 Dec 6;26(1):180.
110. Loi S, Michiels S, Adams S, Loibl S, Budczies J, Denkert C, et al. The journey of tumor-infiltrating lymphocytes as a biomarker in breast cancer: Clinical utility in an era of checkpoint inhibition. Ann Oncol. 2021 Oct 1;32(10):1236–44.
111. Nunes Filho P, Albuquerque C, Pilon Capella M, Debiasi M. Immune checkpoint inhibitors in breast cancer: A narrative review. Oncol Ther. 2023 Mar 14;11(2):171–83.
112. Chen DS, Mellman I. Elements of cancer immunity and the cancer–immune set point. Nature. 2017 Jan;541(7637):321–30.
113. Rebaudi F, De Franco F, Goda R, Obino V, Vita G, Baronti C, et al. The landscape of combining immune checkpoint inhibitors with novel Therapies: Secret alliances against breast cancer. Cancer Treat Rev. 2024 Nov 1;130:102831.
114. Swoboda A, Nanda R. Immune checkpoint blockade for breast cancer. Cancer Treat Res. 2018;173:155–65.
115. Chen L, Mo DC, Hu M, Zhao SJ, Yang QW, Huang ZL. PD-1/PD-L1 inhibitor monotherapy in recurrent or metastatic squamous cell carcinoma of the head and neck: A meta-analysis. Am J Otolaryngol. 2022;43(2):103324.
116. Luke JJ, Rutkowski P, Queirolo P, Del Vecchio M, Mackiewicz J, Chiarion-Sileni V, et al. Pembrolizumab versus placebo as adjuvant therapy in completely resected stage IIB or IIC melanoma (KEYNOTE-716): A randomised, double-blind, phase 3 trial. Lancet Lond Engl. 2022 Apr 30;399(10336):1718–29.
117. Saito Y, Fujiwara Y, Shinchi Y, Mito R, Miura Y, Yamaguchi T, et al. Classification of PD-L1 expression in various cancers and macrophages based on immunohistocytological analysis. Cancer Sci. 2022 Sep;113(9):3255–66.
118. Stergiopoulos S, Getz KA, Blazynski C. Evaluating the completeness of ClinicalTrials.gov. Ther Innov Regul Sci. 2019 May 1;53(3):307–17.
119. Herbst RS, Soria JC, Kowanetz M, Fine GD, Hamid O, Gordon MS, et al. Predictive correlates of response to the anti-PD-L1 antibody MPDL3280A in cancer patients. Nature. 2014 Nov 27;515(7528):563–7.
120. Kwa MJ, Novik Y, Speyer JL, Snuderl M, Cotzia P, Miller K, et al. Nivolumab with chemotherapy as neoadjuvant treatment for inflammatory breast cancer J Clin Oncol. 2022 Jun 1;40(16_suppl):e12633.
121. Tivol EA, Borriello F, Schweitzer AN, Lynch WP, Bluestone JA, Sharpe AH. Loss of CTLA-4 leads to massive lymphoproliferation and fatal multiorgan tissue destruction, revealing a critical negative regulatory role of CTLA-4. Immunity. 1995 Nov 1;3(5):541–7.
122. Waterhouse P, Penninger JM, Timms E, Wakeham A, Shahinian A, Lee KP, et al. Lymphoproliferative disorders with early lethality in mice deficient in Ctla-4. Science. 1995 Nov 10;270(5238):985–8.
123. Sharpe AH, Freeman GJ. The B7–CD28 superfamily. Nat Rev Immunol. 2002 Feb;2(2):116–26.
124. Bindea G, Mlecnik B, Fridman WH, Galon J. The prognostic impact of anti-cancer immune response: A novel classification of cancer patients. Semin Immunopathol. 2011 Jul;33(4):335–40.

125. Hellmann MD, Nathanson T, Rizvi H, Creelan BC, Sanchez-Vega F, Ahuja A, et al. Genomic features of response to combination immunotherapy in patients with advanced non-small-cell lung cancer. Cancer Cell. 2018 May 14;33(5):843–52.e4.
126. Kyte JA, Andresen NK, Russnes HG, Fretland SØ, Falk RS, Lingjærde OC, et al. ICON: A randomized phase IIb study evaluating immunogenic chemotherapy combined with ipilimumab and nivolumab in patients with metastatic hormone receptor positive breast cancer. J Transl Med. 2020 Jul 3;18(1):269.
127. Liu Q, Qi Y, Zhai J, Kong X, Wang X, Wang Z, et al. Molecular and clinical characterization of LAG3 in breast cancer through 2994 samples. Front Immunol. 2021 Jun 29;12:599207.
128. Main O, Marks DK. Immunotherapy in breast cancer: Can we expand and improve the therapeutic index by moving beyond PD-1/PD-L1 blockade? [Internet]. [cited 2025 May 31]. Available from: https://dailynews.ascopubs.org/do/10.1200/ADN.24.201892/full
129. Tawbi HA, Schadendorf D, Lipson EJ, Ascierto PA, Matamala L, Gutiérrez, EC, Rutkowski, P. Relatlimaband nivolumab versus nivolumab in untreated advanced melanoma. N Engl J Med [Internet]. [cited 2025 May 31]. Available from: https://www.nejm.org/doi/10.1056/NEJMoa2109970
130. Geurts V, Kok M. Immunotherapy for metastatic triple negative breast cancer: Current paradigm and future approaches. Curr Treat Options Oncol. 2023 Jun 1;24(6):628–43.
131. Isaacs C, Nanda R, Chien J, Trivedi MS, Stringer-Reasor E, Vaklavas C, et al. Abstract GS5-03: Evaluation of anti-PD-1 Cemiplimab plus anti-LAG-3 REGN3767 in early-stage, high-risk HER2-negative breast cancer: Results from the neoadjuvant I-SPY 2 TRIAL. Cancer Res. 2023 Mar 1;83(5_Supplement):GS5-03.
132. Guo C, Luo Z, Ismtula D, Bi X, Kong H, Wang Y, et al. TIGIT as a novel prognostic marker for immune infiltration in invasive breast cancer. Comb Chem High Throughput Screen. 26(3):639–51.
133. Schmid P, Cortes J, Pusztai L, McArthur H, Kümmel S, Bergh J, et al. Pembrolizumab for early triple-negative breast cancer. N Engl J Med. 2020 Feb 27;382(9):810–21.
134. Cortes J, Rugo HS, Cescon DW, Im SA, Yusof MM, Gallardo C, et al. Pembrolizumab plus chemotherapy in advanced triple-negative breast cancer. N Engl J Med. 2022 Jul 20;387(3):217–26.
135. Li Q, Liu J, Zhang Q, Ouyang Q, Zhang Y, Liu Q, et al. The anti-PD-L1/CTLA-4 bispecific antibody KN046 in combination with nab-paclitaxel in first-line treatment of metastatic triple-negative breast cancer: A multicenter phase II trial. Nat Commun. 2024 Feb 3;15(1):1015.
136. Shaw ML. AJMC [Internet]. 2022 [cited 2025 Jun 3]. I-SPY2 Supports Neoadjuvant Cemiplimab/REGN3767 in Early-Stage, High-Risk Breast Cancer. Available from: https://www.ajmc.com/view/i-spy2-data-on-dual-immune-blockade-support-use-of-investigative-regn3767
137. Lin CC, Garralda E, Schöffski P, Hong DS, Siu LL, Martin M, et al. A phase 2, multicenter, open-label study of anti-LAG-3 ieramilimab in combination with anti-PD-1 spartalizumab in patients with advanced solid malignancies. Oncoimmunology. 13(1):2290787.
138. Fuentes-Antrás J, Guevara-Hoyer K, Baliu-Piqué M, García-Sáenz JÁ, Pérez-Segura P, Pandiella A, et al. Adoptive cell therapy in breast cancer: A current perspective of next-generation medicine. Front Oncol. 2020 Oct 27;10:605633.
139. Marei HE, Bedair K, Hasan A, Al-Mansoori L, Caratelli S, Sconocchia G, et al. Current status and innovative developments of CAR-T-cell therapy for the treatment of breast cancer. Cancer Cell Int. 2025 Dec;25(1):1–23.
140. Seitz CM, Schroeder S, Knopf P, Krahl AC, Hau J, Schleicher S, et al. GD2-targeted chimeric antigen receptor T cells prevent metastasis formation by elimination of breast cancer stem-like cells. Oncoimmunology. 2020;9(1):1683345.
141. Sun M, Shi H, Liu C, Liu J, Liu X, Sun Y. Construction and evaluation of a novel humanized HER2-specific chimeric receptor. Breast Cancer Res. 2014 Jun 11;16(3):R61.
142. Priceman SJ, Tilakawardane D, Jeang B, Aguilar B, Murad JP, Park AK, et al. Regional delivery of chimeric antigen receptor-engineered T cells effectively targets HER2+ breast cancer metastasis to the brain. Clin Cancer Res. 2018 Jan 1;24(1):95–105.
143. Szőőr Á, Tóth G, Zsebik B, Szabó V, Eshhar Z, Abken H, et al. Trastuzumab derived HER2-specific CARs for the treatment of trastuzumab-resistant breast cancer: CAR T cells penetrate and eradicate tumors that are not accessible to antibodies. Cancer Lett. 2020 Aug 1;484:1–8.
144. Dees S, Ganesan R, Singh S, Grewal IS. Emerging CAR-T cell therapy for the treatment of triple-negative breast cancer. Mol Cancer Ther. 2020 Dec 1;19(12):2409–21.
145. Dey A, Ghosh S, Jha S, Hazra S, Srivastava N, Chakraborty U, et al. Recent advancement in breast cancer treatment using CAR T cell therapy: A review. Adv Cancer Biol – Metastasis. 2023 Jul 1;7:100090.
146. Yang YH, Liu JW, Lu C, Wei JF. CAR-T cell therapy for breast cancer: From basic research to clinical application. Int J Biol Sci. 2022 Mar 21;18(6):2609–26.

147. Shimasaki N, Jain A, Campana D. NK cells for cancer immunotherapy. Nat Rev Drug Discov. 2020 Mar;19(3):200–18.
148. Wang W, Liu Y, He Z, Li L, Liu S, Jiang M, et al. Breakthrough of solid tumor treatment: CAR-NK immunotherapy. Cell Death Discov. 2024 Jan 20;10(1):1–16.
149. Liu Y, Zhou Y, Huang KH, Fang X, Li Y, Wang F, et al. Targeting epidermal growth factor-overexpressing triple-negative breast cancer by natural killer cells expressing a specific chimeric antigen receptor Cell Prolif. 2020 Aug;53(8):e12858.
150. Rosenberg SA, Yang JC, Sherry RM, Kammula US, Hughes MS, Phan GQ, et al. Durable complete responses in heavily pretreated patients with metastatic melanoma using T-cell transfer immunotherapy. Clin Cancer Res. 2011 Jul 1;17(13):4550–7.
151. Lee HJ, Kim YA, Sim CK, Heo SH, Song IH, Park HS, et al. Expansion of tumor-infiltrating lymphocytes and their potential for application as adoptive cell transfer therapy in human breast cancer. Oncotarget. 2017 Dec 6;8(69):113345–59.
152. Gautam N, Elleson KM, Ramamoorthi G, Czerniecki BJ. Current state of cell therapies for breast cancer. Cancer J. 2022 Aug;28(4):301.
153. Taefehshokr S, Parhizkar A, Hayati S, Mousapour M, Mahmoudpour A, Eleid L, et al. Cancer immunotherapy: Challenges and limitations. Pathol – Res Pract. 2022 Jan 1;229:153723.
154. Lodge, A. Charles River [Internet]. 2019 [cited 2025 May 31]. Hot Tumors vs. Cold Tumors. Available from: https://www.criver.com/eureka/hot-tumors-vs-cold-tumors
155. Couzin-Frankel J. Autoimmune diseases surface after cancer treatment. Science. 2017 Nov 17;358(6365):852.
156. Nandi D, Sharma D. Integrating immunotherapy with conventional treatment regime for breast cancer patients- an amalgamation of armamentarium. Front Immunol [Internet]. 2024 Nov 1 [cited 2025 May 31];15. Available from: https://www.frontiersin.org/journals/immunology/articles/10.3389/fimmu.2024.1477980/full
157. Pol J, Vacchelli E, Aranda F, Castoldi F, Eggermont A, Cremer I, et al. Trial watch: Immunogenic cell death inducers for anticancer chemotherapy. Oncoimmunology. 2015 Apr;4(4):e1008866.
158. Wei H, Zhao L, Li W, Fan K, Qian W, Hou S, et al. Combinatorial PD-1 blockade and CD137 activation has therapeutic efficacy in murine cancer models and synergizes with cisplatin. PLoS One. 2013 Dec 19;8(12):e84927.
159. Mahoney KM, Rennert PD, Freeman GJ. Combination cancer immunotherapy and new immunomodulatory targets. Nat Rev Drug Discov. 2015 Aug;14(8):561–84.
160. Suntharalingam G, Perry MR, Ward S, Brett SJ, Castello-Cortes A, Brunner MD, et al. Cytokine storm in a phase 1 trial of the anti-CD28 monoclonal antibody TGN1412. N Engl J Med. 2006 Sep 7;355(10):1018–28.
161. Smyth MJ, Ngiow SF, Ribas A, Teng MW. Combination cancer immunotherapies tailored to the tumour microenvironment. Nat Rev Clin Oncol [Internet]. [cited 2025 May 12]. Available from: https://www.nature.com/articles/nrclinonc.2015.209
162. Criscitiello C, Marra A, Morganti S, Zagami P, Gandini S, Esposito A, et al. Clinical outcomes of patients with metastatic breast cancer enrolled in phase I clinical trials. Eur J Cancer. 2021 Nov;157:40–49.

9 Harnessing Probiotics for Personalized Cancer Therapy

A Holistic Approach

Adheena M, Reshma K V, and Jayamurthy Purushothaman
CSIR—National Institute for Interdisciplinary Science and Technology, Thiruvananthapuram, Kerala
Academy of Scientific and Innovative Research (AcSIR), Ghaziabad, India

9.1 INTRODUCTION

Cancer remains a predominant cause of morbidity and mortality globally, bringing widespread mortality and despair to communities across the globe (Sudaarsan & Ghosh, 2024). Over 10 million deaths were reported in 2022. Projections indicate a rise to 29.4 million new cases by 2040, underscoring the escalating global burden (Bray et al., 2024). Lifestyle factors, such as diets rich in processed meats, alcohol consumption, and smoking, have been linked to increased cancer risk (Marino et al., 2024).

Conventional cancer therapy approaches including chemotherapy and radiation therapy have burdened cancer patients with demanding psychological and physical challenges (Liu et al., 2024). These limitations and adverse effects associated with conventional chemotherapeutic agents necessitate the need for more targeted and safer therapeutic options. Personalized medicine as an emerging intervention in healthcare designs treatment to each individual's unique characteristics, such as their genetic makeup, with the goal of delivering the right therapy to the right person at exactly the right time (Jackson & Chester, 2015). The profound variation in treatment responses and the complex challenges posed by the tumor microenvironment have emphasized the need for more personalized and targeted approaches tailored to each individual's prognosis (Binnewies et al., 2018). Recent studies in oncology suggest that the use of probiotics as tools for oncolytic gene expression, drug delivery systems, and in personalized probiotic treatments is emerging as a promising strategy to enhance cancer therapy (Nama et al., 2025).

Probiotics are defined as live microorganisms for promoting a wide range of health benefits, mainly by modulating the gut microbiome through the release of bioactive molecules. Their positive impact on progressive levels of cancer treatment has been well established. Probiotics can boost the effectiveness of cancer immunotherapy, whether given before, during, or after treatment. Additionally, incorporating probiotics into the diets of cancer patients may help reduce the harmful side effects of chemotherapy and offer a promising supportive tool in cancer therapy (Mukherjee et al., 2024). Probiotics have been documented to improve the effects of chemotherapy drugs, lessen treatment-related side effects, and support the holistic well-being of cancer patients. For example, certain strains such as *Bifidobacterium* and *Lactobacillus* have demonstrated the ability to shape the tumor microenvironment by regulating cytokine production and elevating levels of natural killer (NK) cells as well as T lymphocytes (Pei et al., 2024).

DOI: 10.1201/9781003644309-9

The combination of *Streptococcus thermophilus* and *Lactobacillus delbrueckii* has been found to shift tumor-associated macrophages (TAMs), which promote vasculogenesis and angiogenesis of the tumor and promote the survival of cancer cells, from the M2 type to the pro-inflammatory M1 type, demonstrating the potential to develop new strategies for inhibiting tumor growth, as observed in mouse model studies (Pradhan et al., 2019). The most comprehensively studied probiotic strain is *Lactobacillus rhamnosus* GG (LGG), which alleviates the secondary effects of cancer-based therapy (Capurso, 2019). The anti-metastatic and anti-proliferative effects of LGG have also been explored in models of liver, colorectal, breast, and ovarian cancers. LGG has been shown to suppress tumor growth, largely through its ability to positively modulate the immune system (Mendes et al., 2018).

The innovative idea behind using probiotics is rooted in "personalized" or "precision" treatment, which takes into account the unique characteristics of each individual, moving away from the traditional ineffective "one-size-fits-all" approach. A personalized probiotic strategy was recently proposed and tested in animal models for treating intestinal disorders. In this approach, commensal bacteria from the healthy gut microbiota were collected and stored in a "microbiota biobank." After evaluating certain traits, these bacteria were successfully used to treat diseases linked to dysbiosis. The concept is based on the idea that commensal bacteria, when selected in a personalized manner, can better establish themselves in the gut by matching the host's specific genetic makeup (Al-Fakhrany & Elekhnawy, 2024).

This chapter aims to illustrate the latest insights in leveraging personalized medicine to address conventional cancer immunotherapy concerns, envisioning a future where personalized probiotics-based therapies reshape cancer prevention and management while promoting human health.

9.2 PROBIOTICS: MECHANISM OF ACTION AS AN ANTICANCER AGENT

Probiotics could assist as an adjuvant across different cancer types due to their effectiveness in altering enteric flora and strengthening local as well as systemic immunity. They hinder the initiation, growth, and metastasis of tumors induced by transplants or chemicals (Samanta, 2022). Probiotics can inhibit tumor growth or cancer progression through a variety of ways (**Figure 9.1**), such as altering intestinal microbiota, destroying carcinogenic substances, producing antioxidant effects, and modifying systemic and gut-associated immune responses (So et al., 2017).

Numerous studies have highlighted how probiotic metabolites, such as bacteriocins, peptides, and organic acids, interact with key metabolic pathways involved in cancer progression, including those regulating cell proliferation, inflammation, apoptosis, angiogenesis, and metastasis (**Figure 9.1**). Additionally, probiotics contribute to cancer prevention by suppressing pathogenic microbes through competitive exclusion, boosting the synthesis of short-chain fatty acids (SCFAs), decreasing the formation of carcinogenic bile acids, binding to and neutralizing carcinogens, downregulating NF-kappa B-dependent gene products involved in cell proliferation (e.g., cyclin D1, COX-2) and survival (e.g., Bcl-xL, Bcl-3), probiotics also promote apoptosis (Latif et al., 2023).

9.2.1 Altering Gut Microbiome

The human gut microbiome is a complex community of millions of microbes and consists of several strains of bacteria and yeasts residing in the colon. Their biological activity is significant for ensuring host homeostasis. The implication of probiotics has gained significant attention for their ability to positively influence the gut microbiota composition. Probiotics play a significant role in shaping the microbiota within the gut. By inhibiting the growth of pathogenic bacteria, they aid the host in maintaining a healthy intestinal lining (Chandrasekaran et al., 2024).

Modulation of complex gastrointestinal microbiota impacts various biological pathways, including the regulation of inflammatory mediators and the stimulation of immune responses against tumor cells. Additionally, probiotics can promote the production of antimicrobial compounds with

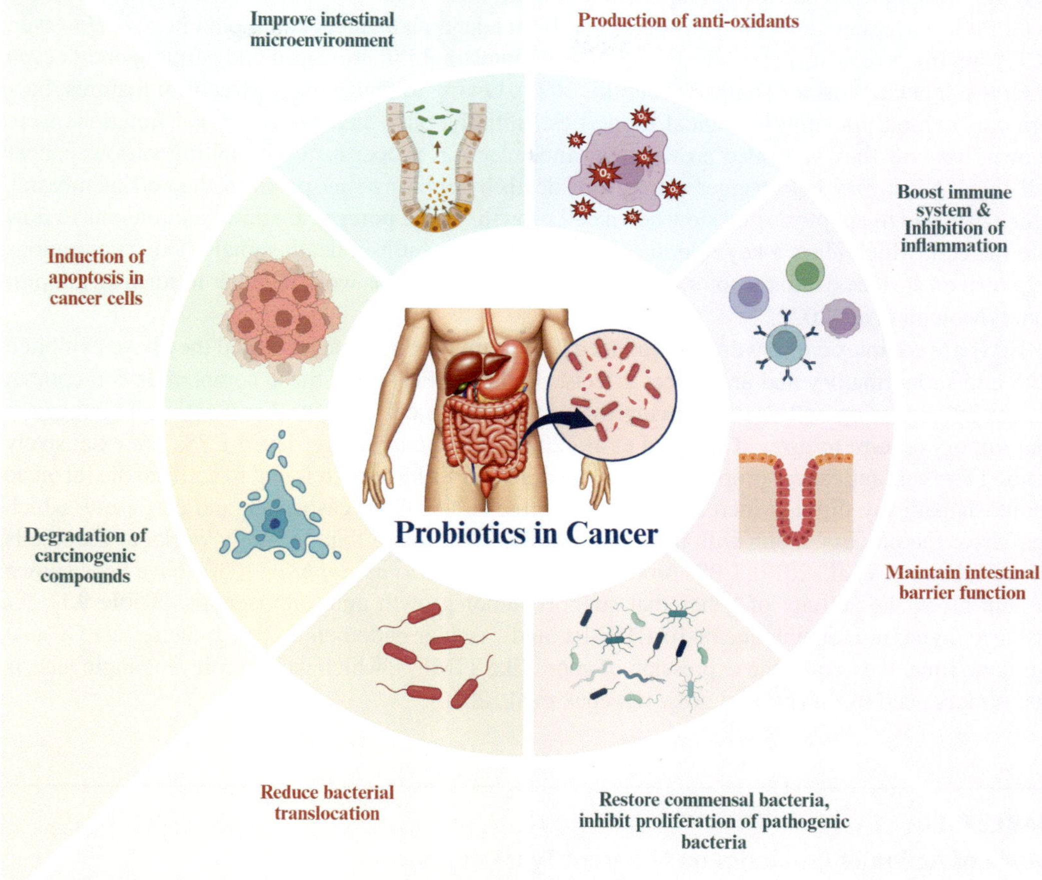

FIGURE 9.1 Multifaceted ways through which probiotics can act as anticancer agents and aid in cancer prevention.

cytotoxic effects on malignant cells and support the synthesis of antioxidant molecules, which help protect host cells from oxidative damage and other harmful effects (Naeem et al., 2024). Sustaining a homeostatic balance of gut microbiota in a stable ecological niche is of prime importance. Through their growth, probiotics elevate the count of beneficial bacteria in the intestine. They further assist in promoting the growth of desirable indigenous microbes (Fassarella et al., 2021).

9.2.2 Production of Anti-oncogenic Components

Various probiotic strains can secrete compounds that have demonstrated anticancer properties. These include bacteriocins, SCFAs, conjugated linoleic acid (CLA), and exopolysaccharides (EPSs), all of which are shown to possess potential anti-oncogenic activity (Sourav et al., 2023). SCFAs are metabolic byproducts synthesized by the microbe through the fermentation of non-digestible carbohydrates. Approximately 95% of the SCFAs generated by the gut microbiota are absorbed by the intestinal epithelium. The effects of SCFAs are primarily mediated through two mechanisms: activation of G-protein-coupled receptors (GPRs) and inhibition of histone deacetylases (HDACs), specifically GPR41, GPR43, and GPR109A (Thoda & Touraki, 2023).

A study conducted in a mouse model of colitis-associated colorectal cancer (CRC), by administering a mixture of SCFAs—acetate, butyrate, and propionate—has shown a significant reduction of tumor development and alleviated colonic inflammation (Tian et al., 2018). Notably, a deficiency in GPR43 was associated with the progression from adenoma to adenocarcinoma *in vivo*. However, SCFA treatment was still effective in suppressing intestinal inflammation and carcinogenesis even in GPR43-deficient mice (Thoda & Touraki, 2023). Owing to their unique structural features, bacteriocins exhibit potential biological properties. Initially, only their antimicrobial functions were known, but now they have also proven their anticancerous properties by inhibiting various cancer cell lines. Nisin may help trigger cancer cell death by creating tiny pores in the cell membrane, which can lead to apoptosis and slow down cell growth. These pores also allow calcium ions to flow into the cell, which plays a key role in activating the cell's built-in death signals. The calcium ions help turn on surface death receptors and caspases. These proteins work together to form an apoptosome (Molujin et al., 2022).

EPSs are complex carbohydrates produced by certain probiotic bacteria, and they have exhibited both anti-inflammatory and anticancer effects. Studies indicate that these compounds can combat cancer by triggering cell death, slowing the growth of cancer cells, and preventing angiogenesis that tumors require to grow (Chattaraj et al., 2025). *Lactobacillus*-retrieved EPSs are extensively studied for their anticancer properties. In many cases, EPSs have been found to activate the intrinsic apoptosis pathway through increased levels of proteins like Bax, caspase-3, and caspase-9, which help drive the process, along with a decrease in Bcl-2, a protein that normally works to keep cells alive (Tukenmez et al., 2019). EPSs produced by *Lactobacillus acidophilus* 10307 have been shown to help block the activity of genes that support tumor growth and angiogenesis (**Table 9.1**), for instance, hypoxia-inducible factor-1α (HIF-1α) and vascular endothelial growth factor (VEGF). At the same time, they boost the expression of genes like TIMP-3, which work to prevent angiogenesis that tumors need to survive and grow (Deepak et al., 2016).

TABLE 9.1
Mode of Action of Probiotics on Different Types of Cancer

Probiotics	Cancer Type	Mode of Action	Reference
Lactobacillus plantarum AS1	Colorectal cancer	Increasing host's immune response, degradation of carcinogens, antitumorigenic production	Legesse Bedada et al. (2020)
Pichia fermentans YSH	Oral squamous cell carcinoma	Induction of genes *BAX* and *CASP*	Shamloo et al. (2020)
Lactobacillus acidophilus	Breast cancer	Activating innate anticancer cell	Maroof et al. (2012)
Lactococcus *lactis* NK34	Lung	Decreases pro-inflammatory cytokines and NO production	Han et al. (2015)
Streptococcus thermophilus and Lactobacillus Delbrueckii	Colorectal cancer	Reducing the activity of gut enzymes, thereby reducing carcinogen level	Guha et al. (2019)
Lactobacillus *gasseri*	Cervical cancer	EPS-mediated apoptosis by stimulating cytokine production, showing anti-inflammatory effects	Sungur et al. (2017)
L. acidophil*us*	Liver	Stimulates immune response, apoptotic role, and inactivate NF-κB inflammatory pathway	El-Deeb et al. (2018)
Lactobacillus casei	Cervical cancer	Upregulation of apoptotic genes (caspase8, caspase9, caspase3, BAX, and BAD), downregulation of BCL-2	Rajoka et al. (2018)

CLAs are a group of linoleic acid isomers metabolized by certain probiotic bacteria that have been proven to hinder cancerous cell multiplication and induce apoptosis by caspase activation (Chattaraj et al., 2025). CLA can influence the expression of genes taking part in apoptosis, including Bcl-2, caspase-3, and caspase-9, as well as genes that respond to cell growth factors. Additionally, CLAs help reduce the production of eicosanoids in colon cells through two main mechanisms. First, they replace arachidonic acid in cell membranes, and second, they interfere with enzyme kinetics such as cyclooxygenase and lipoxygenase, which facilitate the production of eicosanoids (Bassaganya-Riera et al., 2012).

9.2.3 Immunomodulatory Effects

There are several ways through which probiotic bacteria can exert their effects on the immune system. This includes the colonization of epithelial cells, simultaneous induction of mucin secretion, synthesis of various bioactive compounds, pathogen elimination by blocking adherence to the intestinal lining, and limiting pathogen growth through nutrient competition. Probiotics exhibit immunomodulatory effects that differ between individuals, primarily linked to the secretion of cytokines and chemokines by immune cells. They also activate important immune pathways, such as toll-like receptors (TLRs), and can help reduce inflammation by blocking the NF-κB pathway. Additionally, probiotics help regulate other key immune signaling systems like the JAK/STAT and MAPK pathways by releasing cytokines and antimicrobial peptides, boosting both local and overall immune responses.

Multiple clinical and preclinical studies have demonstrated that the co-administration of probiotics can enhance the efficacy of cancer immunotherapies. In a murine cancer model, daily supplementation with *L. rhamnosus* M9 (5×10^9 CFU/day) significantly revitalized gut microbiota composition and augmented the anti-tumor efficacy of anti-PD-1 therapy, leading to increased survival rates (Gao et al., 2021). Similarly, in a melanoma mouse model, *Lactobacillus kefiranofaciens* ZW18 (1×10^9 CFU/day) exhibited the most potent anti-melanoma effects when combined with PD-1 inhibitor treatment. This combination enhanced immune activity by promoting the invasion of cytotoxic CD8+ T cells into the tumor microenvironment, thereby amplifying the therapeutic response (Chandrasekaran et al., 2024).

9.2.4 Probiotics as Apoptosis Inducer

Probiotics have been shown to induce programmed cell death, or apoptosis, achieved through several processes, including intracellular ROS generation, caspase activation, and control of cell cycle progression. ROS are highly reactive molecules that can harm critical cellular structures, including DNA and proteins, often leading to apoptosis. Research has shown that certain probiotics, including *L. rhamnosus* and *Lactobacillus plantarum*, can promote apoptosis in tumor cells by elevating the production of ROS inside the cells (Sun et al., 2023). The activation of caspases, which are the enzymes essential for triggering apoptosis, is done through boosting the levels of pro-apoptotic proteins while reducing the levels of anti-apoptotic proteins (Bax and Bcl-2, respectively) in cancer cells (Gupta et al., 2025).

Lactobacillus casei extract has been found to prevent gastric cancer by preventing cell proliferation and apoptosis through the suppression of NF-κB and mTOR-mediated signaling, in a study conducted with gastric cancer KATO3 cells (Hwang et al., 2013). Certain bacteria, including *L. rhamnosus*, have been observed to promote apoptosis in cancer cells through the upregulation of death receptors like Fas and DR5 on their surfaces. This process activates caspase-8, which starts the extrinsic apoptotic cascade, ultimately leading to caspase-3 activation (Altonsy et al., 2010). Current research suggests that probiotics may be a viable therapeutic option for cancer by stimulating the activation of caspases. However, further investigation is needed to validate the mechanisms at play and understand the clinical significance.

9.3 APPLYING PERSONALIZED PROBIOTIC STRATEGIES ACROSS CANCER TYPES

The rationale for integrating probiotics into cancer therapy rests on their ability to restore microbial homeostasis, enhance anti-tumor immune responses, and mitigate treatment-associated toxicities. Personalized administration of probiotics based on individual microbiota profiling represents a logical step, where probiotics are selected or engineered to correct specific dysbiosis or to amplify beneficial immunological pathways. Recent advances have highlighted the potential of personalized fecal microbiota transplantation (FMT) and customized probiotic supplementation in cancer immunotherapy settings. These findings underscore the pivotal role of microbiome modulation in shaping anti-tumor immunity. Moreover, uncovering the intricate mechanisms underlying probiotic influence on the tumor microenvironment, such as increasing antigen presentation, enhancing cytotoxic T-cell infiltration, or remodeling the tumor-associated microbiota, can drive the development of sophisticated, microbiome-guided, personalized oncology interventions.

Personalized probiotic approaches may involve selecting microbial consortia tailored to an individual's unique immunogenetics, maximizing anti-tumor benefits while minimizing adverse reactions. Additionally, novel bioengineering techniques now enable the creation of designer probiotics capable of delivering therapeutic molecules such as cytokines, enzymes, or tumor antigens directly to the tumor site (Seo et al., 2015). As our understanding of host–microbiota–tumor interactions deepens, integrating microbiome diagnostics and precision probiotics into routine oncology practice may become a cornerstone of next-generation cancer treatment strategies. Different cancers, such as colorectal, breast, lung, and gastric cancers, exhibit distinct interactions with the gut microbiota, influencing tumor behavior, immune responses, and treatment outcomes. Therefore, we have explored the application of personalized probiotic strategies across various types of cancer. By customizing probiotic interventions based on the specific microbial imbalances and immunological needs associated with each cancer type, researchers aim to enhance therapeutic efficacy, reduce side effects, and support overall patient health. This personalized approach represents a significant advancement in oncology, bridging the gap between microbiome science and precision medicine.

9.3.1 Probiotics in Breast Cancer

Breast cancer is a complex, multifaceted disease influenced by a combination of hormonal, genetic, environmental, and microbial factors. Recent findings have explored the pivotal role of gut microbiota in modulating estrogen metabolism, particularly through its interaction with enterohepatic circulation. This process may, in turn, influence the development and progression of hormone-driven breast cancers (Plottel & Blaser, 2011). Several strains of probiotics (**Table 9.2**), including *L. acidophilus*, *L. casei*, and *Bifidobacterium bifidum*, have been demonstrated to modify the gut microbiota, reduce systemic inflammation, and boost anti-tumor immune responses in breast cancer models (Chau et al., 2015). The oral administration of *Lactobacillus reuteri* has demonstrated significant anti-tumor potential by promoting T-cell responses and decreasing pro-inflammatory cytokines such as TNF-α and IL-6, which are commonly elevated in breast cancer in animal models (Lakritz et al., 2014). Additionally, therapies targeting the microbiome have been found to enhance the efficacy of immune checkpoint inhibitors by creating a more favorable tumor microenvironment, including increased infiltration of CD8+ T-cells and improved immune surveillance (Sivan et al., 2015). Therefore, personalized probiotic therapy offers a promising approach, where probiotics are tailored to modulate estrogen metabolism, strengthen systemic immune function, and attenuate chronic inflammation that fuels tumor progression.

Furthermore, clinical trials are increasingly investigating the use of probiotics to alleviate chemotherapy-induced side effects, such as gastrointestinal discomfort and immune suppression, thereby fostering better life experiences for breast cancer patients (Farran et al., 2020). Studies have also suggested that probiotic supplementation could enhance the gut microbiota's diversity,

TABLE 9.2
Selected Probiotic Strategies Explored for Personalized Cancer Treatment across Different Cancer Types

Type of Cancer	Target Pathogen/ Dysbiosis	Probiotic Strains	Reference
Breast cancer 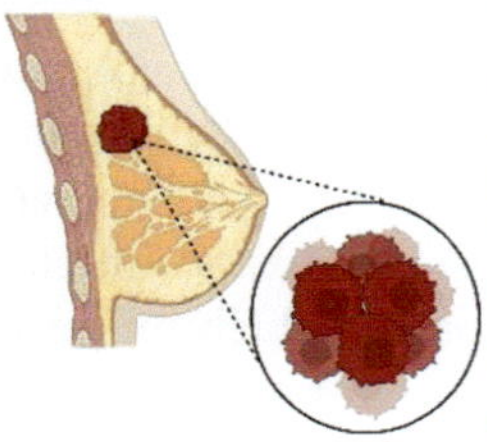	Gut dysbiosis impacting estrogen metabolism	*Lactobacillus acidophilus, Lactobacillus casei, Bifidobacterium bifidum*	Lakritz et al. (2014); Mendoza (2019); Plottel and Blaser (2011); Thu et al. (2023)
	Chronic systemic inflammation	*Lactobacillus reuteri*	Lakritz et al. (2014)
	Immunosuppressive tumor microenvironment	*Bifidobacterium breve*	Sivan et al. (2015)
	Chemotherapy-induced gut toxicity	Mixed *Lactobacillus* and *Bifidobacterium* strains	Farran et al. (2020)
Lung cancer 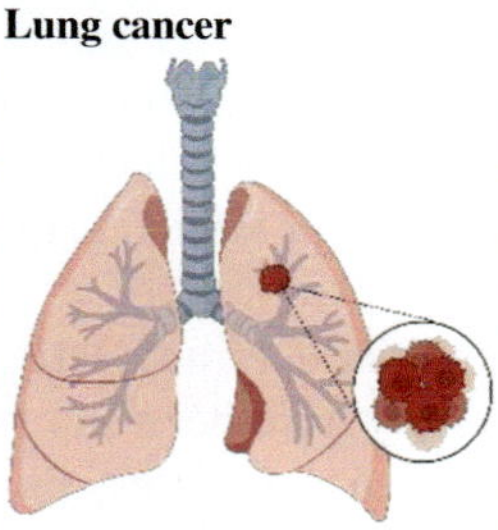	Gut dysbiosis affecting ICI response	*B. breve, Lactobacillus rhamnosus GG, Akkermansia muciniphila*	Matson et al. (2018); Pizzo et al. (2022)
	Impaired systemic immunity	A. muciniphila	Routy et al. (2018)
	Chemotherapy-induced mucositis and diarrhea	*Lactobacillus* spp., *Bifidobacterium* spp.	Mego et al. (2013)
Colorectal cancer 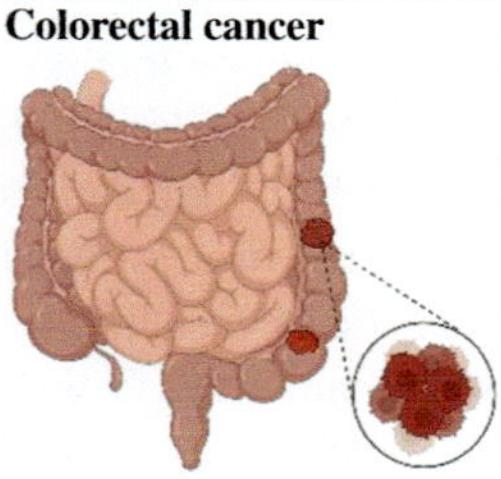	*Fusobacterium nucleatum, Bacteroides fragilis*	*Lactobacillus paracasei*	Chang et al. (2019); Nair et al. (2021)
	Aberrant Notch and Wnt signaling pathways	*Lactobacillus* cocktail (multiple strains)	Darb Emamie et al. (2021)
	Post-surgical infections and gut recovery	*Lactobacillus* spp., *Bifidobacterium* spp.	Zaharuddin et al. (2019)
	Chemotherapy efficacy modulation	*Lactobacillus* spp., *Bifidobacterium* spp.	Gao et al. (2017); Vipperla & O'Keefe (2016)
Pancreatic cancer 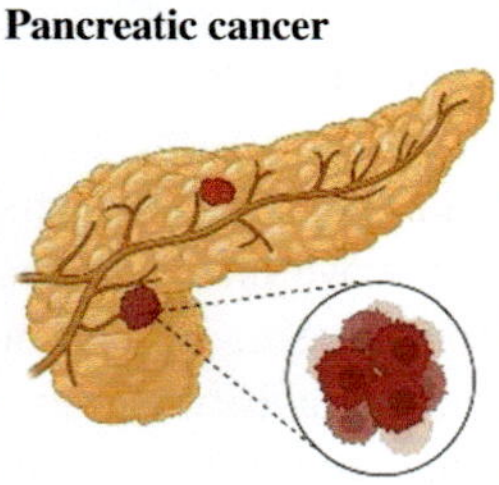	Immunosuppressive tumor microenvironment	A. muciniphila	Han et al. (2024); Zhu et al. (2023)
	Chemotherapy-induced gastrointestinal toxicity	*Lactobacillus plantarum, Bifidobacterium longum*	Li et al. (2024)
	Resistance to checkpoint inhibitors	Microbiota modulation with *Akkermansia* and personalized probiotics	Pushalkar et al. (2018)
Oral cancer 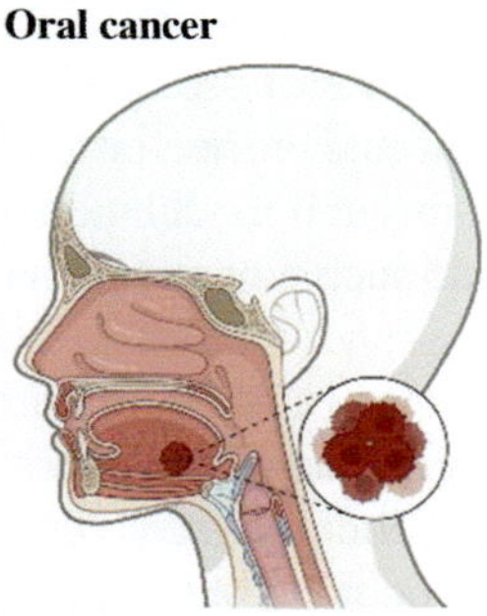	Oral mucositis during therapy	*Lactobacillus* spp., *Bifidobacterium* spp.	Y.-C. Liu et al. (2022)
	Dry mouth (xerostomia)	*Lactobacillus salivarius, Streptococcus thermophilus*	Y.-C. Liu et al. (2022)

potentially reducing the risk of chemotherapy-induced infections and fostering a more resilient immune response (Tremaroli & Bäckhed, 2012). Personalized probiotic regimens based on an individual's microbiota profile could further optimize the therapeutic outcomes by selecting specific strains that enhance estrogen metabolism, improve immune functions, and reduce pro-inflammatory markers in breast cancer patients.

9.3.2 Probiotics in Lung Cancer

The gut–lung axis, which defines the bidirectional interaction between the gut microbiota and the pulmonary immune system, is becoming an increasingly recognized factor in the development and progression of lung cancer. Studies have brought to light that lung cancer patients with a more diverse and balanced gut microbiota demonstrate better clinical responses to immune checkpoint inhibitors (ICIs) compared to those with dysbiotic microbiomes, which are often linked to poorer treatment outcomes (Routy et al., 2018). Probiotic supplementation, particularly with strains such as *Bifidobacterium breve, L. rhamnosus GG*, and *Akkermansia muciniphila*, has been found to restore microbial diversity in the gut (**Table 9.2**), enhance dendritic cell maturation, and stimulate T-cell-mediated anti-tumor immunity, thereby improving cancer immunotherapy outcomes (Gopalakrishnan et al., 2018; Matson et al., 2018). Moreover, personalized probiotics based on comprehensive gut microbiota sequencing could be tailored to selectively enrich beneficial microbial populations that enhance immune responses and potentiate anti-tumor activity against lung cancers.

In addition, probiotics have demonstrated therapeutic potential beyond their immune-modulating effects, particularly in managing the adverse side effects of chemotherapy. They have been shown to reduce chemotherapy-induced mucositis, diarrhea, and other gastrointestinal symptoms, thus improving overall patient quality of life during treatment (Mego et al., 2013). In a recent study, when gut microbiota from patients who responded well to ICIs were transplanted into non-responding lung cancer patients, there was a marked improvement in progression-free survival (Davar et al., 2021). This underscores the potential of microbiome-based personalized treatments in lung cancer, offering a novel approach to improve therapeutic efficacy. Furthermore, ongoing research is focusing on identifying microbial signatures that can predict treatment response, thereby enabling a more personalized approach to selecting specific probiotics that optimize clinical outcomes for lung cancer patients.

9.3.3 Probiotics in Colorectal Cancer

CRC stands as one of the significant cancers linked to gut microbiota imbalances. For CRC patients, the incorporation of probiotics may serve as a simple yet effective strategy to improve survival rates, reduce disease recurrence, and alleviate suffering (Nair et al., 2021). In an innovative study, a probiotic strain of *Lactobacillus paracasei* was found to significantly reduce CRC cell viability. Notably, co-treatment with the chemotherapy drug 5-fluorouracil (5-FU) further enhanced these effects, suggesting the potential of *Lactobacillus* in adjuvant therapy (Chang et al., 2019). Probiotics, especially *Lactobacillus* and *Bifidobacterium* species (**Table 9.2**), have been shown to counteract pro-carcinogenic effects by restoring microbial balance, enhancing the integrity of the mucosal barrier, producing tumor-suppressive metabolites like butyrate, and reducing inflammation through modulation of cytokine production (Vipperla & O'Keefe, 2016). In animal models, probiotic supplementation has been shown to significantly decrease tumor incidence as well.

The use of *Lactobacillus* cocktails in cancer treatment has also gained attention due to their synergistic effects (Nair et al., 2021). In a study, *Lactobacillus* cocktail induced apoptosis by modulating Notch and Wnt signaling pathways, offering a promising strategy for CRC treatment (Darb Emamie et al., 2021). A randomized double-blind placebo-controlled trial also demonstrated that the combination of *Lactobacillus* and *Bifidobacterium* strains was safe for consumption post-surgery

(Zaharuddin et al., 2019). Moreover, the latest insights suggest that gut microbiota composition can determine the outcome of CRC treatments, including chemotherapy (such as 5-fluorouracil) and immunotherapy. Personalized probiotic strategies, based on sequencing individual microbiota profiles, could identify dysbiosis patterns and allow for targeted interventions that exclude carcinogenic bacteria or enhance anti-inflammatory pathways. Clinical trials investigating personalized probiotics in CRC patients undergoing surgery or chemotherapy have yielded promising results, such as reduced infection rates, accelerated recovery of gut function, and improved immune markers (Gao et al., 2017). These findings support the potential of microbiome-guided approaches to improve CRC management and patient outcomes.

9.3.4 Probiotics in Pancreatic Cancer

Pancreatic cancer represents a growing global health challenge, with its incidence projected to reach 18.6 cases per 100,000 individuals by 2050, corresponding to an average annual increase of approximately 1.1% (Li et al., 2025). Despite being only the 10th most common cancer, pancreatic ductal adenocarcinoma (PDAC) ranks as the seventh most common cause of cancer-related deaths worldwide due to its inadequate prognosis and limited treatment options. Emerging evidence suggests that shifts in the oral microbiota have a strong association with the development of pancreatic cancer. Notably, the abundance of *Neisseria elongata* and *Streptococcus mitis* was reported to be significantly reduced in pancreatic cancer patients in contrast to healthy controls, and the combined presence of these bacterial biomarkers could effectively distinguish patients from healthy individuals, highlighting the diagnostic potential of microbiome profiling (Farrell et al., 2012). *L. rhamnosus GG* and *Bifidobacterium longum* are being explored for their capacity to improve gut barrier integrity, reduce systemic inflammation, and promote anti-tumor cytokine production such as interferon-gamma (IFN-γ) and interleukin-12 (IL-12). Furthermore, recent studies have uncovered that the pancreatic tumor microenvironment (TME) is not sterile but harbors its own unique microbiota, which actively shapes immune responses (Pushalkar et al., 2018).

Therefore, probiotics offer a valuable therapeutic avenue to favorably modulate both the gut and tumor-associated microbiota. Personalized probiotic therapies, tailored based on comprehensive microbiome sequencing of individual patients' gut and tumor microbiota, hold the potential to overcome the profound immune suppression that characterizes PDAC and to sensitize tumors to immunotherapies. Furthermore, emerging research suggests that engineered probiotics, capable of secreting anti-inflammatory cytokines or immune checkpoint inhibitors directly within the tumor microenvironment, could represent the next frontier in personalized microbiome-based therapies for pancreatic cancer (Charbonneau et al., 2020). Additionally, probiotics could offer supportive care benefits by alleviating the gastrointestinal toxicities associated with standard chemotherapeutic regimens such as gemcitabine and nab-paclitaxel. These regimens often cause mucositis, diarrhea, and dysbiosis, which not only reduce patient quality of life but also compromise treatment adherence (Guo et al., 2019). Thus, integrating personalized probiotic therapies into standard oncological practice for pancreatic cancer will require rigorous clinical validation through well-designed, randomized controlled trials.

9.3.5 Probiotics in Oral Cancers

Oral cavity malignancies, particularly oral squamous cell carcinoma (OSCC), constitute a major subset of head and neck cancers, accounting for nearly 48% of cases, with approximately 90% being OSCC (Sun et al., 2023). The incidence of oral cancer exhibits significant geographical variability, whereas India reports particularly high rates, largely attributable to cultural practices such as tobacco chewing, betel quid consumption, and poor oral hygiene. Increasing evidence underscores the pivotal role of the oral and gut microbiota in OSCC pathogenesis. Oral dysbiosis—marked by an increased prevalence of pathogenic species like *Porphyromonas gingivalis*, *Fusobacterium nucleatum*, and *Prevotella intermedia*—has been implicated in driving chronic inflammation, promoting epithelial–mesenchymal transition, activating oncogenic pathways such as NF-κB, and suppressing effective anti-tumor immune responses (Perera et al., 2016). Probiotic interventions aimed at restoring oral microbial homeostasis offer a promising preventive and therapeutic strategy. Specific strains like *Lactobacillus salivarius* and *S. thermophilus* have demonstrated the capacity to downregulate inflammatory cytokines (e.g., IL-6, TNF-α), inhibit the formation of carcinogenic biofilms, and bolster local mucosal immunity, thereby reducing the risk of malignant transformation (Stasiewicz & Karpiński, 2022).

Hence, personalized oral probiotic therapies could be developed through precision profiling of an individual's oral microbiome, enabling early detection of dysbiosis and the targeted administration of beneficial bacterial strains to correct microbial imbalances. Moreover, probiotics have shown potential in mitigating treatment-related toxicities. Randomized clinical trials have revealed that administration of probiotic formulations can profoundly reduce the severity and duration of oral mucositis, a common and debilitating complication of chemotherapy and radiotherapy in oral cancer patients (Colella et al., 2023). Probiotics also offer the benefit of alleviating xerostomia (dry mouth) and promoting epithelial healing (**Table 9.2**), which are critical for maintaining oral function and quality of life during cancer therapy. Emerging studies advocate for the integration of oral microbiome sequencing into personalized oncological care pathways. By identifying high-risk microbial signatures, clinicians could employ targeted probiotic strategies not only for prophylaxis but also to enhance responsiveness to immunotherapies and conventional treatments. As the field advances, future research involving multicentric, large-scale randomized controlled trials is essential to validate the clinical efficacy, safety, and optimal administration protocols of personalized probiotic interventions in the management of oral cancers.

9.4 PERSONALIZED PROBIOTICS IN CANCER IMMUNOTHERAPY

Personalized probiotics hold great promise in cancer immunotherapies. The inherent complexities and challenges of cancer immunotherapies necessitate a move toward more specialized treatment strategies. The link between the microbiome and the immune system serves as the foundational basis for understanding the potential of personalized probiotics in cancer immunotherapies. The human microbiome displays significant interindividual variability, which can influence treatment responses and clinical outcomes. Recognizing this variability, personalized probiotic therapies aim to tailor interventions to the specific microbiome composition of each patient, thereby enhancing the efficacy of cancer immunotherapies. This approach is based on the premise that targeted modulation of the microbiome can foster a more favorable environment for promoting anticancer immune responses (Chowdhury et al., 2024).

There are an increasing number of clinical studies that highlight the efficacy of personalized probiotics in cancer immunotherapy. For instance, a study conducted by administering probiotics orally for melanoma patients based on individual gut microbiota composition in combination with immune checkpoint inhibitors showed enhanced anti-tumor immunity and increased infiltration of cytotoxic T lymphocytes into metastatic tumors (Gopalakrishnan et al., 2018). Another study has shown improved response to immunotherapy and modulation of gut microbiota composition in cancer patients when customized probiotics were supplemented (Najmi et al., 2022). Personalized FMT in melanoma patients has shown improved response to anti-PD-1 therapies and overall survival (Miller et al., 2022).

The medical outcomes and translational potential of personalized probiotics in cancer immunotherapy represent promising avenues for enhancing treatment outcomes. As each patient's microbial community is unique, customizing probiotic therapies could completely revolutionize the way cancer patients are treated (**Figure 9.2**), and this will profoundly influence the future of cancer treatment.

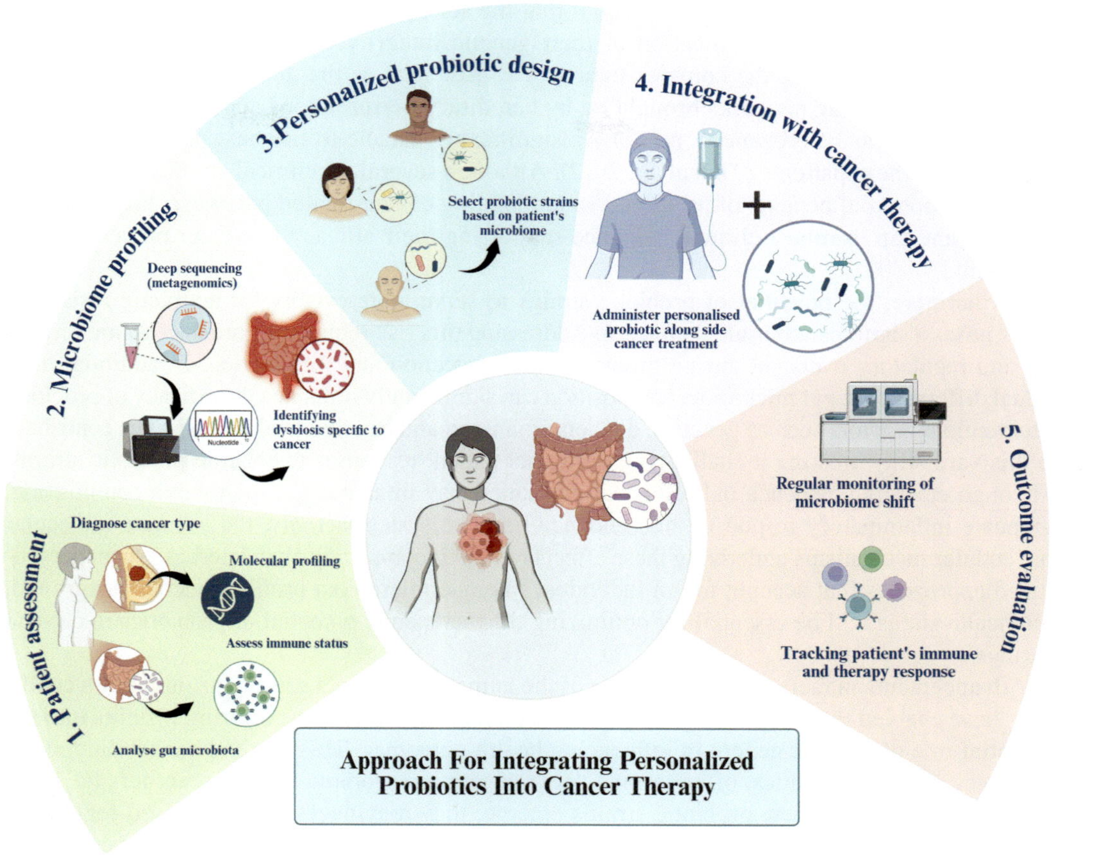

FIGURE 9.2 Approach for integrating personalized probiotics into cancer therapy (1) patient assessment, (2) microbiome profiling, (3) personalized probiotic design, (4) integration with cancer therapy, and (5) outcome evaluation.

9.5 CHALLENGES AND CONSIDERATIONS IN CLINICAL TRANSLATION

Despite the promising potential of probiotics as adjuncts in cancer prevention and therapy, several scientific and clinical challenges must be systematically addressed to ensure their efficacy, safety, and translational applicability. A major limitation lies in the insufficient standardization of probiotic strain identification and characterization, which presents a significant barrier to reproducibility and comparability across studies. Dosage also plays a critical role; administering an inappropriate number of colony-forming units (CFUs) can lead to suboptimal efficacy or unintended side effects, such as gastrointestinal discomfort. The successful clinical use of probiotic-based therapies is thus limited by this lack of standardization, which impedes the determination of optimal dosing regimens and treatment durations for probiotic-based interventions. Moreover, the health benefits conferred by probiotics are often strain-specific, underscoring the importance of precise identification and characterization of probiotic strains used in clinical settings (Guarner et al., 2024).

The clinical application of probiotics necessitates rigorous safety assessments, particularly for vulnerable populations such as immunocompromised individuals. Ensuring the safety of probiotics is a critical prerequisite prior to their commercialization, despite the fact that many probiotic strains are categorized as "Generally Recognized As Safe" (GRAS) microorganisms. As there have been reports of adverse events, including bacteremia and fungemia, in susceptible patients (Hempel et al., 2011), it is essential that the selected strains be preserved in microbial collections, with ongoing verification of their genetic integrity to guarantee consistent quality and safety. Moreover, the complex nature of cancer such as the numerous malfunctions of molecular and genetic networks brought on by hereditary perturbations and environmental disturbances, cellular heterogeneity presents a significant obstacle to the best possible treatment outcomes for these patients (Tian et al., 2012). Although several preclinical studies have demonstrated the potential benefits of probiotics in modulating cancer-related pathways, there remains a significant gap in robust clinical evidence supporting their efficacy in cancer prevention and treatment.

Furthermore, the potential of probiotic strains to serve as reservoirs for antibiotic resistance genes poses a significant biosafety concern. Addressing this risk requires rigorous genomic screening and regulatory oversight during probiotic strain selection and formulation. In addition, individual differences in gut microbiota composition can significantly influence the efficacy of probiotic interventions. Factors such as genetics, diet, environment, and existing health conditions contribute to this variability, making it challenging to predict patient responses to specific probiotic strains. Although emerging evidence indicates that probiotics may influence gut microbiota composition, attenuate inflammatory responses, and enhance immune system activity, the accurate molecular and cellular mechanisms underlying these effects remain incompletely elucidated. As such, personalized approaches that account for an individual's unique microbiota profile, genetic background, and health status will be essential for optimizing the therapeutic potential of probiotics in clinical settings.

Advancements in metagenomic analysis of the human microbiota across various health conditions have enabled the evaluation of microbial abundance and diversity, offering insights into the potential role of specific genera in influencing health outcomes. This method has facilitated the discovery of new probiotics, often termed "next-generation probiotics" by researchers (O'Toole et al., 2017). As these new probiotic strains emerge, they may necessitate a revised regulatory framework and be considered under current discussions surrounding live biotherapeutics. To address the existing challenges in this field, future studies should prioritize the standardization of probiotic strains, enhance their stability and viability, conduct thorough safety evaluations, explore their mechanisms of action in greater depth, and carry out meticulously planned clinical trials. Additionally, the exploration of innovative alternatives such as postbiotics, bacteriophages, and genetically engineered probiotics may open up new avenues for innovative and safe therapeutic strategies.

9.6 FUTURE INSIGHTS INTO MICROBIOME-GUIDED ONCOLOGY FOR PERSONALIZED CANCER TREATMENTS

The growing body of evidence underlines the significance of gut microbiota on cancer progression and treatment responses; however, the precise mechanisms underlying this interaction remain largely unclear. This complexity is attributed to factors such as microbial-derived metabolites, immunological modulation, and intricate interactions with host cellular signaling pathways (Kamel et al., 2024). To close these knowledge gaps, future research should integrate advanced methodologies including metagenomics, metabolomics, and immunoprofiling to unravel the functional dynamics of specific microbial taxa in oncogenesis and therapeutic outcomes. Such multidimensional insights are essential for establishing microbiome-driven frameworks in personalized oncology. Therapeutic modalities such as FMT, as well as incorporating probiotics and postbiotics, are currently under investigation for their ability to restore gut microbial equilibrium and bolster host immune function (Yadav & Chauhan, 2021). Moreover, the innovation of engineered probiotic strains and bacteriophage-based interventions presents promising avenues for selectively modulating tumor-associated microbiota, potentially curtailing cancer progression and enhancing clinical outcomes (Meng et al., 2022).

The emergence of individualized cancer therapies—particularly mRNA-based vaccines—has significantly advanced the capacity to customize treatments based on each patient's unique molecular profile. These vaccines employ tumor-specific neoantigen identification through genomic sequencing, enabling the generation of highly targeted immunotherapies that potentiate anti-tumor immune responses (Li et al., 2024). Incorporating microbiome profiles into these personalized strategies could further optimize therapeutic efficacy by accounting for microbial influences on host immunity and pharmacokinetics. This integrative model offers a promising direction for minimizing adverse effects and maximizing clinical benefit. However, the clinical translation of microbiome-based oncology approaches necessitates standardized protocols for microbial analysis and therapeutic deployment. Moving forward, robust, large-scale clinical trials are necessary to substantiate the therapeutic potential of microbiome-targeted interventions and to formulate regulatory guidelines for their implementation. In parallel, advances in multi-omics platforms and artificial intelligence will be pivotal in delineating host–microbe interactions, thereby enabling the realization of truly personalized, microbiome-guided cancer treatments.

9.7 CONCLUSION

The integration of probiotics into personalized cancer therapy offers a promising and innovative approach to enhancing treatment outcomes. As microbiome-based diagnostics advance, microbiota profiling could become a valuable tool in predicting individual responses to treatments, allowing for the selection of optimal probiotic strains tailored to each patient's needs. This personalized strategy holds the potential to complement conventional therapies, improving efficacy while minimizing treatment-related toxicities. While clinical trials continue to evaluate the safety and effectiveness of combining probiotics with traditional cancer treatments, early evidence suggests that such interventions may positively impact immune profiles, alleviate gastrointestinal toxicity, and potentially improve overall survival rates. Given the increasing evidence and potential benefits, probiotics may emerge as a cost-effective, less invasive option that could revolutionize cancer therapy, offering a unique strategy to improve patient outcomes in the near future.

REFERENCES

Al-Fakhrany, O. M., & Elekhnawy, E. (2024). Next-generation probiotics: The upcoming biotherapeutics. *Molecular Biology Reports*, *51*(1), 505. https://doi.org/10.1007/s11033-024-09398-5

Altonsy, M. O., Andrews, S. C., & Tuohy, K. M. (2010). Differential induction of apoptosis in human colonic carcinoma cells (Caco-2) by Atopobium, and commensal, probiotic and enteropathogenic bacteria: Mediation by the mitochondrial pathway. *International Journal of Food Microbiology*, *137*(2–3), Article 2–3. https://doi.org/10.1016/j.ijfoodmicro.2009.11.015

Bassaganya-Riera, J., Viladomiu, M., Pedragosa, M., De Simone, C., & Hontecillas, R. (2012). Immunoregulatory mechanisms underlying prevention of colitis-associated colorectal cancer by probiotic bacteria. *PLoS ONE*, *7*(4), Article 4. https://doi.org/10.1371/journal.pone.0034676

Binnewies, M., Roberts, E. W., Kersten, K., Chan, V., Fearon, D. F., Merad, M., Coussens, L. M., Gabrilovich, D. I., Ostrand-Rosenberg, S., Hedrick, C. C., Vonderheide, R. H., Pittet, M. J., Jain, R. K., Zou, W., Howcroft, T. K., Woodhouse, E. C., Weinberg, R. A., & Krummel, M. F. (2018). Understanding the tumor immune microenvironment (TIME) for effective therapy. *Nature Medicine*, *24*(5), Article 5. https://doi.org/10.1038/s41591-018-0014-x

Bray, F., Laversanne, M., Sung, H., Ferlay, J., Siegel, R. L., Soerjomataram, I., & Jemal, A. (2024). Global cancer statistics 2022: GLOBOCAN estimates of incidence and mortality worldwide for 36 cancers in 185 countries. *CA: A Cancer Journal for Clinicians*, *74*(3), 229–263. https://doi.org/10.3322/caac.21834

Capurso, L. (2019). Thirty years of *Lactobacillus rhamnosus* GG: A review. *Journal of Clinical Gastroenterology*, *53*(Suppl 1), S1–S41. https://doi.org/10.1097/MCG.0000000000001170

Chandrasekaran, P., Weiskirchen, S., & Weiskirchen, R. (2024). Effects of probiotics on gut microbiota: An overview. *International Journal of Molecular Sciences*, *25*(11), 6022. https://doi.org/10.3390/ijms25116022

Chang, C.-Y., Ho, B.-Y., & Pan, T.-M. (2019). *Lactobacillus paracasei* subsp. *Paracasei* NTU 101-fermented skim milk as an adjuvant to uracil-tegafur reduces tumor growth and improves chemotherapy side effects in an orthotopic mouse model of colorectal cancer. *Journal of Functional Foods*, *55*, 36–47. https://doi.org/10.1016/j.jff.2019.02.025

Charbonneau, M. R., Isabella, V. M., Li, N., & Kurtz, C. B. (2020). Developing a new class of engineered live bacterial therapeutics to treat human diseases. *Nature Communications*, *11*(1), 1738. https://doi.org/10.1038/s41467-020-15508-1

Chattaraj, S., Mitra, D., Chattaraj, A., Chattaraj, M., Kundu, M., Ganguly, A., & Mohapatra, P. K. D. (2025). Antioncogenic potential of probiotics: Challenges and future prospective. *Indian Journal of Microbiology Research*, *10*(1), Article 1. https://doi.org/10.18231/j.ijmr.2023.001

Chau, T.-L., Göktuna, S. I., Rammal, A., Casanova, T., Duong, H.-Q., Gatot, J.-S., Close, P., Dejardin, E., Desmecht, D., Shostak, K., & Chariot, A. (2015). A role for APPL1 in TLR3/4-dependent TBK1 and IKKε activation in macrophages. *The Journal of Immunology*, *194*(8), 3970–3983. https://doi.org/10.4049/jimmunol.1401614

Chowdhury, T., Rushni, Z., Anjum, H., & Mouree, K. R. (2024). Microbial allies: Personalized probiotics and their role in tailoring cancer immunotherapies. *Cancer Plus*, *6*(2), Article 2. https://doi.org/10.36922/cp.3289

Colella, G., Boschetti, C. E., Vitagliano, R., Colella, C., Jiao, L., King-Smith, N., Li, C., Nuoh Lau, Y., Lai, Z., Mohammed, A. I., & Cirillo, N. (2023). Interventions for the prevention of oral mucositis in patients receiving cancer treatment: Evidence from randomised controlled trials. *Current Oncology*, *30*(1), 967–980. https://doi.org/10.3390/curroncol30010074

Darb Emamie, A., Rajabpour, M., Ghanavati, R., Asadolahi, P., Farzi, S., Sobouti, B., & Darbandi, A. (2021). The effects of probiotics, prebiotics and synbiotics on the reduction of IBD complications, a periodic review during 2009-2020. *Journal of Applied Microbiology*, *130*(6), 1823–1838. https://doi.org/10.1111/jam.14907

Davar, D., Dzutsev, A. K., McCulloch, J. A., Rodrigues, R. R., Chauvin, J.-M., Morrison, R. M., Deblasio, R. N., Menna, C., Ding, Q., Pagliano, O., Zidi, B., Zhang, S., Badger, J. H., Vetizou, M., Cole, A. M., Fernandes, M. R., Prescott, S., Costa, R. G. F., Balaji, A. K., … & Zarour, H. M.. (2021). Fecal microbiota transplant overcomes resistance to anti–PD-1 therapy in melanoma patients. *Science*. https://doi.org/10.1126/science.abf3363

Deepak, V., Ramachandran, S., Balahmar, R. M., Pandian, S. R. K., Sivasubramaniam, S. D., Nellaiah, H., & Sundar, K. (2016). In vitro evaluation of anticancer properties of exopolysaccharides from *Lactobacillus acidophilus* in colon cancer cell lines. *In Vitro Cellular & Developmental Biology - Animal*, *52*(2), Article 2. https://doi.org/10.1007/s11626-015-9970-3

El-Deeb, N. M., Yassin, A. M., Al-Madboly, L. A., & El-Hawiet, A. (2018). A novel purified *Lactobacillus acidophilus* 20079 exopolysaccharide, LA-EPS-20079, molecularly regulates both apoptotic and NF-κB inflammatory pathways in human colon cancer. *Microbial Cell Factories*, *17*(1), Article 1. https://doi.org/10.1186/s12934-018-0877-z

Farran, B., Montenegro, R. C., Kasa, P., Pavitra, E., Huh, Y. S., Han, Y.-K., Kamal, M. A., Nagaraju, G. P., & Rama Raju, G. S. (2020). Folate-conjugated nanovehicles: Strategies for cancer therapy. *Materials Science & Engineering. C, Materials for Biological Applications*, *107*, 110341. https://doi.org/10.1016/j.msec.2019.110341

Farrell, J. J., Zhang, L., Zhou, H., Chia, D., Elashoff, D., Akin, D., Paster, B. J., Joshipura, K., & Wong, D. T. W. (2012). Variations of oral microbiota are associated with pancreatic diseases including pancreatic cancer. *Gut*, *61*(4), 582–588. https://doi.org/10.1136/gutjnl-2011-300784

Fassarella, M., Blaak, E. E., Penders, J., Nauta, A., Smidt, H., & Zoetendal, E. G. (2021). Gut microbiome stability and resilience: Elucidating the response to perturbations in order to modulate gut health. *Gut*, *70*(3). https://doi.org/10.1136/gutjnl-2020-321747

Gao, G., Ma, T., Zhang, T., Jin, H., Li, Y., Kwok, L.-Y., Zhang, H., & Sun, Z. (2021). Adjunctive probiotic *Lactobacillus rhamnosus* probio-M9 administration enhances the effect of anti-PD-1 antitumor therapy via restoring antibiotic-disrupted gut microbiota. *Frontiers in Immunology*, *12*, 772532. https://doi.org/10.3389/fimmu.2021.772532

Gao, R., Gao, Z., Huang, L., & Qin, H. (2017). Gut microbiota and colorectal cancer. *European Journal of Clinical Microbiology & Infectious Diseases: Official Publication of the European Society of Clinical Microbiology*, *36*(5), 757–769. https://doi.org/10.1007/s10096-016-2881-8

Gopalakrishnan, V., Spencer, C. N., Nezi, L., Reuben, A., Andrews, M. C., Karpinets, T. V., Prieto, P. A., Vicente, D., Hoffman, K., Wei, S. C., Cogdill, A. P., Zhao, L., Hudgens, C. W., Hutchinson, D. S., Manzo, T., Petaccia de Macedo, M., Cotechini, T., Kumar, T., Chen, W. S., …, & Wargo, J. A. (2018). Gut microbiome modulates response to anti–PD-1 immunotherapy in melanoma patients. *Science*, *359*(6371), 97–103. https://doi.org/10.1126/science.aan4236

Guarner, F., Sanders, M. E., Szajewska, H., Cohen, H., Eliakim, R., Herrera-deGuise, C., Karakan, T., Merenstein, D., Piscoya, A., Ramakrishna, B., Salminen, S., & Melberg, J. (2024). World gastroenterology organisation global guidelines: Probiotics and prebiotics. *Journal of Clinical Gastroenterology, 58*(6), 533–553. https://doi.org/10.1097/MCG.0000000000002002

Guha, D., Banerjee, A., Mukherjee, R., Pradhan, B., Peneva, M., Aleksandrov, G., Suklabaidya, S., Senapati, S., & Aich, P. (2019). A probiotic formulation containing *Lactobacillus bulgaricus* DWT1 inhibits tumor growth by activating pro-inflammatory responses in macrophages. *Journal of Functional Foods, 56*, 232–245. https://doi.org/10.1016/j.jff.2019.03.030

Guo, R., Chen, L.-H., Xing, C., & Liu, T. (2019). Pain regulation by gut microbiota: Molecular mechanisms and therapeutic potential. *British Journal of Anaesthesia, 123*(5), 637–654. https://doi.org/10.1016/j.bja.2019.07.026

Gupta, S., Tomar, A., & Singh, R. (2025). Personalized medicine in oral cancer. *Critical Reviews in Oncology/Hematology, 209*, 104670. https://doi.org/10.1016/j.critrevonc.2025.104670

Han, K. J., Lee, N.-K., Park, H., & Paik, H.-D. (2015). Anticancer and anti-inflammatory activity of probiotic *Lactococcus lactis* NK34. *Journal of Microbiology and Biotechnology, 25*(10), Article 10. https://doi.org/10.4014/jmb.1503.03033

Han, Z.-Y., Fu, Z.-J., Wang, Y.-Z., Zhang, C., Chen, Q.-W., An, J.-X., & Zhang, X.-Z. (2024). Probiotics functionalized with a gallium-polyphenol network modulate the intratumor microbiota and promote antitumor immune responses in pancreatic cancer. *Nature Communications, 15*(1), Article 1. https://doi.org/10.1038/s41467-024-51534-z

Hempel, S., Newberry, S., Ruelaz, A., Wang, Z., Miles, J. N. V., Suttorp, M. J., Johnsen, B., Shanman, R., Slusser, W., Fu, N., Smith, A., Roth, B., Polak, J., Motala, A., Perry, T., & Shekelle, P. G. (2011). Safety of probiotics used to reduce risk and prevent or treat disease. *Evidence Report/Technology Assessment, 200*, 1–645.

Hwang, J. W., Baek, Y.-M., Yang, K. E., Yoo, H.-S., Cho, C.-K., Lee, Y.-W., Park, J., Eom, C.-Y., Lee, Z.-W., Choi, J.-S., & Jang, I.-S. (2013). *Lactobacillus casei* extract induces apoptosis in gastric cancer by inhibiting NF-κB and mTOR-mediated signaling. *Integrative Cancer Therapies, 12*(2), Article 2. https://doi.org/10.1177/1534735412442380

Jackson, S. E., & Chester, J. D. (2015). Personalised cancer medicine. *International Journal of Cancer, 137*(2), 262–266. https://doi.org/10.1002/ijc.28940

Kamel, M., Aleya, S., Alsubih, M., & Aleya, L. (2024). Microbiome dynamics: A paradigm shift in combatting infectious diseases. *Journal of Personalized Medicine, 14*(2), 217. https://doi.org/10.3390/jpm14020217

Lakritz, J. R., Poutahidis, T., Levkovich, T., Varian, B. J., Ibrahim, Y. M., Chatzigiagkos, A., Mirabal, S., Alm, E. J., & Erdman, S. E. (2014). Beneficial bacteria stimulate host immune cells to counteract dietary and genetic predisposition to mammary cancer in mice. *International Journal of Cancer, 135*(3), 529–540. https://doi.org/10.1002/ijc.28702

Latif, A., Shehzad, A., Niazi, S., Zahid, A., Ashraf, W., Iqbal, M. W., Rehman, A., Riaz, T., Aadil, R. M., Khan, I. M., Özogul, F., Rocha, J. M., Esatbeyoglu, T., & Korma, S. A. (2023). Probiotics: Mechanism of action, health benefits and their application in food industries. *Frontiers in Microbiology, 14*, 1216674. https://doi.org/10.3389/fmicb.2023.1216674

Legesse Bedada, T., Feto, T. K., Awoke, K. S., Garedew, A. D., Yifat, F. T., & Birri, D. J. (2020). Probiotics for cancer alternative prevention and treatment. *Biomedicine & Pharmacotherapy, 129*, 110409. https://doi.org/10.1016/j.biopha.2020.110409

Li, T., Lin, C., & Wang, W. (2025). Global, regional, and national burden of pancreatic cancer from 1990 to 2021, its attributable risk factors, and projections to 2050: A systematic analysis of the global burden of disease study 2021. *BMC Cancer, 25*, 189. https://doi.org/10.1186/s12885-025-13597-z

Li, X., You, J., Hong, L., Liu, W., Guo, P., & Hao, X. (2024). Neoantigen cancer vaccines: A new star on the horizon. *Cancer Biology & Medicine, 21*(4), 274–311. https://doi.org/10.20892/j.issn.2095-3941.2023.0395

Liu, B., Zhou, H., Tan, L., Siu, K. T. H., & Guan, X.-Y. (2024). Exploring treatment options in cancer: Tumor treatment strategies. *Signal Transduction and Targeted Therapy, 9*(1), 1–44. https://doi.org/10.1038/s41392-024-01856-7

Liu, Y.-C., Wu, C.-R., & Huang, T.-W. (2022). Preventive effect of probiotics on Oral mucositis induced by cancer treatment: A systematic review and meta-analysis. *International Journal of Molecular Sciences, 23*(21), 13268. https://doi.org/10.3390/ijms232113268

Marino, P., Mininni, M., Deiana, G., Marino, G., Divella, R., Bochicchio, I., Giuliano, A., Lapadula, S., Lettini, A. R., & Sanseverino, F. (2024). Healthy lifestyle and cancer risk: Modifiable risk factors to prevent cancer. *Nutrients, 16*(6), 800. https://doi.org/10.3390/nu16060800

Maroof, H., Hassan, Z. M., Mobarez, A. M., & Mohamadabadi, M. A. (2012). *Lactobacillus acidophilus* could modulate the immune response against breast cancer in murine model. *Journal of Clinical Immunology*, *32*(6), Article 6. https://doi.org/10.1007/s10875-012-9708-x

Matson, V., Fessler, J., Bao, R., Chongsuwat, T., Zha, Y., Alegre, M.-L., Luke, J. J., & Gajewski, T. F. (2018). The commensal microbiome is associated with anti-PD-1 efficacy in metastatic melanoma patients. *Science*, *359*(6371), 104–108. https://doi.org/10.1126/science.aao3290

Mego, M., Holec, V., Drgona, L., Hainova, K., Ciernikova, S., & Zajac, V. (2013). Probiotic bacteria in cancer patients undergoing chemotherapy and radiation therapy. *Complementary Therapies in Medicine*, *21*(6), 712–723. https://doi.org/10.1016/j.ctim.2013.08.018

Mendes, M. C. S., Paulino, D. S., Brambilla, S. R., Camargo, J. A., Persinoti, G. F., & Carvalheira, J. B. C. (2018). Microbiota modification by probiotic supplementation reduces colitis associated colon cancer in mice. *World Journal of Gastroenterology*, *24*(18), 1995–2008. https://doi.org/10.3748/wjg.v24.i18.1995

Mendoza, L. (2019). Potential effect of probiotics in the treatment of breast cancer. *Oncology Reviews*, *13*(2), 422. https://doi.org/10.4081/oncol.2019.422

Meng, Z., Ye, Z., Zhu, P., Zhu, J., Fang, S., Qiu, T., Li, Y., & Meng, L. (2022). New developments and opportunities of microbiota in treating breast cancers. *Frontiers in Microbiology*, *13*. https://doi.org/10.3389/fmicb.2022.818793

Miller, W. H., Routy, B., Jamal, R., Ernst, D. S., Logan, D., Esfahani, K., Belanger, K., Elkrief, A., Lapointe, R., Thebault, P., Ponce, M., Parvathy, S. N., Messaoudene, M., Silverman, M., Maleki, S., & Lenehan, J. G. (2022). Fecal microbiota transplantation followed by anti–PD-1 treatment in patients with advanced melanoma. *Journal of Clinical Oncology*, *40*(16_suppl), 9533–9533. https://doi.org/10.1200/JCO.2022.40.16_suppl.9533

Molujin, A. M., Abbasiliasi, S., Nurdin, A., Lee, P.-C., Gansau, J. A., & Jawan, R. (2022). Bacteriocins as potential therapeutic approaches in the treatment of various cancers: A review of in vitro studies. *Cancers*, *14*(19), Article 19. https://doi.org/10.3390/cancers14194758

Mukherjee, S., Kumar, D., & Guha, D. (2024). Insights of probiotics as an alternative medicine for cancer therapy, mechanism, and applications. *Medicine in Microecology*, *22*, 100111. https://doi.org/10.1016/j.medmic.2024.100111

Naeem, H., Hassan, H. U., Shahbaz, M., Imran, M., Memon, A. G., Hasnain, A., Murtaza, S., Alsagaby, S. A., Al Abdulmonem, W., Hussain, M., Abdelgawad, M. A., Ghoneim, M. M., & Al Jbawi, E. (2024). Role of probiotics against human cancers, inflammatory diseases, and other complex malignancies. *Journal of Food Biochemistry*, *2024*, 1–6632209. https://doi.org/10.1155/2024/6632209

Nair, A., Anto, E. M., & Purushothaman, J. (2021). Probiotics in Colon Cancer: A Therapeutic Approach. In N. K. Vishvakarma, G. P. Nagaraju, & D. Shukla (Eds.), *Colon Cancer Diagnosis and Therapy* (pp. 421–434). Springer International Publishing. https://doi.org/10.1007/978-3-030-64668-4_18

Najmi, M., Tran, T., Witt, R. G., & Nelson, K. C. (2022). Modulation of the gut microbiome to enhance immunotherapy response in metastatic melanoma patients: A clinical review. *Dermatology and Therapy*, *12*(11), 2489–2497. https://doi.org/10.1007/s13555-022-00810-1

Nama, A. S. A., Sandeepa, G. M., Buddolla, V., & Mastan, A. (2025). Advances in understanding therapeutic mechanisms of probiotics in cancer management, with special emphasis on breast cancer: A comprehensive review. *European Journal of Pharmacology*, *995*, 177410. https://doi.org/10.1016/j.ejphar.2025.177410

O'Toole, P. W., Marchesi, J. R., & Hill, C. (2017). Next-generation probiotics: The spectrum from probiotics to live biotherapeutics. *Nature Microbiology*, *2*(5), 1–6. https://doi.org/10.1038/nmicrobiol.2017.57

Pei, B., Peng, S., Huang, C., & Zhou, F. (2024). *Bifidobacterium* modulation of tumor immunotherapy and its mechanism. *Cancer Immunology, Immunotherapy: CII*, *73*(5), 94. https://doi.org/10.1007/s00262-024-03665-x

Perera, M., Al-Hebshi, N. N., Speicher, D. J., Perera, I., & Johnson, N. W. (2016). Emerging role of bacteria in oral carcinogenesis: A review with special reference to perio-pathogenic bacteria. *Journal of Oral Microbiology*, *8*, 32762. https://doi.org/10.3402/jom.v8.32762

Pizzo, F., Maroccia, Z., Hammarberg Ferri, I., & Fiorentini, C. (2022). Role of the microbiota in lung cancer: Insights on prevention and treatment. *International Journal of Molecular Sciences*, *23*(11), Article 11. https://doi.org/10.3390/ijms23116138

Plottel, C. S., & Blaser, M. J. (2011). Microbiome and malignancy. *Cell Host & Microbe*, *10*(4), 324–335. https://doi.org/10.1016/j.chom.2011.10.003

Pradhan, B., Guha, D., Naik, A. K., Banerjee, A., Tambat, S., Chawla, S., Senapati, S., & Aich, P. (2019). Probiotics *L. acidophilus* and *B. clausii* modulate gut microbiota in Th1- and Th2-biased mice to ameliorate Salmonella Typhimurium-induced diarrhea. *Probiotics and Antimicrobial Proteins*, *11*(3), 887–904. https://doi.org/10.1007/s12602-018-9436-5

Pushalkar, S., Hundeyin, M., Daley, D., Zambirinis, C. P., Kurz, E., Mishra, A., Mohan, N., Aykut, B., Usyk, M., Torres, L. E., Werba, G., Zhang, K., Guo, Y., Li, Q., Akkad, N., Lall, S., Wadowski, B., Gutierrez, J., Kochen Rossi, J. A., …, & Miller, G. (2018). The pancreatic cancer microbiome promotes oncogenesis by induction of innate and adaptive immune suppression. *Cancer Discovery*, *8*(4), 403–416. https://doi.org/10.1158/2159-8290.CD-17-1134

Rajoka, M. S. R., Zhao, H., Lu, Y., Lian, Z., Li, N., Hussain, N., Shao, D., Jin, M., Li, Q., & Shi, J. (2018). Anticancer potential against cervix cancer (HeLa) cell line of probiotic *Lactobacillus casei* and *Lactobacillus paracasei* strains isolated from human breast milk. *Food & Function*, *9*(5), Article 5. https://doi.org/10.1039/C8FO00547H

Routy, B., Le Chatelier, E., Derosa, L., Duong, C. P. M., Alou, M. T., Daillère, R., Fluckiger, A., Messaoudene, M., Rauber, C., Roberti, M. P., Fidelle, M., Flament, C., Poirier-Colame, V., Opolon, P., Klein, C., Iribarren, K., Mondragón, L., Jacquelot, N., Qu, B., …, & Zitvogel, L. (2018). Gut microbiome influences efficacy of PD-1-based immunotherapy against epithelial tumors. *Science (New York, N.Y.)*, *359*(6371), 91–97. https://doi.org/10.1126/science.aan3706

Samanta, S. (2022). Potential impacts of prebiotics and probiotics on cancer prevention. *Anti-Cancer Agents in Medicinal Chemistry*, *22*(4), Article 4. https://doi.org/10.2174/1871520621999201210220442

Seo, B.-B., Choi, H., Koh, J.-T., & Song, S.-C. (2015). Sustained BMP-2 delivery and injectable bone regeneration using thermosensitive polymeric nanoparticle hydrogel bearing dual interactions with BMP-2. *Journal of Controlled Release*, *209*, 67–76. https://doi.org/10.1016/j.jconrel.2015.04.023

Shamloo, H. B., Shahabi, A., Aghazadeh, Z., & Yari Khosroushahi, A. (2020). *Pichia fermentans* originates apoptosis in human oral squamous cell carcinoma by over-expressing BAX and CASP 9 genes. *Cytotechnology*, *72*(3), Article 3. https://doi.org/10.1007/s10616-020-00392-w

Sivan, A., Corrales, L., Hubert, N., Williams, J. B., Aquino-Michaels, K., Earley, Z. M., Benyamin, F. W., Lei, Y. M., Jabri, B., Alegre, M.-L., Chang, E. B., & Gajewski, T. F. (2015). Commensal *Bifidobacterium* promotes antitumor immunity and facilitates anti-PD-L1 efficacy. *Science (New York, N.Y.)*, *350*(6264), 1084–1089. https://doi.org/10.1126/science.aac4255

Sourav, C., Debasis, M., Abhishek, C., Manasi, C., Meghna, K., Arindam, G., & Pradeep, K. (2023). Antioncogenic potential of probiotics: Challenges and future prospective. *Indian Journal of Pharmacy and Pharmacology*, *2023*, 18793. https://doi.org/10.18231/j.ijmr.2023.001

So, S.S.Y., Wan, M.L.Y., & El-Nezami, H. (2017). Probiotics-mediated suppression of cancer. *Current Opinion in Oncology*, *29*(1). https://doi.org/10.1097/CCO.0000000000000342

Stasiewicz, M., & Karpiński, T. M. (2022). The oral microbiota and its role in carcinogenesis. *Seminars in Cancer Biology*, *86*, 633–642. https://doi.org/10.1016/j.semcancer.2021.11.002

Sudaarsan, A. S. K., & Ghosh, A. R. (2024). Appraisal of postbiotics in cancer therapy. *Frontiers in Pharmacology*, *15*. https://doi.org/10.3389/fphar.2024.1436021

Sun, R., Dou, W., Liu, W., Li, J., Han, X., Li, S., Wu, X., Wang, F., Xu, X., & Li, J. (2023). Global, regional, and national burden of oral cancer and its attributable risk factors from 1990 to 2019. *Cancer Medicine*, *12*(12), 13811–13820. https://doi.org/10.1002/cam4.6025

Sungur, T., Aslim, B., Karaaslan, C., & Aktas, B. (2017). Impact of Exopolysaccharides (EPSs) of *Lactobacillus gasseri* strains isolated from human vagina on cervical tumor cells (HeLa). *Anaerobe*, *47*, 137–144. https://doi.org/10.1016/j.anaerobe.2017.05.013

Thoda, C., & Touraki, M. (2023). Probiotic-derived bioactive compounds in colorectal cancer treatment. *Microorganisms*, *11*(8), Article 8. https://doi.org/10.3390/microorganisms11081898

Thu, M. S., Ondee, T., Nopsopon, T., Farzana, I. A. K., Fothergill, J. L., Hirankarn, N., Campbell, B. J., & Pongpirul, K. (2023). Effect of probiotics in breast cancer: A systematic review and meta-analysis. *Biology*, *12*(2), Article 2. https://doi.org/10.3390/biology12020280

Tian, Q., Price, N. D., & Hood, L. (2012). Systems cancer medicine: Towards realization of predictive, preventive, personalized and participatory (P4) medicine. *Journal of Internal Medicine*, *271*(2), 111–121. https://doi.org/10.1111/j.1365-2796.2011.02498.x

Tian, Y., Xu, Q., Sun, L., Ye, Y., & Ji, G. (2018). Short-chain fatty acids administration is protective in colitis-associated colorectal cancer development. *The Journal of Nutritional Biochemistry*, *57*, 103–109. https://doi.org/10.1016/j.jnutbio.2018.03.007

Tremaroli, V., & Bäckhed, F. (2012). Functional interactions between the gut microbiota and host metabolism. *Nature*, *489*(7415), 242–249. https://doi.org/10.1038/nature11552

Tukenmez, U., Aktas, B., Aslim, B., & Yavuz, S. (2019). The relationship between the structural characteristics of lactobacilli-EPS and its ability to induce apoptosis in colon cancer cells in vitro. *Scientific Reports*, *9*(1), Article 1. https://doi.org/10.1038/s41598-019-44753-8

Vipperla, K., & O'Keefe, S. J. (2016). Diet, microbiota, and dysbiosis: A 'recipe' for colorectal cancer. *Food & Function*, *7*(4), 1731–1740. https://doi.org/10.1039/c5fo01276g

Yadav, M., & Chauhan, N. S. (2021). Microbiome therapeutics: Exploring the present scenario and challenges. *Gastroenterology Report*, *10*, goab046. https://doi.org/10.1093/gastro/goab046

Zaharuddin, L., Mokhtar, N. M., Muhammad Nawawi, K. N., & Raja Ali, R. A. (2019). A randomized double-blind placebo-controlled trial of probiotics in post-surgical colorectal cancer. *BMC Gastroenterology*, *19*(1), 131. https://doi.org/10.1186/s12876-019-1047-4

Zhu, Z., Yi, B., Tang, Z., Chen, X., Li, M., Xu, T., Zhao, Z., & Tang, C. (2023). *Lactobacillus casei* combined with *Lactobacillus reuteri* alleviate pancreatic cancer by inhibiting TLR4 to promote macrophage M1 polarization and regulate gut microbial homeostasis. *BMC Cancer*, *23*(1), 1044. https://doi.org/10.1186/s12885-023-11557-z

10 Mitochondrial Dysfunction in Gliomas

Pathophysiological Insights and Therapeutic Targets

Charles Emmanuel Jebaraj Walter[#] *and Tina Sara Biju*[#]
Sri Ramachandra Institute of Higher Education and Research (DU), Chennai, India

Zioni Sangeetha Shankaran
Sree Balaji Medical College and Hospital, Chennai, India

Lawrence D. Cruze
Sri Ramachandra Institute of Higher Education and Research (DU), Chennai, India

Thanka Johnson and Jezra Emmanuel Walter
Sree Balaji Medical College and Hospital, Chennai, India

Christhunesa Soundararajan Christudass
Christian Medical College, Vellore, India

10.1 INTRODUCTION

Gliomas are the most prevalent form of primary brain tumor, characterized by glial cell origin and great variability of clinical presentation and prognosis (1). Gliomas are classified by the World Health Organization (WHO) according to histopathological features and molecular markers into various subtypes, i.e., astrocytomas, oligodendrogliomas, and glioblastomas, with disparate genetic composition and responsiveness to treatment (2). Gliomas, including the high-grade forms like glioblastoma (GB), even with advancements in the traditional treatment modalities like surgery, radiotherapy, and chemotherapy, are difficult to treat owing to their malignant behavior and resistance to conventional therapy.

Recent studies have highlighted the pivotal role of mitochondrial dysfunction in glioma pathophysiologic processes. Mitochondria are essential organelles that play a role in energy production, handling of reactive oxygen species (ROS), and induction of apoptosis. Structural and functional alterations of mitochondria have been implicated in tumor growth, impacting

[#] These authors share the first authorship.

DOI: 10.1201/9781003644309-10

a series of processes including metabolic reprogramming, evasion of programmed cell death, and increased invasiveness (3). Notably, glioma cells are often described by metabolic disturbances, particularly by an adaptation to glycolysis rather than oxidative phosphorylation (OXPHOS) so-called Warburg effect even in the presence of oxygen. Such metabolic reprogramming allows for fast cell growth and also provides resistance to therapeutic interventions (4,5).

In this era of precision oncology, the determination of the molecular bases that cause the initiation and growth of gliomas is central to the quest for the identification of new targets for therapy. Mitochondria have emerged as promising targets, with ideas conceived to exploit mitochondrial vulnerabilities to selectively destroy tumor cells (6). Mechanisms involving mitochondrial metabolism inhibition, mitochondrial apoptosis induction, and mitochondrial DNA (mtDNA) mutation targeting are being investigated, with the potential to be directions toward improved and personalized therapies of glioma. In this chapter, we will explain the complex relationship between mitochondrial dysfunction and glioma pathophysiology and the function of mitochondrial alterations in tumor progression and drug resistance. The current and future mitochondrial-targeted therapeutic approaches in the setting of precision neuro-oncology, with the goal of giving an integrated description of how mitochondrial information can enlighten and refine glioma models of treatment, are also focused.

10.2 GLIOMAS IN THE ERA OF PRECISION NEURO-ONCOLOGY

Gliomas, the most common primary brain neoplasms, have imposing therapeutic challenges based on their heterogeneity and malignant biology. Precision neuro-oncology has transformed its treatment through the personalization of therapies with respect to the patient-specific tumor molecular profiles, thus increasing the diagnostic specificity and therapeutic efficacy (7). One of the most significant developments in this field is the inclusion of molecular profiling in the model of glioma classification by the WHO in 2016, and the revised one in 2021 includes important genetic alterations, such as isocitrate dehydrogenase (IDH) mutations, 1p/19q codeletion, and Telomerase Reverse Transcriptase (TERT) promoter mutations, in the diagnostic criteria (8). For instance, IDH mutations, seen in approximately 70% of lower-grade gliomas, are associated with a unique hypermethylation phenotype and better prognosis. Similarly, the 1p/19q codeletion is identified as a characteristic of oligodendrogliomas, indicating improved efficacy with the use of certain chemotherapeutic drugs (8,9). Targeted agents have evolved to exploit these molecular findings.

Mutant IDH inhibitors, such as ivosidenib and vorasidenib, have managed to reduce the oncometabolite D-2-hydroxyglutarate, thereby inhibiting glioma growth (10). Clinical trials have shown that vorasidenib significantly improves progression-free survival in IDH-mutant glioma patients by 27.7 months compared to placebo by 11.1 months (11,12). In addition, gliomas with the BRAF V600E mutation have been shown to be sensitive to BRAF and MEK inhibitor combination, such as dabrafenib and trametinib, emphasizing the use of molecular profiling in the direction of therapeutic strategies (13). Despite these advances, challenges persist in the application of precision medicine to gliomas. The blood–brain barrier (BBB) hinders the delivery of the majority of therapeutic agents, and intratumoral heterogeneity makes treatment approaches challenging (14). In addition, continued expansion of glioma genomes necessitates continued monitoring to modulate therapeutic approaches as necessary.

10.3 MITOCHONDRIAL BIOLOGY IN NEURAL TISSUES

Mitochondria are essential organelles of neural tissue required for maintenance of the high-energy requirements and intricate processes of neurons, such as axonal and dendritic development, synaptic function, and axonal regeneration (15). In addition to their well-established function in adenosine triphosphate (ATP) production by OXPHOS, mitochondria are also essential for calcium homeostasis, ROS regulation, and control of apoptotic pathways, all of which are required for neuronal development, function, and survival (16).

10.3.1 Energy Generation and Metabolic Adjustments

Neurons, with their polarized morphology and synaptic function, need to consume a lot of energy to sustain ionic gradients, generate action potentials, and release neurotransmitters. These needs are addressed by mitochondria through the production of ATP by OXPHOS, an activity that is especially relevant considering the brain's utilization of about 20% of the body's total energy despite its weight of only about 2% of body weight (17). During differentiation of neurons, there is a shift in metabolism from glycolysis to OXPHOS, which is paralleled by an increase in mitochondrial mass and activity, showing the organelle's role in supporting neuronal maturation and function (18).

10.3.2 Mitochondrial Dynamics: Fission, Fusion, and Trafficking

Mitochondria are dynamic organelles that are constantly undergoing fission and fusion events, which are important in maintaining mitochondrial integrity and function. Fusion permits the intermixing of mitochondrial contents, thus diluting damaged components and facilitating repair mechanisms, whereas fission is important in mitochondrial biogenesis and elimination of defective mitochondria through mitophagy. In neurons, the precise targeting of mitochondria to axons, dendrites, and synaptic terminals is essential for localized energy supply and buffering of calcium levels (19,20). Alterations in mitochondrial dynamics can lead to defective synaptic function and have also been implicated in a variety of neurodegenerative diseases.

Calcium homeostasis and signaling mitochondria are also important in the regulation of intracellular calcium levels, serving as stores that take up and release calcium ions based on neuronal activity (21,22). This is important for synaptic plasticity and transmission because calcium signaling has an effect on gene expression and neurotransmitter release. Abnormality in the regulation of mitochondrial calcium may lead to synaptic pathology and play a role in the pathogenesis of neurological disorders.

10.3.3 Mitochondrial Contribution to Neurogenesis and Neural Maturation

Advances in research emphasize the crucial role of mitochondria in neurogenesis and neural development. Neural Stem Cell (NSCs) depend on mitochondrial function to attain a balance between self-renewal and differentiation. Mitochondrial biogenesis and the transition to OXPHOS are seen in differentiation, supplying the energy requirements of the developing neurons (23,24). Impairment in mitochondrial function during such pivotal stages can negatively impact neuronal development and has been associated with neurodevelopmental disorders.

10.3.4 Implications for Neurological Disorders

Mitochondrial dysfunction is a unifying factor for several neurological diseases, including Alzheimer's, Parkinson's disease, and amyotrophic lateral sclerosis (ALS) (25). Mitochondrial dynamics, abnormal bioenergetics, and increased oxidative stress are key factors in neuronal degeneration in these pathologies. A detailed understanding of the intricacies surrounding mitochondrial biology in neural tissues is essential for the development of effective, targeted therapeutic approaches aimed at preserving or restoring neuronal function.

10.3.5 Mitochondrial Dysfunction in Glioma Progression

Mitochondrial dysfunction has emerged as a defining characteristic of glioma pathogenesis, with wide-ranging implications for tumor initiation, growth, and therapeutic resistance. In gliomas, particularly GB, which is the most aggressive form, mitochondria are structurally and functionally compromised in harmony with the neoplastic cell's metabolic and molecular needs (26). These adaptations are not random events but are ongoing processes that enhance the malignant profile of gliomas. At the molecular level, glioma cells show recurrent alterations in mtDNA, such as mutations, deletions, and copy number changes. These alterations compromise OXPHOS, disrupt the integrity of the electron transport chain (ETC), and result in an imbalanced generation of ATP and ROS (24,27). For example, it has been reported that mtDNA mutations in the constituents of Complex I and Complex IV are commonly observed in high-grade gliomas, which are associated with poor prognosis and metabolic reprogramming (28–31).

Moreover, glioma mitochondria are master regulators of cell death and bioenergetics. By controlling the mitochondrial permeability transition pore (mPTP), glioma cells suppress apoptosis and are resistant to chemotherapy. Disturbance of pro- and anti-apoptotic BCL-2 family proteins also maintains mitochondrial membrane stability and promotes cell survival (32,33). Remarkably, the increased BCL-xL and MCL-1 expression in GB is associated with mitochondrial resistance and therapy resistance, as reported by Shang et al. in 2020 (34). Gliomas also capitalize on mitochondrial dysfunction to adapt to hypoxic and nutrient-poor microenvironments. Under such conditions, hypoxia-inducible factors (HIFs) control mitochondrial function, inhibit OXPHOS genes, and promote glycolysis (35). Concurrently, glioma cells maintain some OXPHOS activity, which offers metabolic flexibility (36). This double-edged mechanism allows glioma cells to thrive in fluctuating oxygen levels—a characteristic of the intratumoral environment. In addition, oncometabolite accumulation generated by aberrant mitochondria—like 2-hydroxyglutarate (2-HG) in IDH1/2 mutated gliomas—is reprogramming epigenetic landscapes. 2-HG represses α-ketoglutarate–dependent dioxygenase activity on histone and DNA demethylation (37,38). The epigenetic modifications disrupt differentiation pathways and the gliomagenesis process. Of particular note, such IDH mutations were discovered as early drivers in low-grade glioma formation as well as in secondary GB progression (38). The cellular metabolism in glioma cells is presented in **Figure 10.1**.

At its core is the interaction of mitochondrial failure and glioma stem-like cells (GSCs), adding another level of complexity. GSCs possess more mitochondrial mass and are highly reliant on mitochondrial function for tumorigenicity and survival. Mitochondrial dysfunction in GSCs is detrimental to their tumorigenicity, and this implies that mitochondrial integrity is at the core of the glioma hierarchy and its development.

10.4 METABOLIC REPROGRAMMING AND ONCOMETABOLISM

Metabolic reprogramming is a key feature of gliomas, enabling tumor cells to meet their bioenergetic, biosynthetic, and redox demands in an extremely heterogeneous and often adverse microenvironment. Unlike healthy neural cells that are geared to use OXPHOS for ATP production, glioma cells exhibit drastic metabolic changes that include augmented glycolysis, altered tricarboxylic acid (TCA) cycle kinetics, and oncometabolite accumulation—all playing a pivotal role in tumor growth, drug resistance, and immune evasion.

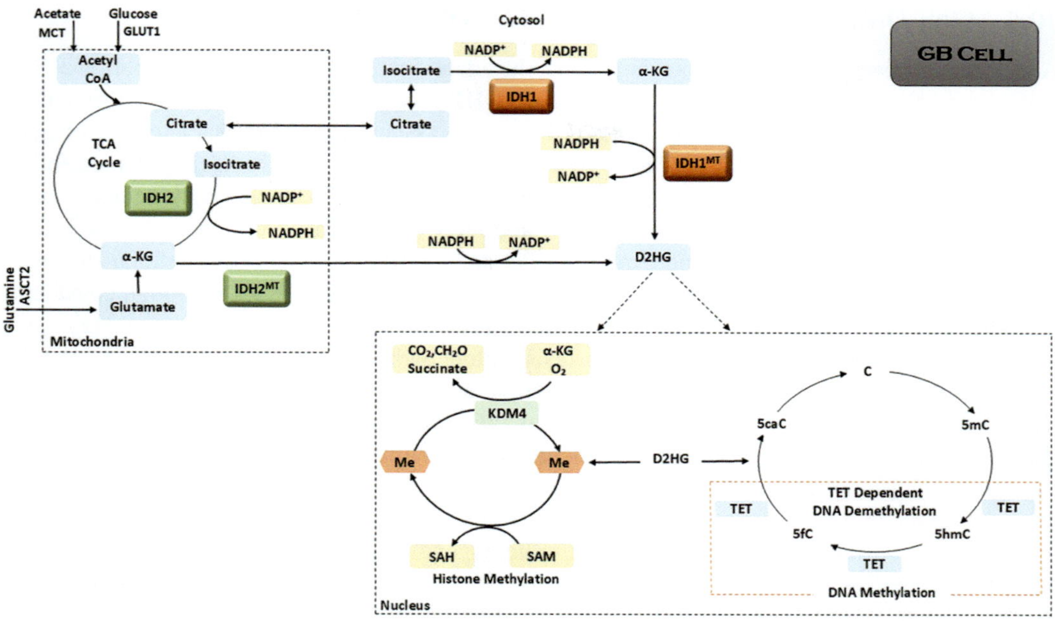

FIGURE 10.1 Cellular metabolism of glioma cells. Mutant IDH1/2 drives D2HG-mediated epigenetic reprogramming in gliomas.

10.4.1 The Warburg Effect and Its Extensions

Glioma cells show mainly the Warburg phenotype, with the catabolism of glucose to lactate in both normoxic and aerated conditions—a phenomenon referred to as aerobic glycolysis. Such an oncogenic metabolic adaptation, governed by oncogenic pathways (e.g., PI3K/AKT/mTOR, MYC), allows for quick ATP production and supplies precursors for the building of nucleotides, amino acids, and lipids (39). Upregulation of glycolytic enzymes such as hexokinase 2 (HK2), pyruvate kinase M2 (PKM2), and lactate dehydrogenase A (LDHA) has been documented in GB and has been associated with poor survival outcomes and aggressive tumor behavior (40). In spite of the glycolytic bias, glioma cells possess functional mitochondria and perform OXPHOS under certain conditions. Such metabolic plasticity enables adaptation to fluctuating oxygen and nutrient levels—a property particularly important in the heterogeneous tumor environment. In certain glioma subpopulations, most notably GSCs, there is a dependence on mitochondrial respiration, which is necessary for self-renewal and tumor initiation (41).

10.4.2 TCA Cycle Rewiring and Glutamine Dependence

Aside from glycolysis, gliomas also exhibit extensive rewiring of the TCA cycle. Among the most striking aspects is glutamine addiction. Glutamine is a significant source of carbon and nitrogen, replenishing TCA intermediates by anaplerotic reactions (42). Glutaminase (GLS) is overexpressed in glioma cells, which hydrolyzes glutamine to glutamate, activating α-ketoglutarate production and supporting ATP generation and biosynthesis. Inhibition of GLS inhibits glioma cell growth, which makes it of therapeutic interest (43). Besides, the biosynthesis processes of β-oxidation and fatty acid synthesis are also regulated in gliomas to promote membrane biosynthesis and redox homeostasis. GB tissues are said to exhibit overexpression of fatty acid synthase (FASN) and carnitine palmitoyltransferase 1A (CPT1A) and are shown to be associated with increased survival in stress conditions (44).

10.5 ONCOMETABOLITES: A REVIEW OF 2-HYDROXYGLUTARATE

A central discovery in glioma metabolism is the identification of the oncometabolite 2-HG, which occurs as a byproduct of IDH mutations. IDH1/2 mutations are present in greater than 70% of lower-grade gliomas and secondary GB and are associated with a characteristic epigenetic and metabolic phenotype (45). Mutant IDH catalyzes the Nicotinamide Adenine Dinucleotide Phosphate (NADPH)-dependent reduction of α-ketoglutarate to 2-HG, an aberrant metabolite that acts as a competitive inhibitor of α-ketoglutarate(α-KG)-dependent dioxygenases (38,45). The reaction results in DNA and histone hypermethylation, contributes to defective cellular differentiation, and contributes to genomic instability, thereby promoting oncogenesis through epigenetic reprogramming.

2-HG also impacts cellular redox homeostasis, mitochondrial metabolism, and NAD+ metabolism. Inhibiting IDH mutant enzyme has shown potential in the clinic with drugs such as ivosidenib and vorasidenib for IDH-mutant gliomas (46). These discoveries represent a paradigm shift in precision oncology by converting oncometabolic vulnerabilities into therapeutic targets. Lactate is an effector molecule that is traditionally regarded as a glycolytic waste product; it is now shown to be a potent signaling molecule in gliomas. Increased lactate levels acidify the tumor microenvironment, promoting invasion, angiogenesis, and immunosuppression. Lactate dehydrogenase-dependent lactate production also controls histone lactylation, which in turn controls gene expression linked to tumor growth (47–49). Monocarboxylate transporters (MCT1/4), which facilitate lactate export/import, are overexpressed in GB and represent potential metabolic checkpoints (50,51).

10.6 MITOCHONDRIA-MEDIATED RESISTANCE TO THERAPY

The treatment resistance remains a major challenge in glioma management, particularly GB, with constantly low median survival rates on intensive multimodal treatments. While genetic and epigenetic alterations contribute to the avoidance of treatments, recent evidence is highlighting the central role of mitochondria in mediating radiotherapy, chemotherapy, and immunotherapy resistance. Mitochondria regulate diverse processes critical for glioma cell survival—such as apoptosis modulation, metabolic adaptation, and redox buffering—thus conferring tumor resistance to treatment insult.

10.6.1 Avoidance of Mitochondrial Apoptosis in Gliomas

One of the key roles played by mitochondria is the regulation of intrinsic (mitochondria-dependent) apoptosis, which within gliomas can be dysregulated. Regulation of mitochondrial outer membrane permeabilization (MOMP), a central event leading to the release of cytochrome c and subsequent caspase activation, is governed by BCL-2 family proteins (52). Glioma overexpression of anti-apoptotic proteins, including BCL-2, BCL-XL, and MCL-1, stops the process of apoptosis initiated as a result of DNA damage or oxidative stress promoted by chemoradiotherapy. Notably, GSCs express high levels of these anti-apoptotic factors and are extremely resistant to temozolomide (TMZ), the alkylating agent of choice (53). Pharmacologic inhibition of BCL-XL or MCL-1 has been shown to exhibit synergistic activity with TMZ or radiation in preclinical glioma models, re-sensitizing for apoptosis, such as the study conducted by Karpel-Massler et al. in 2015, suggesting that the combination of TIC10/ONC201 with the BH3-mimetic, ABT-263, resulted in tumor regression in vivo (54). Another study by Yang et al. in 2015 suggested that ABT-737 also sensitized glioma cells to TMZ-induced apoptosis (55). Even phytochemicals, such as resveratrol, were found to inhibit X-linked inhibitor of apoptotic proteins in glioma models (56).

10.6.2 Mitochondrial DNA (mtDNA) and Genomic Instability

Mitochondria also have a separate genome (mtDNA) that is subject to mutation by virtue of the absence of protective histones and the presence of limited repair machinery. Deletions and alterations within mtDNA in gliomas can interfere with ETC activity, thereby generating altered ROS and inducing metabolic reprogramming (57). These mitochondrial genome alterations are a survival advantage in the form of enhanced resistance to oxidative stress and to therapeutic interventions. Moreover, mtDNA copy number discrepancies and mutations within the ETC complexes (most notably Complex I and IV) were associated with radiation and hypoxia-resistant death in glioma models (58,59). Selective killing strategies targeting mitochondria with pro-oxidant agents (such as elesclomol, mitocans) have been suggested to take advantage of this susceptibility (60).

10.6.3 Reactive Oxygen Species and Antioxidant Defense

Therapeutic drugs such as TMZ and radiation induce cytotoxicity primarily by enhancing the generation of ROS and oxidative DNA damage. Glioma cells possess robust antioxidant defense mechanisms in their mitochondria—e.g., glutathione (GSH), superoxide dismutase 2 (SOD2), and peroxiredoxins (PRDXs)—that effectively detoxify ROS, thus reducing the therapeutic effectiveness (61–63). GSCs, specifically, have high mitochondrial membrane potential ($\Delta\Psi m$) and low ROS levels by upregulating antioxidant regulators like NRF2 and SOD2, making them resistant to oxidative damage (64). Inhibition of the antioxidant pathway sensitizes glioma cells to treatment, a strategy now under preclinical investigation.

10.6.4 Mitochondria and Temozolomide Resistance

Glioma temozolomide resistance is polyfactorial and involves DNA repair pathways such as MGMT upregulation and mismatch repair deficiency. Mitochondrial dynamics contribute to TMZ resistance (65), as demonstrated by Zhang et al. in 2023, who showed that high Ca^2+ levels and activation of the JNK–STAT3 pathway contributed to TMZ resistance, and that blocking either JNK or STAT3 makes cells more susceptible to TMZ (66). Dysregulation of the balance between mitochondrial fission–fusion, governed by proteins such as DRP1 and MFN2, influences mitochondrial bioenergetics and apoptotic priming (67–69). It has been shown that mitochondrial fission is associated with increased TMZ resistance, and inhibition of DRP1 could reverse drug sensitivity (67–69). In addition, mitochondrial membrane potential alterations and ATP-dependent drug efflux by ABC transporters (namely ABCG2) have been associated with reduced TMZ accumulation and activity. In 2021, Giddings et al. created MCJ mimetics that are able to inhibit mitochondrial respiration and overcome chemoresistance safely in vitro and in vivo models (70).

10.7 MITOCHONDRIA AND RADIOTHERAPY RESISTANCE

Hypoxic niche glioma cells exhibit reduced ROS production following exposure to radiation caused by defective oxygen-dependent damage facilitation. This is compensated for by mitochondria that increase levels of antioxidant enzymes and regulate ETC activity (71). Furthermore, radiation-resistant glioma cells exhibit a disrupted mitochondrial morphology as well as a higher level of expression of the fusion proteins MFN1/2, responsible for metabolic resistance, and cell death evasion (72). Disrupting mitochondrial bioenergetics with ETC complex inhibitors (e.g., IACS-010759, metformin) may have the potential to sensitize GB cells to radiation by augmenting oxidative stress and disrupting ATP production (73).

Clinical Significance and Targeting Specificity: The mitochondrial origin of therapy resistance offers novel possibilities for precision neuro-oncology. Pharmacologic agents that hit mitochondrial apoptosis (e.g., BH3 mimetics), regulation of ROS (e.g., GSH inhibitors), or metabolic activity (e.g., ETC inhibitors) have the potential to specifically erode the survival apparatus of glioma cells (74). In addition, co-administration of such agents with conventional therapies or immune checkpoint inhibitors could bypass resistance and enhance therapeutic efficacy. Mitochondria-directed therapies like Mito-CP, MitoQ, and mitochondrial uncouplers are of particular interest (75). Notably, responder stratification based on mitochondrial gene expression and functional phenotypic profiling in patient tumor models is possible and may inform personalized treatment regimens—aligned with the principles of precision medicine (76).

10.8 REDOX IMBALANCE AND OXIDATIVE STRESS IN GLIOMAS

Gliomas, especially the high-grade types such as GB, exhibit extensive oxidative stress and redox homeostasis disruption, conditions that enhance tumor growth, drug resistance, and immune evasion. ROS, such as superoxide anions, hydrogen peroxide, and hydroxyl radicals, are mainly generated by mitochondrial OXPHOS and NADPH oxidase activity (77,78). Whereas low-to-moderate ROS levels are employed as secondary messengers in cell proliferation and angiogenesis, high ROS levels induce oxidative damage to DNA, lipids, and proteins, requiring tight redox control (79). The glioma cells compensate for this oxidative stress by modifying their antioxidant mechanisms, which ironically facilitate tumor survival, growth, and resistance to conventional therapies.

Mitochondria are the central hubs of redox regulation in gliomas. As sites of OXPHOS, mitochondria are also the primary sources of intracellular ROS. In glioma cells, particularly GSCs, mitochondrial function is altered to maintain a favorable redox balance. These cells exhibit an elevated mitochondrial membrane potential and increased expression of antioxidant enzymes, including manganese SOD2, GPX, thioredoxin (TRX), and PRDXs (72,80). These enzymes collectively mitigate oxidative damage and buffer intracellular ROS levels, enabling the survival of malignant cells in oxidative microenvironments, such as the hypoxic tumor core. High SOD2 expression has been correlated with poor prognosis and therapeutic resistance in glioma patients (63,81).

The GSH pathway is a significant antioxidant defense mechanism in gliomas. GSH, produced by the glutamate-cysteine ligase (GCL) pathway, neutralizes ROS directly and is a cofactor for GPX enzymes (82). Gliomas have a tendency to overexpress enzymes for GSH biosynthesis and cystine/glutamate antiporters such as SLC7A11 (xCT) to drive cystine import and GSH production. This pathway is pivotal in detoxifying ROS produced by treatments such as radiation and TMZ (83,84). Therefore, targeting SLC7A11 has been promising in sensitizing glioma cells to ROS-inducing treatments. In addition, the GPX4 enzyme—highly GSH-dependent—neutralizes lipid hydroperoxides and inhibits ferroptotic cell death, adding an extra layer of redox protection (85). Targeting the SLC7A11–GSH–GPX4 axis is being explored as a precision oncology strategy to break glioma redox homeostasis and increase treatment efficiency. Other transporters such as SLC1A5 (glutamine transporter), SLC25A10 (dicarboxylate transporter), and SLC3A2 (amino acid transport complex subunit) play roles in the redox status and metabolic flexibility of glioma cells (86). Their cooperative regulation enhances uptake of cystine, glutamine, and malate to sustain the production of antioxidants and generation of NADPH, integrating redox homeostasis with metabolic reprogramming.

At the genomic level, oxidative stress triggers mutagenesis, genomic instability, and oncogene activation. For example, 8-hydroxy-2′-deoxyguanosine (8-OHdG), a DNA damage marker of oxidative damage, is commonly upregulated in gliomas and correlated with IDH1 mutations, MGMT promoter methylation, and aberrant DNA repair (87,88). ROS-induced damage also triggers pro-survival signaling pathways, such as PI3K/AKT, MAPK/ERK, and HIF-1α pathways, all of which are involved in glioma cell proliferation and drug resistance (89). Notably, redox state also underlies the tumor immune microenvironment. High ROS in glioma cells inhibits T-cell activation and enhances immunosuppressive macrophage polarization (90). Additionally, GSH-replete tumor cells are resistant to immune checkpoint blockade owing to decreased immunogenicity. Therefore, modification of redox balance not only affects tumor cell survival but also affects the efficacy of immunotherapy (91).

Mitochondrial redox adaptation is closely linked to the metabolic reprogramming observed in gliomas. By enhancing NADPH production through the pentose phosphate pathway (PPP) and IDH activity, glioma cells gain a reductive intracellular environment favorable to proliferation and survival (92). IDH1(R132H) mutation in low-grade gliomas reduces NADPH levels and disrupts redox homeostasis, the result being a paradox in that such tumors become hypersensitive to oxidative stress, although they are generally indolent (93). From the therapeutic point of view, redox modulation is an attractive precision approach. Pro-oxidant medicines, such as elesclomol, a copper-chelating ROS inducer, or mitochondria-targeted ROS enhancers (e.g., Mito-CP, MitoQ), selectively augment oxidative stress in glioma cells without harming normal tissue (94,95). Clinical methods of sensitizing gliomas by employing redox modulators in combination with standard treatments (e.g., TMZ, radiotherapy) are under active investigation. Moreover, nanoparticles and drug delivery systems that employ tumor-specific redox gradients provide new opportunities for glioma-selective therapy.

10.9 MITOCHONDRIAL DYNAMICS AND MITOPHAGY IN TUMOR ADAPTATION

Mitochondria are dynamic organelles continually remodeling morphologically through fission, fusion, biogenesis, and selective degradation (mitophagy). Taken together as mitochondrial dynamics, these processes are essential to maintaining mitochondrial integrity, bioenergetic function, and cell survival. In gliomas, such as GB, mitochondrial dynamics are drastically reorganized to enable tumor cell adaptation to metabolic stress, hypoxia, and therapeutic pressure. Dysregulation of these processes not only fuels tumor growth but also therapy resistance, immune evasion, and GSC maintenance. Mitochondrial fission, regulated primarily by dynamin-related protein 1 (DRP1), causes fragmentation of mitochondria, a hallmark of proliferating and stress-acclimated cancer, including GB, cells (96,97). DRP1 is usually upregulated or hyperactivated in GB, allowing mitochondrial fragmentation to power mitotic division, ROS detoxification, and apoptosis resistance (98). DRP1 overexpression is intriguingly correlated with poor prognosis and high tumor grade (99). Phosphorylation of Dynamin-related protein 1 (DRP1) at Serine 616 (Ser616), a specific phosphorylation site on Drp1promotes its recruitment to the mitochondrial outer membrane, where it assembles into complexes with adaptors like Mitochondrial fission protein 1 (FIS1), Mitochondrial fission factor (MFF), and Mitochondrial dynamics proteins of 49 and 51 kDa (MID49/51) to cause fission (100). Inhibition of DRP1 by drugs like Mdivi-1 has been shown to suppress glioma cell proliferation and increase cells' sensitivity to chemotherapy (101).

Mitochondrial fusion, mediated by mitofusins (MFN1, MFN2) and optic atrophy 1 (OPA1), allows merging of mitochondrial contents and thus preservation of mtDNA integrity and OXPHOS maintenance (102,103). In GB, the fusion process is often disrupted, leading to metabolic reprogramming to glycolysis and increased tolerance to ROS. However, within a particular subgroup of glioma cells—most importantly, GSCs—the fusion machinery is preserved or reactivated, essential for the maintenance of mitochondrial function and stemness in hypoxia (104,105). Reduced expression of MFN2 and OPA1 has been found in high-grade gliomas and is associated with dedifferentiation, resistance to therapy, and immune evasion (106).

Mitophagy, selective autophagic degradation of damaged or dysfunctional mitochondria, is a quality control process. Glioma cells utilize mitophagy to survive oxidative stress, starvation, and hypoxia (107). The PINK1–Parkin pathway is the core of mitophagy: mitochondrial depolarization causes PINK1 to accumulate on the outer membrane, which recruits and activates the E3 ubiquitin ligase Parkin, triggering the ubiquitination of mitochondrial proteins and recruitment of autophagosomes (108,109). Although PINK1 and Parkin expression are low in normal brain tissue, a number of glioma studies have described context-specific reactivation of mitophagy under stress conditions.

Autophagic degradation of damaged mitochondria prevents cytotoxic ROS accumulation and apoptosis (110).

Outside the described PINK1–Parkin pathway, glioma cells participate in receptor-mediated mitophagy through proteins such as BNIP3, NIX, and FUNDC1, especially under hypoxia (111). BNIP3 is a HIF-1α-regulated, hypoxia-inducible protein; its overexpression has been correlated with hypoxia-induced tumor aggressiveness and metabolic plasticity. BNIP3-induced mitophagy not only inhibits apoptosis induced by mitochondrial stimuli but also induces metabolic plasticity by inducing cells to glycolysis, thereby ensuring tumor survival in hypoxic microenvironments (112).

Notably, mitophagy and mitochondrial dynamics intersect with glioma stemness and drug resistance. GSCs have elevated mitochondrial fission and high mitophagic flux, which enable them to be resistant to radiation-induced mitochondrial damage and remain quiescent or initiate differentiation based on environmental signals (113). These processes are controlled in part by oncogenic pathways such as PI3K/AKT, mTOR, and c-MYC, which control DRP1, MFNs, and autophagy proteins directly or indirectly (114). Furthermore, aberrant mitochondrial dynamics contribute to epigenetic reprogramming by metabolite flux, affecting histone acetylation, DNA methylation, and immune checkpoint expression (115). Therapeutically, the targeting of mitochondrial dynamics and mitophagy presents new opportunities for the treatment of gliomas. DRP1 inhibitors (e.g., Mdivi-1), autophagy regulators (e.g., chloroquine, hydroxychloroquine), and HIF-1α/BNIP3 pathway inhibitors are studied for their capacity to disrupt mitochondrial homeostasis and render glioma cells vulnerable to radiation, TMZ, and redox stress (116–118). Combination therapies targeting both energy metabolism and mitochondrial quality control are especially promising the overcoming therapy resistance and eliminating GSCs.

10.10 GLIOMA STEM CELLS AND MITOCHONDRIAL PLASTICITY

GSCs are special cells in brain tumors that can start new tumors and are resistant to treatments, making them hard to eliminate. These cells can change how they produce energy, which helps them survive in difficult conditions. Depending on the availability of oxygen and nutrients, GSCs can switch between two main energy-making processes—glycolysis and OXPHOS. This flexibility is closely linked to how their mitochondria (the energy factories of the cell) function, allowing GSCs to continue producing energy even when under stress (119).

Research has shown that GSCs rely significantly on mitochondria to produce energy, especially when there is a lack of oxygen or nutrients (120). Analysis of GSCs taken from patients reveals that many genes related to OXPHOS are more active in these cells, giving them a survival edge in stressful conditions (121). GSCs have more and stronger mitochondria compared to other tumor cells, helping them maintain their 'stem-like' status and their ability to initiate new tumors.

Several important proteins regulate this mitochondrial flexibility, including PGC-1α and Mitochondrial Transcription Factor A (TFAM), along with proteins that help change the shape of mitochondria, like DRP1 (122,123). These proteins are essential for GSCs to divide and retain their unique features. Disrupting DRP1 or PGC-1α affects mitochondrial function, making it harder for GSCs to form cells and making them more sensitive to chemotherapy (124). Mitochondrial adaptability in GSCs is not just about energy production. It also plays a role in controlling gene expression and helping GSCs dodge the immune system. Mitochondria produce substances that influence how genes are regulated, affecting qualities such as invasiveness and treatment resistance. Changes in mitochondrial function can also alter how GSCs avoid detection by the immune system.

Recent research indicates that GSCs use a pathway called the mitochondrial unfolded protein response (UPRmt) such as ATF5 to stay alive during stress (125). This pathway helps maintain mitochondrial health and protects GSCs from cell death. Additionally, GSCs employ a process called mitophagy, which removes damaged mitochondria to ensure the remaining ones stay functional. From a treatment perspective, targeting the adaptability of mitochondria in GSCs is being actively explored. Some drugs, like CPI-613, metformin, and IACS-010759, have shown potential in disrupting energy production in GSCs in preclinical studies (126). Researchers are looking for ways to specifically target and destroy these GSCs without harming normal brain cells. Overall, the ability of GSCs to manage their energy needs is a key feature that helps them resist treatments and contribute to tumor diversity. Targeting mitochondrial networks in these cells represents a promising strategy for developing new therapies for brain tumors.

10.11 CROSSTALK WITH THE NEURO-TUMOR MICROENVIRONMENT

The glioma microenvironment is a dynamic, heterogeneous niche shaped by bidirectional cross-talk between the tumor cells and surrounding neural, immune, and stromal elements. This complex neuro-tumor interface supports glioma expansion, immune evasion, and drug resistance by spatially and temporally regulated molecular signals (127). Mitochondria are central to mediating this cross-talk, affecting not just the intrinsic glioma cell biology but also influencing their behavior during interactions with neurons, glial, endothelial cells, and infiltrating immune cells.

One of the most striking features of the glioma microenvironment is that it is neurobiologically oriented. Glioma cells harness neuronal activity to promote their invasive growth and proliferation (128). The exocytosis of activity-regulated synaptic vesicles from the neurons sustains glioma growth through the secretion of neuroligin-3 (NLGN3), which promotes PI3K-mTOR signaling pathways to render the tumors more aggressive (129). Glioma cells also form functional pseudo-synapses with neurons through α-amino-3-hydroxy-5-methyl-4-isoxazolepropionic acid (AMPA)-type glutamate receptors, essentially becoming integral to neuronal circuits to hijack excitatory signaling pathways (130). This electrochemical interaction puts high metabolic burdens on the tumor cells, which is correlated with enhanced mitochondrial activity and enhanced calcium buffer capacities.

In addition, glioma cells release glutamate and other excitotoxic neurotransmitters through the system Xc− antiporter, leading to excitotoxic neuronal cell death and facilitating the establishment of peritumoral vacated niches that allow for infiltration (131). Mitochondrial calcium regulation by the mitochondrial calcium uniporter (MCU) also contributes to this invasive process by controlling cytoskeletal dynamics and mitochondrial ATP production in response to alterations in calcium (132). Astrocytes, a prevailing glial population, are reprogrammed by glioma-derived factors to gain a pro-tumorigenic phenotype. Tumor-associated astrocytes release cytokines (e.g., IL-6 and TGF-β) and extracellular vesicles that promote glioma stemness and metabolic reprogramming (133). Mitochondrial transfer from astrocytes to glioma cells through tunneling nanotubes has been documented, particularly under stress conditions like hypoxia or chemotherapy, as a mitochondrial rescue mechanism favoring tumor cell survival (134). Such intercellular mitochondrial transfer is a pivotal axis of metabolic symbiosis at the neuro-tumor interface. **Figure 10.2** represents the intricate tumor microenvironment in advanced-stage glial tumors

Endothelial cells and pericytes also support glioma growth by preserving endothelial cell function via angiocrine signaling and metabolic cross-talk. Glioma cells promote aberrant angiogenesis through the secretion of vascular endothelial growth factor (VEGF) and angiopoietins, which result in leaky and dysfunctional vasculature that worsens hypoxia (135). Mitochondrial adaptation to hypoxic stress activates HIF-1α and induces pseudopalisading death, a histological feature of high-grade gliomas (136). Additionally, mitochondrial metabolism in tumor cells evolves to hypoxia through increased reductive glutaminolysis and disturbed NAD+/NADH homeostasis that supports growth even in oxygen-deprived areas (137). The immunological environment of gliomas is influenced by both mitochondrial processes and metabolic signaling pathways. Lactate, succinate, and ROS produced by tumors drive macrophages toward an immunosuppressive M2-like phenotype, simultaneously hindering the efficacy of cytotoxic T lymphocytes (138). In glioma cells, mitochondrial ROS induces the expression of PD-L1 through the NF-κB/STAT3 signaling pathway, which further suppresses anti-tumor immune responses (139). Moreover, mtDNA released from compromised glioma cells can activate the cGAS-STING pathway in microglia and dendritic cells,

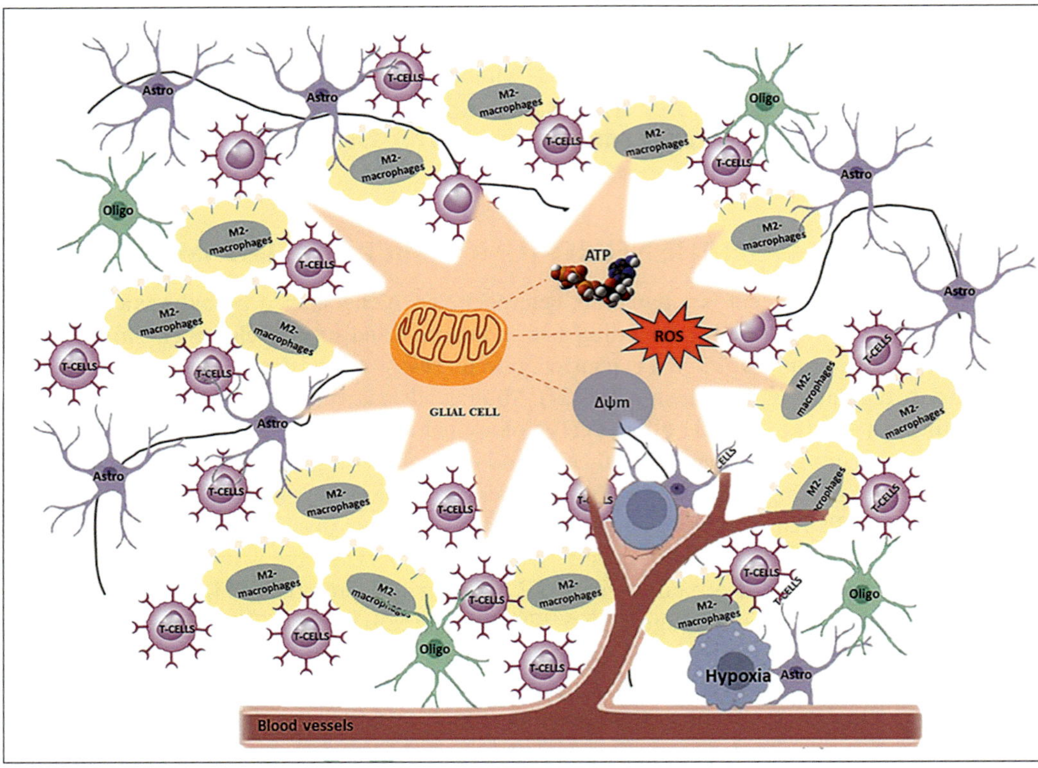

FIGURE 10.2 Crosstalk between glioma and neuro-tumor microenvironment.

paradoxically fostering chronic inflammation that facilitates tumor progression (140). Nevertheless, under specific circumstances, mitochondrial-damage-associated molecular patterns (mtDAMPs) may reinstate innate immune responses and provide a potential therapeutic opportunity for immune reprogramming (141).

Tumor–neuron communication also regulates synaptic pruning and axonal remodeling. Glioma cells upregulate complement component expression and recruit microglia to remodel neuronal circuits, thus facilitating niche expansion and immune evasion. This remodeling of the neural environment is a more general level of neuroplastic manipulation, in which mitochondria play a pivotal role in directing ATP-dependent processes, ROS-mediated signaling, and apoptosis resistance during tumor invasion (142). Therapeutically, it has been promising to target the neuro-tumor microenvironment in preclinical models. In addition, mitochondrial immunometabolism-targeting agents like IDO1 inhibitors or modulators of mitochondrial ROS are under investigation for their ability to reprogram the immune environment and enhance immunotherapy (143). **Table 10.1** summarizes the key mitochondrial functions altered in gliomas, underscoring their role in tumor progression and therapy resistance.

10.12 TARGETING MITOCHONDRIA: THERAPEUTIC APPROACHES AND INNOVATIONS

Therapeutic modulation of mitochondria in gliomas stands at the frontier of molecular specificity, from the non-selective cytotoxicity of previous strategies to organelle-directed intervention. Beyond the traditional methods of oxidative stress induction or apoptosis modulators, a new generation of breakthroughs takes advantage of the complex mitochondrial machinery to engineer therapies that

TABLE 10.1
Mitochondrial Functions Altered in Gliomas

Function	Normal Role	Alteration in Gliomas	Implication	Supporting Databases/ References
Oxidative phosphorylation (OXPHOS)	Primary ATP production via electron transport chain	Downregulated; shift toward glycolysis (Warburg effect)	Enhanced proliferation and survival under hypoxic conditions	(144,145)
Reactive oxygen species (ROS) regulation	Maintains redox balance Signaling	Elevated ROS levels due to mitochondrial dysfunction	DNA damage, genomic instability, and promotion of tumorigenesis	(146,147)
Mitochondrial dynamics (fission/fusion)	Maintains mitochondrial integrity and function	Imbalance favoring fission over fusion	Mitochondrial fragmentation, promoting apoptosis resistance	(72,148)
Apoptosis regulation	Initiates intrinsic apoptosis via cytochrome c release	Overexpression of anti-apoptotic proteins (e.g., Bcl-2, Bcl-xL); inhibition of pro-apoptotic factors	Resistance to cell death; therapy resistance	(149,150)
Mitochondrial DNA (mtDNA) integrity	Encodes essential components for OXPHOS	Mutations and deletions in mtDNA	Impaired respiratory function; increased ROS production	(27,151)
Calcium homeostasis	Regulates intracellular calcium levels	Disrupted calcium uptake and release	Altered signaling pathways; contributes to tumor progression	(152,153)
Mitochondrial biogenesis	Generates new mitochondria to meet energy demands	Dysregulated biogenesis pathways	Mitochondrial dysfunction; metabolic reprogramming	(72,154)
Mitophagy	Removes damaged mitochondria via autophagy	Impaired mitophagy processes	Accumulation of dysfunctional mitochondria; increased oxidative stress	(155)
Lipid metabolism	Synthesizes and degrades lipids for energy and membrane formation	Dysregulated lipid metabolism; accumulation of lipid droplets	Supports rapid tumor growth and therapy resistance	(44,156)
Mitochondrial transport	Distributes mitochondria to areas of high energy demand	Altered mitochondrial trafficking within tumor cells	Affects cellular energy distribution and tumor invasiveness	(134)
Mitochondrial unfolded protein response (UPRmt)	Maintains protein homeostasis within mitochondria	Activation of UPRmt due to mitochondrial stress	Promotes tumor cell survival under stress conditions	(157,158)

(*Continued*)

TABLE 10.1 (*Continued*)
Mitochondrial Functions Altered in Gliomas

Function	Normal Role	Alteration in Gliomas	Implication	Supporting Databases/ References
Mitochondrial permeability transition pore (mPTP) regulation	Regulates mitochondrial membrane permeability	Dysregulated mPTP opening leading to cell death resistance	Contributes to therapy resistance and tumor survival	(159,160)
Mitochondrial-nuclear communication	Coordinates mitochondrial and nuclear gene expression	Disrupted signaling pathways between mitochondria and nucleus	Alters gene expression profiles supporting tumor progression	(161,162)
Mitochondrial ribosome function	Synthesizes mitochondrial-encoded proteins	Mutations in mitochondrial ribosomal RNA	Impaired protein synthesis affecting OXPHOS	(163,164)

interfere with cancer progression without harming normal neural tissue (165). A field of new interest is selective inhibition of the mitochondrial translation machinery, with attention to targeting the mitochondrial ribosomes (mitoribosomes) that have different structural features than their cytoplasmic counterparts (166). Mitochondrial ribosome-targeting compounds like tigecycline, an antibiotic molecule that impairs mitoribosome activity, have exhibited preclinical effectiveness through induction of energy depletion and inhibition of viability of glioma cells, specifically in resistant and stem-like populations (167).

Another emerging strategy involves the targeting of mitochondrial import machinery and the outer membrane (TOMM) and inner membrane (TIMM) complexes (168,169). Abnormally regulated nuclear-encoded mitochondrial protein import in glioma causes tumor resistance and metabolic plasticity. Targeting of the TOM20–TIM23 axis disrupts mitochondrial proteostasis and disassembly of organelle integrity, demonstrating enhanced glioma cell sensitivity to metabolic inhibitors and DNA-damaging agents (169). Furthermore, the mPTP is also an actionable node in therapy-resistant gliomas. mPTP opening leads to mitochondrial swelling and cell death, but glioma cells frequently prevent pore opening (170). Modulators like cyclosporin A analogs (e.g., NIM811) and sanglifehrin A can render tumor cells sensitive to apoptosis by lifting this blockade (171). Significantly, this treatment selectively increases cytotoxicity under conditions of nutrient starvation or hypoxia—a common feature of the glioma microenvironment.

There are also unique vulnerabilities in mitochondrial lipid metabolism. Cardiolipin, a mitochondrial inner membrane-specific phospholipid, plays a critical role in the maintenance of cristae structure and ETC function in mammalian cells (172). Disruption of cardiolipin synthesis enzymes such as TAZ (tafazzin) destabilizes mitochondrial membranes and abolishes energy production. Pharmacologic agents or RNA-based inhibitors of lipid remodeling proteins have been promising for glioma xenograft models with reduced tumorigenicity and impaired mitochondrial respiration (173). In addition, epitranscriptomic regulation of mitochondrial RNAs (mtRNAs) is gaining increasing importance. Emerging results indicate that such modifications as m6A methylation of mtRNAs control mitochondrial protein translation and stress adaptation (174). Mitochondrial tRNA-modifying enzymes NSUN3 and TRMT61B are overexpressed in a range of tumors, such as gliomas with an unfavorable prognosis (175). Small molecule inhibitors of these RNA-modifying enzymes are in the early stages of development, making organelle-specific translational regulation a therapeutic target. Specifically targeted photodynamic and photothermal therapies (PDT/PTT) have been created, employing light-activated agents with a preference for accumulation in

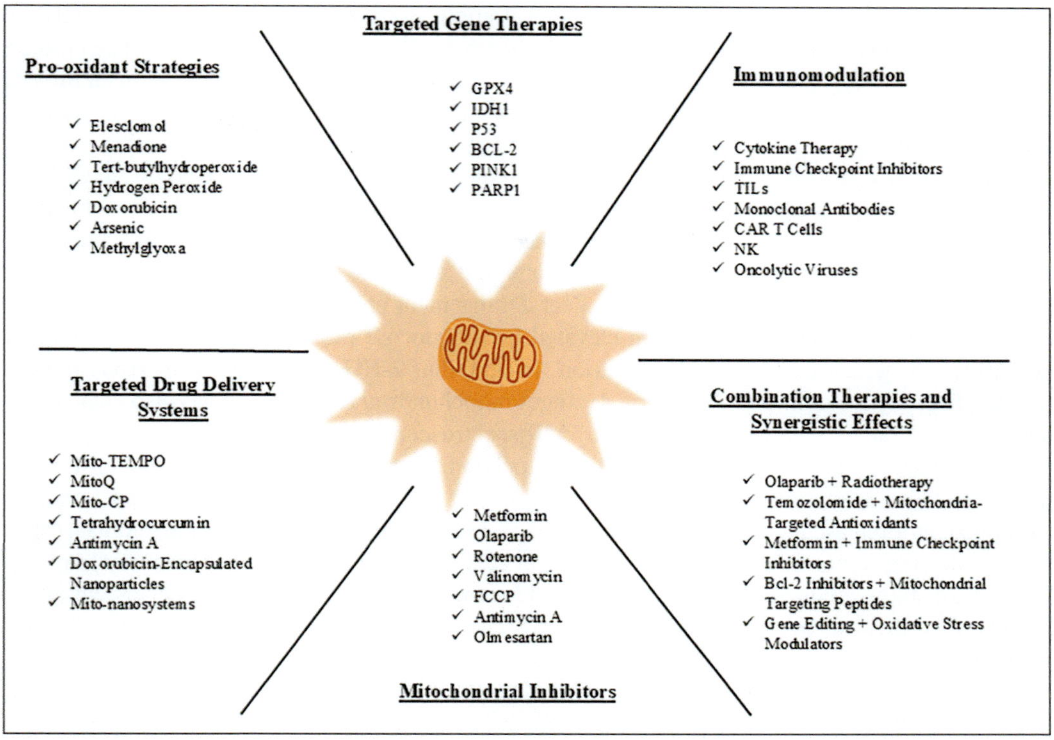

FIGURE 10.3 Various mitochondria-targeted therapy approaches.

mitochondrial areas and the generation of lethal ROS or heat upon light activation (176,177). New mitochondrial-targeting units paired with porphyrins or nanoparticles exhibit improved efficacy in glioma cell death with high spatial selectivity and limited collateral damage to nearby healthy brain tissue (178–180).

Lastly, immunometabolic reprogramming by mitochondrial modulation is gaining traction. As glioma cells are busy rewiring mitochondrial metabolism to avoid immune recognition, new strategies focus on reprogramming immune cells specifically, tumor-infiltrating macrophages and T cells—by enhancing their mitochondrial well-being (181). Delivery of mitochondrial uncouplers, PGC1α agonists, or NAD+ precursors (e.g., nicotinamide riboside) into immune cells has been shown to enhance antitumor immunity, increase T-cell longevity, and break immune exhaustion (182). These innovative interventions highlight a paradigm shift toward a mitochondrial-centered therapy paradigm encompassing not just tumor bioenergetics, but immune modulation, epitranscriptomics, and structural organelle vulnerability (183). As the art advances, the convergence of mitochondrial pharmacology, nanomedicine, and immune-oncology holds immense promise for glioma therapy in the context of precision oncology. **Figure 10.3** represents the various mitochondria-targeted therapy approaches.

10.13 MITOCHONDRIAL BIOMARKERS FOR PRECISION ONCOLOGY

In the rapidly evolving arena of precision neuro-oncology, the identification and utilization of mitochondrial biomarkers offer promising avenues for early diagnosis, prognostic stratification, treatment, and response prediction in gliomas. Unlike conventional markers limited to surface antigens or gene mutations, mitochondrial biomarkers capture the dynamic alterations in metabolism and bioenergetics that underlie the pathophysiology of gliomas. One of the most potent mitochondrial biomarkers of gliomas is mtDNA copy number variation. Both increased and decreased mtDNA content have been reported during the process of glioma grading, with variation having been linked to response to therapy and tumor aggressiveness (27). Decreased mtDNA content has been linked, for example, with increased glycolytic dependency and poor prognosis, whereas mtDNA-high tumors have increased oxidative metabolism and drug resistance (27). Moreover, mtDNA mutations, particularly in genes encoding complex I subunits (e.g., MT-ND1, MT-ND5), have been linked with impaired electron transport, elevated ROS production, and glioma aggressiveness (184).

Another novel class of mitochondrial biomarkers includes mitochondrial metabolites and oncometabolites. Changes in levels of citrate, fumarate, and succinate detectable with high-resolution magnetic resonance spectroscopy (MRS) reflect derangement of mitochondrial metabolism (185). These metabolites, in combination with elevated lactate/glucose ratios, are non-invasive imaging biomarkers of metabolic glioma classification. In addition, 2-HG accumulation in IDH1-mutant gliomas, irrespective of its nuclear origin, deranges mitochondrial function and has also been incorporated into clinical diagnostic algorithms by MR spectroscopy.

Proteogenomic analysis has now revealed mitochondria-associated proteins of diagnostic and prognostic value in gliomas. AIFM1 (apoptosis-inducing factor mitochondria-associated 1), a pro-apoptotic factor released with mitochondrial damage, is overexpressed in high-grade gliomas, especially pediatric glioma, as reported by Smith et al. in 2011 and correlates with poor survival (186,187). Similarly, a study conducted by Arif et al. in 2017 showed that VDAC1 (voltage-dependent anion channel 1), critical to mitochondrial metabolite exchange, is overexpressed in GB and supports metabolic flux under stress, serving as a biomarker and potential target (188).

Mitochondrial lipidomic alterations also provide a novel aspect for biomarker discovery. Altered levels of acyl-carnitines, cardiolipin, and phosphatidylethanolamine have also been found in glioma tissue, reflecting mitochondrial membrane remodeling and status of fatty acid oxidation (189). They can be quantified using mass spectrometry and investigated as either serum- or cerebrospinal fluid (CSF)-derived biomarkers. Mitochondrial components in the bloodstream—cell-free mtDNA (cf-mtDNA) and protein-bound mitochondrial extracellular vesicles—are emerging into focus for liquid biopsy (190). High plasma and CSF cf-mtDNA in glioma patients have been linked with tumor load and resistance to treatment (191,192). Furthermore, exosomes with mitochondrial enzymes like pyruvate dehydrogenase or NDUFS1 may represent the intratumoral metabolic state and inform the adjustment of therapy (193). Interestingly, mitochondrial biomarkers are prognostic but are also being utilized to predict response to treatment. Expression levels of mitochondrial chaperones like TRAP1 and HSP60, which ensure mitochondrial proteostasis, were identified to be associated with temozolomide and radiotherapy resistance (194). Overexpression of TRAP1, for instance, is predictive of refractoriness to alkylating agents and is being investigated in therapeutic stratification models (195). Incorporation of mitochondrial biomarkers into multi-omics platforms—integrating genomics, transcriptomics, metabolomics, and epigenomics—is now maximizing the accuracy of glioma classification. Mitochondria-based classifiers are now being created that link metabolic signatures to histopathological and molecular subtypes, eventually paving the way for the development of personalized therapies. **Table 10.2** presents the mitochondrial biomarkers in gliomas.

10.14 FUTURE DIRECTIONS IN MITOCHONDRIA-BASED NEURO-ONCOLOGY

The intersection of mitochondrial biology and neuro-oncology has opened up a previously unseen new frontier for glioma research and treatment. With our growing understanding of mitochondrial processes in tumor metabolism, redox homeostasis, apoptosis, and immune escape, the future of glioma treatment is ever more focused on these organelles as vulnerabilities for therapy. The mitochondrial-focusing perspective is revolutionizing the paradigm from the traditional cytotoxic broad-brush approaches to precision-guided and tumor-targeting therapies. One of the most promising directions is next-generation mitochondrial-targeted therapies. These comprise optimized small molecules that can selectively impair mitochondrial function in glioma cells without

TABLE 10.2
Mitochondrial Biomarkers in Gliomas

Biomarker	Biological Role	Type of Alteration in Gliomas	Clinical Relevance	Supporting Databases/ References
mtDNA copy number	Maintains mitochondrial genome stability and OXPHOS function	Increased or decreased copy number depending on glioma grade; linked to metabolic rewiring	Prognostic marker; low mtDNA associated with poor survival	(27,196,197)
MT-ND1, MT-ND5 (complex I subunits)	Electron transport chain function (NADH dehydrogenase activity)	Mutations lead to impaired respiration, ROS accumulation	Associated with tumor aggressiveness and radioresistance	(198,199)
COX4I1 (complex IV Isoform 1)	Cytochrome c oxidase function; oxygen sensing	Upregulated in hypoxic glioma regions	Predicts hypoxia-driven therapy resistance and poor prognosis	(200)
AIFM1 (apoptosis-inducing factor, mitochondrial)	Induces caspase-independent apoptosis under mitochondrial stress	Overexpressed in high-grade gliomas	Indicator of apoptosis dysregulation and adverse outcome	(201,202)
VDAC1 (voltage-dependent anion channel 1)	Regulates mitochondrial membrane potential and metabolite flux	Overexpressed in GB tissues; supports high metabolic demand	Marker of metabolic adaptability; therapeutic target candidate	(203,204)
TRAP1 (TNF-receptor-associated protein 1)	Mitochondrial chaperone regulating folding and ROS defense	Overexpressed in therapy-resistant gliomas	Predicts temozolomide resistance and shorter progression-free survival	(205,206)
Cardiolipin remodeling enzymes (TAZ, PLA2G6)	Maintain mitochondrial inner membrane integrity and cristae structure	Dysregulated cardiolipin metabolism in glioma mitochondria	Potential marker for mitochondrial membrane dysfunction and therapy sensitivity	(207,208)
cf-mtDNA (cell-free mitochondrial DNA)	Released into circulation from stressed or apoptotic cells	Elevated levels detected in glioma patients' plasma and CSF	Non-invasive biomarker for tumor burden and therapy monitoring	(191,209)

damaging normal neural tissue (210). Compounds like mito-metformin, MitoQ, and mitochondria-targeted honokiol analogs are being designed for increased BBB penetration and tumor selectivity. Furthermore, mitochondria-penetrating peptides (MPPs) and lipophilic cations (e.g., triphenylphosphonium-conjugated drugs) are being optimized to deliver payloads specifically into the mitochondrial matrix of glioma cells, allowing targeted modulation of respiration, membrane potential, or redox balance (211).

The concomitant advancement in therapeutic strategies is complemented by single-cell multi-omics technologies, which are revolutionizing the study of heterogeneity of mitochondria within the glioma microenvironment. Single-cell transcriptomics, proteomics, and metabolomics are integrated into these technologies to define mitochondrial states within different tumor subpopulations, i.e., GSCs with resistance to therapy. The global profiling has revealed subclones with specific mitochondrial dependencies, thus promising insights into precision stratification based on mitochondrial phenotypes rather than broad tumor features. Increasing evidence also supports the development of mitochondrial-based immunotherapeutics. Experiments indicate that modulating mitochondrial function in glioma cells can influence their immunogenicity, antigen presentation, and responsiveness to immune checkpoint blockade. New strategies to target mitochondrial stress pathways—such as ATF4/CHOP, UPRmt (unfolded protein response-mitochondria), and mitochondrial ROS signaling—are being explored to reverse immune suppression in the tumor microenvironment (157,212). In addition, mtDNA released from stressed tumor cells can function as a damage-associated molecular pattern (DAMP) to trigger innate immune activation through cGAS-STING signaling—a promising axis to increase immunotherapy responsiveness. Another expanding frontier is the use of AI-powered mitochondrial biomarker discovery. Through machine learning on high-throughput datasets from The Cancer Genome Atlas (TCGA), Genotype-Tissue Expression project (GTEx), and proteogenomic research, scientists are discovering mitochondrial gene signaling pathways (213).

10.15 CONCLUSION

Mitochondria, originally considered largely as cellular batteries, have come to be dynamic regulators of glioma pathophysiology—interacting with metabolism, redox signaling, stemness, treatment resistance, and immune modulation. Mitochondrial reprogramming in gliomas, particularly GB, is no longer a secondary effect but a prime regulator of tumor aggressiveness and treatment resistance. The chapter has highlighted the multi-dimensional roles of mitochondrial biology in tumor progression, with a focus on how compromised OXPHOS, metabolic plasticity, defective mitophagy, and redox imbalance provide the basis for glioma survival in hostile microenvironmental conditions. The incorporation of mitochondrial biomarkers into the realm of neuro-oncology is driving a new era of precision medicine. Individual mitochondrial proteins, genetic signatures, and metabolic intermediates yield strong diagnostic and prognostic information and are potential therapeutic targets. In addition, recent breakthroughs—spanning drug delivery systems for mitochondria and peptide conjugates to mitochondrial genome editing technologies—underscore the translational potential of this work. However, despite promising developments, significant lacunae and deficiencies remain. Current mitochondria-targeted therapies are not necessarily selective and may produce off-target toxicity in non-tumor cells, particularly neurons and astrocytes, as mitochondria-dependent. Additionally, the majority of mitochondrial modulators are at the preclinical or phase I trial stage, with limited data on long-term efficacy, penetration across the BBB, and tumor selectivity across heterogeneous patient populations.

One of the most significant limitations is our ignorance of mitochondrial heterogeneity in gliomas, especially in the GSC compartment. While technical advances in single-cell and spatial omics have begun to reveal metabolic zonation and the heterogeneity of mitochondrial states in tumors, their clinical potential is yet to be realized. Additionally, the functional interplay between mitochondrial dysfunction and epigenetic regulation in gliomas is yet to be exhaustively explored—most importantly, how mitochondrial metabolites influence chromatin remodeling, histone modification, and DNA methylation in response to IDH mutations or therapeutic resistance.

Another key gap is the lack of comprehensive integration of mitochondrial biology with immuno-oncology. Although mitochondrial stress and redox imbalance are proven to control tumor immune escape mechanisms, there is a deficiency of adequate clarity regarding how mitochondrial manipulation could be harnessed to enhance immune-based therapies, such as CAR-T cells and immune checkpoint inhibitors. Technical constraints are strong barriers. Lack of access to efficient in vivo imaging probes to monitor continuously mitochondrial activity in gliomas does not allow tracking of therapeutic response, as well as patient stratification. Similarly, current in vitro and in vivo glioma models often do not mirror the whole complexity of human mitochondrial dynamics and interactions between tumor and microenvironment, particularly the neurovascular unit.

In the coming years, systems-level integration of mitochondrial science with genomics, immunology, and neuroscience will be essential. Future mitochondria-centered neuro-oncology will be established by designing personalized metabolic blueprints using patient-derived organoids, imaging platforms, and artificial intelligence-powered biomarker discovery pipelines. Therapeutically, multimodality strategies incorporating redox modification, metabolic interference, and immuno-programming will probably deliver better outcomes than mono-targeted therapies. Mitochondria not only appear as a target but as a therapeutic axis that intersects with several glioma biology hallmarks. Moving beyond current constraints through interdisciplinarity and harnessing next-generation cutting-edge technology will be essential to unlocking the full clinical potential of mitochondria-targeted strategies. As our understanding continues to expand, mitochondria can very much be the key to shattering the long-standing therapeutic stalemate in glioma therapy—promising hope for extended mechanism-based intervention in precision neuro-oncology.

REFERENCES

1. Chen R, Smith-Cohn M, Cohen AL, Colman H. Glioma subclassifications and their clinical significance. Neurotherapeutics. 2017 Apr;14(2):284–97. https://doi.org/10.1007/s13311-017-0519-x
2. Torp SH, Solheim O, Skjulsvik AJ. The WHO 2021 Classification of Central Nervous System tumours: A practical update on what neurosurgeons need to know-a minireview. Acta Neurochir (Wien). 2022 Sep;164(9):2453–64. http://dx.doi.org/10.1007/s00701-022-05301-y
3. Liu Y'e, Sun Y, Guo Y, Shi X, Chen X, Feng W, et al. An overview: The diversified role of mitochondria in cancer metabolism. Int J Biol Sci. 2023 Jan 16;19(3):897–915. http://dx.doi.org/10.7150/ijbs.81609
4. Duraj T, García-Romero N, Carrión-Navarro J, Madurga R, Mendivil AO de, Prat-Acin R, et al. Beyond the Warburg effect: Oxidative and glycolytic phenotypes coexist within the metabolic heterogeneity of glioblastoma. Cells. 2021 Jan 20;10(2):202. http://dx.doi.org/10.3390/cells10020202
5. Agnihotri S, Zadeh G. Metabolic reprogramming in glioblastoma: The influence of cancer metabolism on epigenetics and unanswered questions. Neuro Oncol. 2016 Feb;18(2):160–72. http://dx.doi.org/10.1093/neuonc/nov125
6. Nguyen C, Pandey S. Exploiting mitochondrial vulnerabilities to trigger apoptosis selectively in cancer cells. Cancers (Basel). 2019 Jun 29;11(7):916. http://dx.doi.org/10.3390/cancers11070916
7. Krzyszczyk P, Acevedo A, Davidoff EJ, Timmins LM, Marrero-Berrios I, Patel M, et al. The growing role of precision and personalized medicine for cancer treatment. Technology. 2018 Sep-Dec;6(3–4):79–100. http://dx.doi.org/10.1142/S2339547818300020
8. Park YW, Vollmuth P, Foltyn-Dumitru M, Sahm F, Ahn SS, Chang JH, et al. The 2021 WHO classification for gliomas and implications on imaging diagnosis: Part 1 – Key points of the fifth edition and summary of imaging findings on adult-type diffuse gliomas. J Magn Reson Imaging. 2023 Sep;58(3):677–89. https://doi.org/10.1002/jmri.28743
9. Kayabolen A, Yilmaz E, Bagci-Onder T. IDH mutations in glioma: Double-edged sword in clinical applications? Biomedicines. 2021 Jul 10;9(7):799. http://dx.doi.org/10.3390/biomedicines9070799
10. Solomou G, Finch A, Asghar A, Bardella C. Mutant IDH in gliomas: Role in cancer and treatment options. Cancers (Basel). 2023 May 23;15(11). http://dx.doi.org/10.3390/cancers15112883
11. Dipasquale A, Franceschi E, Lombardi G, Simonelli M. Vorasidenib in IDH mutant WHO grade 2 gliomas: Time to stop sitting on the fence? Neurooncol Adv. 2024 Jan;6(1):vdae003. http://dx.doi.org/10.1093/noajnl/vdae003
12. Mellinghoff IK, van den Bent MJ, Blumenthal DT, Touat M, Peters KB, Clarke J, et al. Vorasidenib in IDH1- or IDH2-mutant low-grade glioma. N Engl J Med. 2023 Aug 17;389(7):589–601. http://dx.doi.org/10.1056/NEJMoa2304194
13. Steininger J, Buszello C, Oertel R, Meinhardt M, Schmid S, Engellandt K, et al. Efficacy of BRAF/MEK-inhibitor therapy for epithelioid glioblastoma with a novel BRAFV600 mutation. Acta Neuropathol Commun. 2024 Aug 6;12(1):124. http://dx.doi.org/10.1186/s40478-024-01834-8
14. Bhowmik A, Khan R, Ghosh MK. Blood brain barrier: A challenge for effectual therapy of brain tumors. Biomed Res Int. 2015 Mar 19;2015:320941. http://dx.doi.org/10.1155/2015/320941
15. Rangaraju V, Lewis TL Jr, Hirabayashi Y, Bergami M, Motori E, Cartoni R, et al. Pleiotropic mitochondria: The influence of mitochondria on neuronal development and disease. J Neurosci. 2019 Oct 16;39(42):8200–8. http://dx.doi.org/10.1523/JNEUROSCI.1157-19.2019
16. Bhatti JS, Bhatti GK, Reddy PH. Mitochondrial dysfunction and oxidative stress in metabolic disorders – A step towards mitochondria based therapeutic strategies. Biochim Biophys Acta Mol Basis Dis. 2017 May;1863(5):1066–77. https://doi.org/10.1016/j.bbadis.2016.11.010

17. Song N, Mei S, Wang X, Hu G, Lu M. Focusing on mitochondria in the brain: From biology to therapeutics. Transl Neurodegener. 2024 Apr 17;13(1):23. http://dx.doi.org/10.1186/s40035-024-00409-w
18. Zhang S, Zhao J, Quan Z, Li H, Qing H. Mitochondria and other organelles in neural development and their potential as therapeutic targets in neurodegenerative diseases. Front Neurosci. 2022 Apr 5;16:853911. http://dx.doi.org/10.3389/fnins.2022.853911
19. Ferree A, Shirihai O. Mitochondrial dynamics: The intersection of form and function. Adv Exp Med Biol. 2012;748:13–40. http://dx.doi.org/10.1007/978-1-4614-3573-0_2
20. Quintana-Cabrera R, Scorrano L. Determinants and outcomes of mitochondrial dynamics. Mol Cell. 2023 Mar 16;83(6):857–76. https://doi.org/10.1016/j.molcel.2023.02.012
21. Bagur R, Hajnóczky G. Intracellular Ca^{2}+ sensing: Its role in calcium homeostasis and signaling. Mol Cell. 2017 Jun 15;66(6):780–8. http://dx.doi.org/10.1016/j.molcel.2017.05.028
22. Gleichmann M, Mattson MP. Neuronal calcium homeostasis and dysregulation. Antioxid Redox Signal. 2011 Apr 1;14(7):1261–73. http://dx.doi.org/10.1089/ars.2010.3386
23. Beckervordersandforth R. Mitochondrial metabolism-mediated regulation of adult neurogenesis. Brain Plast. 2017 Nov 9;3(1):73–87. http://dx.doi.org/10.3233/BPL-170044
24. Zong Y, Li H, Liao P, Chen L, Pan Y, Zheng Y, et al. Mitochondrial dysfunction: Mechanisms and advances in therapy. Signal Transduct Target Ther. 2024 May 15;9(1):124. https://doi.org/10.1038/s41392-024-01839-8
25. Klemmensen MM, Borrowman SH, Pearce C, Pyles B, Chandra B. Mitochondrial dysfunction in neurodegenerative disorders. Neurotherapeutics. 2024 Jan;21(1):e00292. http://dx.doi.org/10.1016/j.neurot.2023.10.002
26. Arismendi-Morillo G, Castellano-Ramírez A, N. Seyfried T. Functional and therapeutic implications of mitochondrial network and mitochondria-associated membranes: The glioma's case. In: Glioma – Contemporary Diagnostic and Therapeutic Approaches. IntechOpen; 2019. http://dx.doi.org/10.5772/intechopen.77224
27. Mohamed Yusoff AA, Mohd Khair SZN, Abd Radzak SM. Mitochondrial DNA copy number alterations: Key players in the complexity of glioblastoma (review). Mol Med Rep. 2025 Mar;31(3). http://dx.doi.org/10.3892/mmr.2025.13443
28. Mohamed Yusoff AA, Mohd Nasir KN, Haris K, Mohd Khair SZN, Abdul Ghani ARI, Idris Z, et al. Detection of somatic mutations in the mitochondrial DNA control region D-loop in brain tumors: The first report in Malaysian patients. Oncol Lett. 2017 Nov;14(5):5179–88. http://dx.doi.org/10.3892/ol.2017.6851
29. Yeung KY, Dickinson A, Donoghue JF, Polekhina G, White SJ, Grammatopoulos DK, et al. The identification of mitochondrial DNA variants in glioblastoma multiforme. Acta Neuropathol Commun. 2014 Jan 2;2(1):1. http://dx.doi.org/10.1186/2051-5960-2-1
30. Lloyd RE, Keatley K, Littlewood DTJ, Meunier B, Holt WV, An Q, et al. Identification and functional prediction of mitochondrial complex III and IV mutations associated with glioblastoma. Neuro Oncol. 2015 Jul;17(7):942–52. http://dx.doi.org/10.1093/neuonc/nov020
31. Griguer CE, Cantor AB, Fathallah-Shaykh HM, Gillespie GY, Gordon AS, Markert JM, et al. Prognostic relevance of cytochrome C oxidase in primary glioblastoma multiforme. PLoS One. 2013 Apr 10;8(4):e61035. http://dx.doi.org/10.1371/journal.pone.0061035
32. Brunelle JK, Letai A. Control of mitochondrial apoptosis by the Bcl-2 family. J Cell Sci. 2009 Feb 15;122(Pt 4):437–41. http://dx.doi.org/10.1242/jcs.031682
33. Rasola A, Bernardi P. The mitochondrial permeability transition pore and its adaptive responses in tumor cells. Cell Calcium. 2014 Dec;56(6):437–45. http://dx.doi.org/10.1016/j.ceca.2014.10.003
34. Shang E, Nguyen TTT, Shu C, Westhoff MA, Karpel-Massler G, Siegelin MD. Epigenetic targeting of Mcl-1 is synthetically lethal with Bcl-xL/Bcl-2 inhibition in model systems of glioblastoma. Cancers (Basel). 2020 Aug 1;12(8):2137. https://doi.org/10.3390/cancers12082137
35. Mudassar F, Shen H, O'Neill G, Hau E. Targeting tumor hypoxia and mitochondrial metabolism with anti-parasitic drugs to improve radiation response in high-grade gliomas. J Exp Clin Cancer Res. 2020 Oct 7;39(1):208. http://dx.doi.org/10.1186/s13046-020-01724-6
36. Rai Y, Tiwari AK, Pandey R, Dwarakanath BS, Bhatt AN. Hyper-energy metabolism of oxidative phosphorylation and enhanced glycolysis contributes to radioresistance in glioma cells. Free Radic Res. 2025 Feb;59(2):117–28. http://dx.doi.org/10.1080/10715762.2025.2456740
37. Xu W, Yang H, Liu Y, Yang Y, Wang P, Kim SH, et al. Oncometabolite 2-hydroxyglutarate is a competitive inhibitor of α-ketoglutarate-dependent dioxygenases. Cancer Cell. 2011 Jan 18;19(1):17–30. http://dx.doi.org/10.1016/j.ccr.2010.12.014
38. Chou FJ, Liu Y, Lang F, Yang C. D-2-hydroxyglutarate in glioma biology. Cells. 2021 Sep 7;10(9):2345. http://dx.doi.org/10.3390/cells10092345

39. Wigerup C, Påhlman S, Bexell D. Therapeutic targeting of hypoxia and hypoxia-inducible factors in cancer. Pharmacol Ther. 2016 Aug;164:152–69. https://doi.org/10.1016/j.pharmthera.2016.04.009
40. Qiao Q, Hu S, Wang X. The regulatory roles and clinical significance of glycolysis in tumor. Cancer Commun (Lond). 2024 Jul;44(7):761–86. http://dx.doi.org/10.1002/cac2.12549
41. Iranmanesh Y, Jiang B, Favour OC, Dou Z, Wu J, Li J, et al. Mitochondria's role in the maintenance of cancer stem cells in glioblastoma. Front Oncol. 2021 Feb 22;11:582694. http://dx.doi.org/10.3389/fonc.2021.582694
42. Obara-Michlewska M, Szeliga M. Targeting glutamine addiction in gliomas. Cancers (Basel). 2020 Jan 29;12(2):310. http://dx.doi.org/10.3390/cancers12020310
43. Maus A, Peters GJ. Glutamate and α-ketoglutarate: Key players in glioma metabolism. Amino Acids. 2017 Jan;49(1):21–32. http://dx.doi.org/10.1007/s00726-016-2342-9
44. Kou Y, Geng F, Guo D. Lipid metabolism in glioblastoma: From DE Novo synthesis to storage. Biomedicines. 2022 Aug 11;10(8):1943. http://dx.doi.org/10.3390/biomedicines10081943
45. Reiter-Brennan C, Semmler L, Klein A. The effects of 2-hydroxyglutarate on the tumorigenesis of gliomas. Contemp Oncol (Pozn). 2018 Dec 31;22(4):215–22. http://dx.doi.org/10.5114/wo.2018.82642
46. Miller JJ. Targeting IDH-mutant glioma. Neurotherapeutics. 2022 Oct;19(6):1724–32. http://dx.doi.org/10.1007/s13311-022-01238-3
47. Pérez-Tomás R, Pérez-Guillén I. Lactate in the tumor microenvironment: An essential molecule in cancer progression and treatment. Cancers (Basel). 2020 Nov 3;12(11):3244. http://dx.doi.org/10.3390/cancers12113244
48. Zhang D, Tang Z, Huang H, Zhou G, Cui C, Weng Y, et al. Metabolic regulation of gene expression by histone lactylation. Nature. 2019 Oct;574(7779):575–80. http://dx.doi.org/10.1038/s41586-019-1678-1
49. Gu J, Zhou J, Chen Q, Xu X, Gao J, Li X, et al. Tumor metabolite lactate promotes tumorigenesis by modulating MOESIN lactylation and enhancing TGF-β signaling in regulatory T cells. Cell Rep. 2022 Jul 19;40(3):111122. http://dx.doi.org/10.1016/j.celrep.2022.111122
50. Koltai T, Fliegel L. Exploring monocarboxylate transporter inhibition for cancer treatment. Explor Target Antitumor Ther. 2024 Feb 23;5(1):135–69. http://dx.doi.org/10.37349/etat.2024.00210
51. Miranda-Gonçalves V, Honavar M, Pinheiro C, Martinho O, Pires MM, Pinheiro C, et al. Monocarboxylate transporters (MCTs) in gliomas: Expression and exploitation as therapeutic targets. Neuro Oncol. 2013 Feb;15(2):172–88. http://dx.doi.org/10.1093/neuonc/nos298
52. Indran IR, Tufo G, Pervaiz S, Brenner C. Recent advances in apoptosis, mitochondria and drug resistance in cancer cells. Biochim Biophys Acta. 2011 Jun;1807(6):735–45. https://doi.org/10.1016/j.bbabio.2011.03.010
53. Ortiz R, Perazzoli G, Cabeza L, Jiménez-Luna C, Luque R, Prados J, et al. Temozolomide: An updated overview of resistance mechanisms, nanotechnology advances and clinical applications. Curr Neuropharmacol. 2021;19(4):513–37. http://dx.doi.org/10.2174/1570159X18666200626204005
54. Karpel-Massler G, Bâ M, Shu C, Halatsch ME, Westhoff MA, Bruce JN, et al. TIC10/ONC201 synergizes with Bcl-2/Bcl-xL inhibition in glioblastoma by suppression of Mcl-1 and its binding partners in vitro and in vivo. Oncotarget. 2015 Nov 3;6(34):36456–71. http://dx.doi.org/10.18632/oncotarget.5505
55. Yang MC, Loh JK, Li YY, Huang WS, Chou CH, Cheng JT, et al. Bcl2L12 with a BH3-like domain in regulating apoptosis and TMZ-induced autophagy: A prospective combination of ABT-737 and TMZ for treating glioma. Int J Oncol. 2015 Mar;46(3):1304–16. http://dx.doi.org/10.3892/ijo.2015.2838
56. Lopez PLC, Filippi-Chiela EC, Silva AO, Cordero EAA, Garcia-Santos D, Pelegrini AL, et al. Sensitization of glioma cells by X-linked inhibitor of apoptosis protein knockdown. Oncology. 2012 Jun 29;83(2):75–82. https://doi.org/10.1159/000337978
57. Scheid AD, Beadnell TC, Welch DR. The second genome: Effects of the mitochondrial genome on cancer progression. Adv Cancer Res. 2019 Feb 27;142:63–105. http://dx.doi.org/10.1016/bs.acr.2019.01.001
58. Sravya P, Nimbalkar VP, Kanuri NN, Sugur H, Verma BK, Kundu P, et al. Low mitochondrial DNA copy number is associated with poor prognosis and treatment resistance in glioblastoma. Mitochondrio. 2020 Nov;55:154–63. http://dx.doi.org/10.1016/j.mito.2020.10.001
59. van Gisbergen MW, Voets AM, Starmans MHW, de Coo IFM, Yadak R, Hoffmann RF, et al. How do changes in the mtDNA and mitochondrial dysfunction influence cancer and cancer therapy? Challenges, opportunities and models. Mutat Res Rev Mutat Res. 2015 Apr;764:16–30. https://doi.org/10.1016/j.mrrev.2015.01.001
60. Modica-Napolitano JS, Weissig V. Treatment strategies that enhance the efficacy and selectivity of mitochondria-targeted anticancer agents. Int J Mol Sci. 2015 Jul 29;16(8):17394–421. http://dx.doi.org/10.3390/ijms160817394

61. Sharapov MG, Novoselov VI. Catalytic and signaling role of peroxiredoxins in carcinogenesis. Biochemistry (Mosc). 2019 Feb;84(2):79–100. http://dx.doi.org/10.1134/S0006297919020019
62. Ortega AL, Mena S, Estrela JM. Glutathione in cancer cell death. Cancers (Basel). 2011 Mar 11;3(1):1285–310. http://dx.doi.org/10.3390/cancers3011285
63. Chien CH, Chuang JY, Yang ST, Yang WB, Chen PY, Hsu TI, et al. Enrichment of superoxide dismutase 2 in glioblastoma confers to acquisition of temozolomide resistance that is associated with tumor-initiating cell subsets. J Biomed Sci. 2019 Oct 19;26(1):77. http://dx.doi.org/10.1186/s12929-019-0565-2
64. Kasai S, Shimizu S, Tatara Y, Mimura J, Itoh K. Regulation of Nrf2 by mitochondrial reactive oxygen species in physiology and pathology. Biomolecules. 2020 Feb 17;10(2):320. http://dx.doi.org/10.3390/biom10020320
65. Singh N, Miner A, Hennis L, Mittal S. Mechanisms of temozolomide resistance in glioblastoma – A comprehensive review. Canc Drug Resist. 2021 Mar 19;4:17–43. http://dx.doi.org/10.20517/cdr.2020.79
66. Zhang H, Chen Y, Liu X, Deng H. Multi-omics analyses reveal mitochondrial dysfunction contributing to temozolomide resistance in glioblastoma cells. Biomolecules. 2023 Sep 19;13(9). https://doi.org/10.3390/biom13091408
67. Liu YJ, McIntyre RL, Janssens GE, Houtkooper RH. Mitochondrial fission and fusion: A dynamic role in aging and potential target for age-related disease. Mech Ageing Dev. 2020 Mar;186(111212):111212. https://doi.org/10.1016/j.mad.2020.111212
68. Xie Q, Wu Q, Horbinski CM, Flavahan WA, Yang K, Zhou W, et al. Mitochondrial control by DRP1 in brain tumor initiating cells. Nat Neurosci. 2015 Apr;18(4):501–10. http://dx.doi.org/10.1038/nn.3960
69. Lu Z, Sun GF, He KY, Zhang Z, Han XH, Qu XH, et al. Targeted inhibition of branched-chain amino acid metabolism drives apoptosis of glioblastoma by facilitating ubiquitin degradation of Mfn2 and oxidative stress. Biochim Biophys Acta Mol Basis Dis. 2024 Jun;1870(5):167220. http://dx.doi.org/10.1016/j.bbadis.2024.167220
70. Giddings EL, Champagne DP, Wu MH, Laffin JM, Thornton TM, Valenca-Pereira F, et al. Mitochondrial ATP fuels ABC transporter-mediated drug efflux in cancer chemoresistance. Nat Commun. 2021 May 14;12(1):2804. http://dx.doi.org/10.1038/s41467-021-23071-6
71. Jing X, Yang F, Shao C, Wei K, Xie M, Shen H, et al. Role of hypoxia in cancer therapy by regulating the tumor microenvironment. Mol Cancer. 2019 Nov 11;18(1):157. http://dx.doi.org/10.1186/s12943-019-1089-9
72. Chen L, Zhang H, Shang C, Hong Y. The role and applied value of mitochondria in glioma-related research. CNS Neurosci Ther. 2024 Dec;30(12):e70121. http://dx.doi.org/10.1111/cns.70121
73. Pujalte-Martin M, Belaïd A, Bost S, Kahi M, Peraldi P, Rouleau M, et al. Targeting cancer and immune cell metabolism with the complex I inhibitors metformin and IACS-010759. Mol Oncol. 2024 Jul;18(7):1719–38. http://dx.doi.org/10.1002/1878-0261.13583
74. Armstrong JS. Mitochondrial medicine: Pharmacological targeting of mitochondria in disease. Br J Pharmacol. 2007 Aug;151(8):1154–65. http://dx.doi.org/10.1038/sj.bjp.0707288
75. Sulaimon LA, Afolabi LO, Adisa RA, Ayankojo AG, Afolabi MO, Adewolu AM, et al. Pharmacological significance of MitoQ in ameliorating mitochondria-related diseases. Adv Redox Res. 2022 Jul;5(100037):100037. https://doi.org/10.1016/j.arres.2022.100037
76. Tufail M, Hu JJ, Liang J, He CY, Wan WD, Huang YQ, et al. Predictive, preventive, and personalized medicine in breast cancer: Targeting the PI3K pathway. J Transl Med. 2024 Jan 3;22(1):15. http://dx.doi.org/10.1186/s12967-023-04841-w
77. Liu S, Dong L, Shi W, Zheng Z, Liu Z, Meng L, et al. Potential targets and treatments affect oxidative stress in gliomas: An overview of molecular mechanisms. Front Pharmacol. 2022 Jul 22;13:921070. http://dx.doi.org/10.3389/fphar.2022.921070
78. de Almeida AJPO, de Oliveira JCPL, da Silva Pontes LV, de Souza Júnior JF, Gonçalves TAF, Dantas SH, et al. ROS: Basic concepts, sources, cellular signaling, and its implications in aging pathways. Oxid Med Cell Longev. 2022 Oct 19;2022:1225578. http://dx.doi.org/10.1155/2022/1225578
79. Hong Y, Boiti A, Vallone D, Foulkes NS. Reactive oxygen species signaling and oxidative stress: Transcriptional regulation and evolution. Antioxidants (Basel). 2024 Mar 1;13(3):312. http://dx.doi.org/10.3390/antiox13030312
80. Marí M, Morales A, Colell A, García-Ruiz C, Fernández-Checa JC. Mitochondrial glutathione, a key survival antioxidant. Antioxid Redox Signal. 2009 Nov;11(11):2685–700. http://dx.doi.org/10.1089/ARS.2009.2695

81. Chang KY, Hsu TI, Hsu CC, Tsai SY, Liu JJ, Chou SW, et al. Specificity protein 1-modulated superoxide dismutase 2 enhances temozolomide resistance in glioblastoma, which is independent of O6-methylguanine-DNA methyltransferase. Redox Biol. 2017 Oct;13:655–64. https://doi.org/10.1016/j.redox.2017.08.005
82. Lewerenz J, Hewett SJ, Huang Y, Lambros M, Gout PW, Kalivas PW, et al. The cystine/glutamate antiporter system x(c)(-) in health and disease: From molecular mechanisms to novel therapeutic opportunities. Antioxid Redox Signal. 2013 Feb 10;18(5):522–55. http://dx.doi.org/10.1089/ars.2011.4391
83. Polewski MD, Reveron-Thornton RF, Cherryholmes GA, Marinov GK, Aboody KS. SLC7A11 Overexpression in glioblastoma is associated with increased cancer stem cell-like properties. Stem Cells Dev. 2017 Sep 1;26(17):1236–46. http://dx.doi.org/10.1089/scd.2017.0123
84. Liu X, Zhang Y, Zhuang L, Olszewski K, Gan B. NADPH debt drives redox bankruptcy: SLC7A11/xCT-mediated cystine uptake as a double-edged sword in cellular redox regulation. Genes Dis. 2021 Nov;8(6):731–45. https://doi.org/10.1016/j.gendis.2020.11.010
85. Hu CL, Nydes M, Shanley KL, Morales Pantoja IE, Howard TA, Bizzozero OA. Reduced expression of the ferroptosis inhibitor glutathione peroxidase-4 in multiple sclerosis and experimental autoimmune encephalomyelitis. J Neurochem. 2019 Feb;148(3):426–39. http://dx.doi.org/10.1111/jnc.14604
86. Kahya U, Köseer AS, Dubrovska A. Amino acid transporters on the guard of cell genome and epigenome. Cancers (Basel). 2021 Jan 2;13(1):125. http://dx.doi.org/10.3390/cancers13010125
87. Tuna G, Bekar NED, İşlekel S, İşlekel GH. Urinary 8-hydroxy-2′-deoxyguanosine levels are elevated in patients with IDH1-wildtype glioblastoma and are associated with tumor recurrence in gliomas. DNA Repair (Amst). 2023 Apr;124(103463):103463. http://dx.doi.org/10.1016/j.dnarep.2023.103463
88. Lian M, Zhang X, Wang H, Liu H, Chen W, Guo S. Increased 8-hydroxydeoxyguanosine in high-grade gliomas is associated with activation of autophagy. Int J Neurosci. 2014 Dec;124(12):926–34. http://dx.doi.org/10.3109/00207454.2014.891998
89. Khan AQ, Rashid K, AlAmodi AA, Agha MV, Akhtar S, Hakeem I, et al. Reactive oxygen species (ROS) in cancer pathogenesis and therapy: An update on the role of ROS in anticancer action of benzophenanthridine alkaloids. Biomed Pharmacother. 2021 Nov;143:112142. https://doi.org/10.1016/j.biopha.2021.112142
90. Yang YC, Zhu Y, Sun SJ, Zhao CJ, Bai Y, Wang J, et al. ROS regulation in gliomas: Implications for treatment strategies. Front Immunol. 2023 Dec 7;14:1259797. http://dx.doi.org/10.3389/fimmu.2023.1259797
91. Zhang Z, Xu X, Du J, Chen X, Xue Y, Zhang J, et al. Redox-responsive polymer micelles co-encapsulating immune checkpoint inhibitors and chemotherapeutic agents for glioblastoma therapy. Nat Commun. 2024 Feb 6;15(1):1118. http://dx.doi.org/10.1038/s41467-024-44963-3
92. Trejo-Solís C, Escamilla-Ramírez Á, Gómez-Manzo S, Castillo-Rodriguez RA, Palomares-Alonso F, Castillo-Pérez C, et al. The pentose phosphate pathway (PPP) in the glioma metabolism: A potent enhancer of malignancy. Biochimie. 2025 Jan 31;232:117–26. http://dx.doi.org/10.1016/j.biochi.2025.01.013
93. Biedermann J, Preussler M, Conde M, Peitzsch M, Richter S, Wiedemuth R, et al. Mutant IDH1 differently affects redox state and metabolism in glial cells of normal and tumor origin. Cancers (Basel). 2019 Dec 16;11(12):2028. http://dx.doi.org/10.3390/cancers11122028
94. Cheng G, Karoui H, Hardy M, Kalyanaraman B. Redox-crippled MitoQ potently inhibits breast cancer and glioma cell proliferation: A negative control for verifying the antioxidant mechanism of MitoQ in cancer and other oxidative pathologies. Free Radic Biol Med. 2023 Aug 20;205:175–87. https://doi.org/10.1016/j.freeradbiomed.2023.06.009
95. Zheng P, Zhou C, Lu L, Liu B, Ding Y. Elesclomol: A copper ionophore targeting mitochondrial metabolism for cancer therapy. J Exp Clin Cancer Res. 2022 Sep 12;41(1):271. http://dx.doi.org/10.1186/s13046-022-02485-0
96. Zerihun M, Sukumaran S, Qvit N. The Drp1-mediated mitochondrial fission protein interactome as an emerging core player in mitochondrial dynamics and cardiovascular disease therapy. Int J Mol Sci. 2023 Mar 17;24(6). http://dx.doi.org/10.3390/ijms24065785
97. Adhikary A, Mukherjee A, Banerjee R, Nagotu S. DRP1: At the Crossroads of dysregulated mitochondrial dynamics and altered cell signaling in cancer cells. ACS Omega. 2023 Dec 5;8(48):45208–23. http://dx.doi.org/10.1021/acsomega.3c06547
98. Deng Y, Ngo DTM, Holien JK, Lees JG, Lim SY. Mitochondrial dynamin-related protein Drp1: A new player in cardio-oncology. Curr Oncol Rep. 2022 Dec;24(12):1751–63. http://dx.doi.org/10.1007/s11912-022-01333-w
99. Huang TL, Chang CR, Chien CY, Huang GK, Chen YF, Su LJ, et al. DRP1 contributes to head and neck cancer progression and induces glycolysis through modulated FOXM1/MMP12 axis. Mol Oncol. 2022 Jul;16(13):2585–606. http://dx.doi.org/10.1002/1878-0261.13212

100. Wu NS, Ma IC, Lin YF, Ko HJ, Loh JK, Hong YR. The mystery of phospho-Drp1 with four adaptors in cell cycle: When mitochondrial fission couples to cell fate decisions. Cell Cycle. 2023 Nov;22(21-22):2485–503. http://dx.doi.org/10.1080/15384101.2023.2289753
101. Qian W, Wang J, Roginskaya V, McDermott LA, Edwards RP, Stolz DB, et al. Novel combination of mitochondrial division inhibitor 1 (mdivi-1) and platinum agents produces synergistic pro-apoptotic effect in drug resistant tumor cells. Oncotarget. 2014 Jun 30;5(12):4180–94. http://dx.doi.org/10.18632/oncotarget.1944
102. Song Z, Ghochani M, McCaffery JM, Frey TG, Chan DC. Mitofusins and OPA1 mediate sequential steps in mitochondrial membrane fusion. Mol Biol Cell. 2009 Aug;20(15):3525–32. http://dx.doi.org/10.1091/mbc.e09-03-0252
103. Sidarala V, Zhu J, Levi-D'Ancona E, Pearson GL, Reck EC, Walker EM, et al. Mitofusin 1 and 2 regulation of mitochondrial DNA content is a critical determinant of glucose homeostasis. Nat Commun. 2022 Apr 29;13(1):2340. https://doi.org/10.1038/s41467-022-29945-7
104. Cortes Ballen AI, Amosu M, Ravinder S, Chan J, Derin E, Slika H, et al. Metabolic reprogramming in glioblastoma multiforme: A review of pathways and therapeutic targets. Cells. 2024 Sep 19;13(18):1574. http://dx.doi.org/10.3390/cells13181574
105. Gimple RC, Bhargava S, Dixit D, Rich JN. Glioblastoma stem cells: Lessons from the tumor hierarchy in a lethal cancer. Genes Dev. 2019 Jun 1;33(11–12):591–609. http://dx.doi.org/10.1101/gad.324301.119
106. Kriel J, Müller-Nedebock K, Maarman G, Mbizana S, Ojuka E, Klumperman B, et al. Coordinated autophagy modulation overcomes glioblastoma chemoresistance through disruption of mitochondrial bioenergetics. Sci Rep. 2018 Jul 9;8(1):10348. http://dx.doi.org/10.1038/s41598-018-28590-9
107. Wang XL, Feng ST, Wang YT, Yuan YH, Li ZP, Chen NH, et al. Mitophagy, a form of selective autophagy, plays an essential role in mitochondrial dynamics of Parkinson's disease. Cell Mol Neurobiol. 2022 Jul;42(5):1321–39. http://dx.doi.org/10.1007/s10571-021-01039-w
108. Bayne AN, Trempe JF. Mechanisms of PINK1, ubiquitin and Parkin interactions in mitochondrial quality control and beyond. Cell Mol Life Sci. 2019 Dec;76(23):4589–611. http://dx.doi.org/10.1007/s00018-019-03203-4
109. Lin DC, Xu L, Chen Y, Yan H, Hazawa M, Doan N, et al. Genomic and functional analysis of the E3 ligase PARK2 in glioma. Cancer Res. 2015 May 1;75(9):1815–27. http://dx.doi.org/10.1158/0008-5472.CAN-14-1433
110. Jin SM, Youle RJ. PINK1- and Parkin-mediated mitophagy at a glance. J Cell Sci. 2012 Feb 15;125(Pt 4):795–9. http://dx.doi.org/10.1242/jcs.093849
111. Li Y, Zheng W, Lu Y, Zheng Y, Pan L, Wu X, et al. BNIP3L/NIX-mediated mitophagy: Molecular mechanisms and implications for human disease. Cell Death Dis. 2021 Dec 20;13(1):14. http://dx.doi.org/10.1038/s41419-021-04469-y
112. Song C, Pan S, Zhang J, Li N, Geng Q. Mitophagy: A novel perspective for insighting into cancer and cancer treatment. Cell Prolif. 2022 Dec;55(12):e13327. http://dx.doi.org/10.1111/cpr.13327
113. Sessions DT, Kashatus DF. Mitochondrial dynamics in cancer stem cells. Cell Mol Life Sci. 2021 Apr;78(8):3803–16. http://dx.doi.org/10.1007/s00018-021-03773-2
114. Glaviano A, Foo ASC, Lam HY, Yap KCH, Jacot W, Jones RH, et al. PI3K/AKT/mTOR signaling transduction pathway and targeted therapies in cancer. Mol Cancer. 2023 Aug 18;22(1):138. http://dx.doi.org/10.1186/s12943-023-01827-6
115. Xu X, Peng Q, Jiang X, Tan S, Yang Y, Yang W, et al. Metabolic reprogramming and epigenetic modifications in cancer: From the impacts and mechanisms to the treatment potential. Exp Mol Med. 2023 Jul;55(7):1357–70. http://dx.doi.org/10.1038/s12276-023-01020-1
116. Bordt EA, Clerc P, Roelofs BA, Saladino AJ, Tretter L, Adam-Vizi V, et al. The putative Drp1 inhibitor mdivi-1 is a reversible mitochondrial complex I inhibitor that modulates reactive oxygen species. Dev Cell. 2017 Mar 27;40(6):583–94.e6. http://dx.doi.org/10.1016/j.devcel.2017.02.020
117. Geng Y, Kohli L, Klocke BJ, Roth KA. Chloroquine-induced autophagic vacuole accumulation and cell death in glioma cells is p53 independent. Neuro Oncol. 2010 May;12(5):473–81. http://dx.doi.org/10.1093/neuonc/nop048
118. Dong F, Yin H, Zheng Z. Hypoxia-inducible factor-1α regulates BNIP3-dependent mitophagy and mediates metabolic reprogramming through histone lysine lactylation modification to affect glioma proliferation and invasion. J Biochem Mol Toxicol. 2025 Feb;39(2):e70069. https://doi.org/10.1002/jbt.70069
119. Papadaki S, Magklara A. Regulation of metabolic plasticity in cancer stem cells and implications in cancer therapy. Cancers (Basel). 2022 Nov 30;14(23):5912. https://doi.org/10.3390/cancers14235912

120. Bogataj U, Novak M, Galun SK, Fon Tacer K, Vittori M, Van Noorden CJF, et al. Heterogenous mitochondrial ultrastructure and metabolism of human glioblastoma cells: Differences between stem-like and differentiated cancer cells in response to chemotherapy. bioRxiv. 2025. https://doi.org/10.1101/2025.02.17.638633
121. Noh JK, Woo SR, Kong M, Lee MK, Lee JW, Lee YC, et al. Gene signature predicting recurrence in oral squamous cell carcinoma is characterized by increased oxidative phosphorylation. Mol Oncol. 2023 Jan;17(1):134–49. http://dx.doi.org/10.1002/1878-0261.13328
122. Bruns I, Sauer B, Burger MC, Eriksson J, Hofmann U, Braun Y, et al. Disruption of peroxisome proliferator-activated receptor γ coactivator (PGC)-1α reverts key features of the neoplastic phenotype of glioma cells. J Biol Chem. 2019 Mar 1;294(9):3037–50. http://dx.doi.org/10.1074/jbc.RA118.006993
123. Lee H, Park J, Tran Q, Kim D, Hong Y, Cho H, et al. Mitochondrial transcription factor A (TFAM) is upregulated in glioma. Mol Med Rep. 2017 Jun;15(6):3781–6. http://dx.doi.org/10.3892/mmr.2017.6467
124. Zhang L, Cao H, Tao H, Yang J, Gong W, Hu Q. Effect of the interference with DRP1 expression on the biological characteristics of glioma stem cells. Exp Ther Med. 2021 Jul;22(1):696. http://dx.doi.org/10.3892/etm.2021.10128
125. Gu LF, Chen JQ, Lin QY, Yang YZ. Roles of mitochondrial unfolded protein response in mammalian stem cells. World J Stem Cells. 2021 Jul 26;13(7):737–52. http://dx.doi.org/10.4252/wjsc.v13.i7.737
126. Shang E, Nguyen TTT, Westhoff MA, Karpel-Massler G, Siegelin MD. Targeting cellular respiration as a therapeutic strategy in glioblastoma. Oncotarget. 2023 May 4;14:419–25. http://dx.doi.org/10.18632/oncotarget.28424
127. Sharma P, Aaroe A, Liang J, Puduvalli VK. Tumor microenvironment in glioblastoma: Current and emerging concepts. Neurooncol Adv. 2023 Jan;5(1):vdad009. http://dx.doi.org/10.1093/noajnl/vdad009
128. Virtuoso A, Giovannoni R, De Luca C, Gargano F, Cerasuolo M, Maggio N, et al. The glioblastoma microenvironment: Morphology, metabolism, and molecular signature of glial dynamics to discover metabolic rewiring sequence. Int J Mol Sci. 2021 Mar 24;22(7):3301. http://dx.doi.org/10.3390/ijms22073301
129. Venkatesh HS, Johung TB, Caretti V, Noll A, Tang Y, Nagaraja S, et al. Neuronal activity promotes glioma growth through neuroligin-3 secretion. Cell. 2015 May 7;161(4):803–16. http://dx.doi.org/10.1016/j.cell.2015.04.012
130. Venkataramani V, Yang Y, Schubert MC, Reyhan E, Tetzlaff SK, Wißmann N, et al. Glioblastoma hijacks neuronal mechanisms for brain invasion. Cell. 2022 Aug 4;185(16):2899–917.e31. https://doi.org/10.1016/j.cell.2022.06.054
131. Moriarty C, Gupta N, Bhattacharya D. Role of glutamate excitotoxicity in glioblastoma growth and its implications in treatment. Cell Biol Int. 2025 May;49(5):421–34. http://dx.doi.org/10.1002/cbin.70005
132. D'Angelo D, Rizzuto R. The mitochondrial calcium uniporter (MCU): Molecular identity and role in human diseases. Biomolecules. 2023 Aug 25;13(9):1304. http://dx.doi.org/10.3390/biom13091304
133. Matias D, Balça-Silva J, da Graça GC, Wanjiru CM, Macharia LW, Nascimento CP, et al. Microglia/astrocytes-glioblastoma crosstalk: Crucial molecular mechanisms and microenvironmental factors. Front Cell Neurosci. 2018 Aug 3;12:235. http://dx.doi.org/10.3389/fncel.2018.00235
134. Marabitti V, Vulpis E, Nazio F, Campello S. Mitochondrial transfer as a strategy for enhancing cancer cell fitness: Current insights and future directions. Pharmacol Res. 2024 Oct;208(107382):107382. https://doi.org/10.1016/j.phrs.2024.107382
135. Hovis G, Chandra N, Kejriwal N, Hsieh KJY, Chu A, Yang I, et al. Understanding the role of endothelial cells in glioblastoma: Mechanisms and novel treatments. Int J Mol Sci. 2024 Jun 1;25(11):6118. http://dx.doi.org/10.3390/ijms25116118
136. Huang X, Zhao L, Peng R. Hypoxia-inducible factor 1 and mitochondria: An intimate connection. Biomolecules. 2022 Dec 27;13(1):50. http://dx.doi.org/10.3390/biom13010050
137. Miki K, Yagi M, Hatae R, Otsuji R, Miyazaki T, Goto K, et al. Glutaminolysis is associated with mitochondrial pathway activation and can be therapeutically targeted in glioblastoma. Cancer Metab. 2024 Nov 19;12(1):35. http://dx.doi.org/10.1186/s40170-024-00364-0
138. Wang ZH, Peng WB, Zhang P, Yang XP, Zhou Q. Lactate in the tumour microenvironment: From immune modulation to therapy. EBioMedicine. 2021 Nov;73(103627):103627. http://dx.doi.org/10.1016/j.ebiom.2021.103627
139. Atkinson GP, Nozell SE, Benveniste ETN. NF-kappaB and STAT3 signaling in glioma: Targets for future therapies. Expert Rev Neurother. 2010 Apr;10(4):575–86. http://dx.doi.org/10.1586/ern.10.21
140. Liu Y, Zhang B, Duan R, Liu Y. Mitochondrial DNA leakage and cGas/STING pathway in microglia: Crosstalk between neuroinflammation and neurodegeneration. Neuroscience. 2024 Jun 7;548:1–8. http://dx.doi.org/10.1016/j.neuroscience.2024.04.009

141. Sandhbor P, John G, Bhat S, Goda JS. Immune response recalibration using immune therapy and biomimetic nano-therapy against high-grade gliomas and brain metastases. Asian J Pharm Sci. 2025 Apr;20(2):101021. https://doi.org/10.1016/j.ajps.2025.101021
142. Nejo T, Krishna S, Jimenez C, Yamamichi A, Young JS, Lakshmanachetty S, et al. Glioma-neuronal circuit remodeling induces regional immunosuppression. bioRxiv. 2023. http://dx.doi.org/10.1101/2023.08.04.548295
143. Hosseinalizadeh H, Mahmoodpour M, Samadani AA, Roudkenar MH. The immunosuppressive role of indoleamine 2, 3-dioxygenase in glioblastoma: Mechanism of action and immunotherapeutic strategies. Med Oncol. 2022 Jun 18;39(9):130. http://dx.doi.org/10.1007/s12032-022-01724-w
144. Lu J, Tan M, Cai Q. The Warburg effect in tumor progression: Mitochondrial oxidative metabolism as an anti-metastasis mechanism. Cancer Lett. 2015 Jan 28;356(2 Pt A):156–64. http://dx.doi.org/10.1016/j.canlet.2014.04.001
145. Zhao J, Ma X, Gao P, Han X, Zhao P, Xie F, et al. Advancing glioblastoma treatment by targeting metabolism. Neoplasia. 2024 May;51(100985):100985. https://doi.org/10.1016/j.neo.2024.100985
146. Zhao Y, Ye X, Xiong Z, Ihsan A, Ares I, Martínez M, et al. Cancer metabolism: The role of ROS in DNA damage and induction of apoptosis in cancer cells. Metabolites. 2023 Jun 27;13(7). http://dx.doi.org/10.3390/metabo13070796
147. Rinaldi M, Caffo M, Minutoli L, Marini H, Abbritti RV, Squadrito F, et al. ROS and brain gliomas: An overview of potential and innovative therapeutic strategies. Int J Mol Sci. 2016 Jun 22;17(6):984. https://doi.org/10.3390/ijms17060984
148. Shaaban AH, Soliman Wadan AH, El-Sadek MZ, Mostafa SA. Mitochondrial dynamics regulators in cancer metabolism and progression. Mitochondrial Commun. 2025 Apr. https://doi.org/10.1016/j.mitoco.2025.04.001
149. Qian S, Wei Z, Yang W, Huang J, Yang Y, Wang J. The role of BCL-2 family proteins in regulating apoptosis and cancer therapy. Front Oncol. 2022 Oct 12;12:985363. http://dx.doi.org/10.3389/fonc.2022.985363
150. Valdés-Rives SA, Casique-Aguirre D, Germán-Castelán L, Velasco-Velázquez MA, González-Arenas A. Apoptotic signaling pathways in glioblastoma and therapeutic implications. Biomed Res Int. 2017 Nov 12;2017:7403747. http://dx.doi.org/10.1155/2017/7403747
151. Nissanka N, Moraes CT. Mitochondrial DNA damage and reactive oxygen species in neurodegenerative disease. FEBS Lett. 2018 Mar;592(5):728–42. http://dx.doi.org/10.1002/1873-3468.12956
152. Kumari N, Pullaguri N, Rath SN, Bajaj A, Sahu V, Ealla KKR. Dysregulation of calcium homeostasis in cancer and its role in chemoresistance. Canc Drug Resist. 2024 Mar 15;7:11. http://dx.doi.org/10.20517/cdr.2023.145
153. Maklad A, Sharma A, Azimi I. Calcium signaling in brain cancers: Roles and therapeutic targeting. Cancers (Basel). 2019 Jan 26;11(2):145. http://dx.doi.org/10.3390/cancers11020145
154. Popov LD. Mitochondrial biogenesis: An update. J Cell Mol Med. 2020 May;24(9):4892–9. http://dx.doi.org/10.1111/jcmm.15194
155. Lee J, Giordano S, Zhang J. Autophagy, mitochondria and oxidative stress: Cross-talk and redox signalling. Biochem J. 2012 Jan 15;441(2):523–40. http://dx.doi.org/10.1042/BJ20111451
156. Fu Y, Zou T, Shen X, Nelson PJ, Li J, Wu C, et al. Lipid metabolism in cancer progression and therapeutic strategies. MedComm. 2021 Mar;2(1):27–59. http://dx.doi.org/10.1002/mco2.27
157. Inigo JR, Chandra D. The mitochondrial unfolded protein response (UPRmt): Shielding against toxicity to mitochondria in cancer. J Hematol Oncol. 2022 Jul 21;15(1):98. http://dx.doi.org/10.1186/s13045-022-01317-0
158. Zhang X, Fan Y, Tan K. A bird's eye view of mitochondrial unfolded protein response in cancer: Mechanisms, progression and further applications. Cell Death Dis. 2024 Sep 11;15(9):667. https://doi.org/10.1038/s41419-024-07049-y
159. Kalani K, Yan SF, Yan SS. Mitochondrial permeability transition pore: A potential drug target for neurodegeneration. Drug Discov Today. 2018 Dec;23(12):1983–9. http://dx.doi.org/10.1016/j.drudis.2018.08.001
160. Waseem M, Wang BD. Promising strategy of mPTP modulation in cancer therapy: An emerging progress and future insight. Int J Mol Sci. 2023 Mar 14;24(6). http://dx.doi.org/10.3390/ijms24065564
161. Wiese M, Bannister AJ. Two genomes, one cell: Mitochondrial-nuclear coordination via epigenetic pathways. Mol Metab. 2020 Aug;38(100942):100942. http://dx.doi.org/10.1016/j.molmet.2020.01.006
162. Li Y, Li W, Hoffman AR, Cui J, Hu JF. The nucleus/mitochondria-shuttling LncRNAs function as new epigenetic regulators of mitophagy in cancer. Front Cell Dev Biol. 2021 Sep 8;9:699621. https://doi.org/10.3389/fcell.2021.699621

163. Kim HJ, Maiti P, Barrientos A. Mitochondrial ribosomes in cancer. Semin Cancer Biol. 2017 Dec;47:67–81. http://dx.doi.org/10.1016/j.semcancer.2017.04.004
164. Wu H, Zhu X, Zhou H, Sha M, Ye J, Yu H. Mitochondrial ribosomal proteins and cancer. Medicina (Kaunas). 2025 Jan 9;61(1). http://dx.doi.org/10.3390/medicina61010096
165. Jiang H, Zuo J, Li B, Chen R, Luo K, Xiang X, et al. Drug-induced oxidative stress in cancer treatments: Angel or devil? Redox Biol. 2023 Jul;63(102754):102754. http://dx.doi.org/10.1016/j.redox.2023.102754
166. Sighel D, Notarangelo M, Aibara S, Re A, Ricci G, Guida M, et al. Inhibition of mitochondrial translation suppresses glioblastoma stem cell growth. Cell Rep. 2021 Apr 27;35(4):109024. http://dx.doi.org/10.1016/j.celrep.2021.109024
167. Baker MJ, Frazier AE, Gulbis JM, Ryan MT. Mitochondrial protein-import machinery: Correlating structure with function. Trends Cell Biol. 2007 Sep;17(9):456–64. https://doi.org/10.1016/j.tcb.2007.07.010
168. Haastrup MO, Vikramdeo KS, Singh S, Singh AP, Dasgupta S. The journey of mitochondrial protein import and the roadmap to follow. Int J Mol Sci. 2023 Jan 27;24(3):2479. https://doi.org/10.3390/ijms24032479
169. Yablonska S, Ganesan V, Ferrando LM, Kim J, Pyzel A, Baranova OV, et al. Mutant huntingtin disrupts mitochondrial proteostasis by interacting with TIM23. Proc Natl Acad Sci USA. 2019 Aug 13;116(33):16593–602. http://dx.doi.org/10.1073/pnas.1904101116
170. Robichaux DJ, Harata M, Murphy E, Karch J. Mitochondrial permeability transition pore-dependent necrosis. J Mol Cell Cardiol. 2023 Jan;174:47–55. http://dx.doi.org/10.1016/j.yjmcc.2022.11.003
171. Han X, Yoon SH, Ding Y, Choi TG, Choi WJ, Kim YH, et al. Cyclosporin A and sanglifehrin A enhance chemotherapeutic effect of cisplatin in C6 glioma cells. Oncol Rep. 2010 Apr;23(4):1053–62. https://doi.org/10.3892/or_00000732
172. Jiang Z, Shen T, Huynh H, Fang X, Han Z, Ouyang K. Cardiolipin regulates mitochondrial ultrastructure and function in mammalian cells. Genes (Basel). 2022 Oct 18;13(10):1889. http://dx.doi.org/10.3390/genes13101889
173. Weng X, Gonzalez M, Angelia J, Piroozmand S, Jamehdor S, Behrooz AB, et al. Lipidomics-driven drug discovery and delivery strategies in glioblastoma. Biochim Biophys Acta Mol Basis Dis. 2025 Mar;1871(3):167637. https://doi.org/10.1016/j.bbadis.2024.167637
174. Chokkalla AK, Mehta SL, Vemuganti R. Epitranscriptomic regulation by m6A RNA methylation in brain development and diseases. J Cereb Blood Flow Metab. 2020 Dec;40(12):2331–49. http://dx.doi.org/10.1177/0271678X20960033
175. Añazco-Guenkova AM, Miguel-López B, Monteagudo-García Ó, García-Vílchez R, Blanco S. The impact of tRNA modifications on translation in cancer: Identifying novel therapeutic avenues. NAR Cancer. 2024 Mar;6(1):zcae012. http://dx.doi.org/10.1093/narcan/zcae012
176. Branco F, Cunha J, Mendes M, Vitorino C, Sousa JJ. Peptide-hitchhiking for the development of nanosystems in glioblastoma. ACS Nano. 2024 Jul 2;18(26):16359–94. https://doi.org/10.1021/acsnano.4c01790
177. Hirschberg H, Sun CH, Tromberg BJ, Yeh AT, Madsen SJ. Enhanced cytotoxic effects of 5-aminolevulinic acid-mediated photodynamic therapy by concurrent hyperthermia in glioma spheroids. J Neurooncol. 2004 Dec;70(3):289–99. https://doi.org/10.1007/s11060-004-9161-7
178. Li M, Zheng K, Liu X. Mitochondria-targeting phthalocyanines and porphyrins for enhanced photodynamic tumor therapy. ChemistrySelect. 2023 Mar 13;8(10). http://dx.doi.org/10.1002/slct.202205022
179. Buck AC, Maarman GJ, Dube A, Bardien S. Mitochondria targeted nanoparticles for the treatment of mitochondrial dysfunction-associated brain disorders. Front Bioeng Biotechnol. 2025 Mar 12;13:1563701. https://doi.org/10.3389/fbioe.2025.1563701
180. Dahifale A, Agnihotri TG, Jain A, Jain A. Quality-by-design-engineered mitochondrial targeted nanoparticles for glioblastoma therapy. RSC Adv. 2024 Oct 23;14(46):34100–18. http://dx.doi.org/10.1039/d4ra04748f
181. Anwer MS, Abdel-Rasol MA, El-Sayed WM. Emerging therapeutic strategies in glioblastsoma: Drug repurposing, mechanisms of resistance, precision medicine, and technological innovations. Clin Exp Med. 2025 Apr 13;25(1):117. http://dx.doi.org/10.1007/s10238-025-01631-0
182. Koh JH, Kim JY. Role of PGC-1α in the mitochondrial NAD+ pool in metabolic diseases. Int J Mol Sci. 2021 Apr 27;22(9):4558. http://dx.doi.org/10.3390/ijms22094558
183. Chen K, Ernst P, Kim S, Si Y, Varadkar T, Ringel MD, et al. An innovative mitochondrial-targeted gene therapy for cancer treatment. bioRxivorg. 2024. http://dx.doi.org/10.1101/2024.03.24.584499
184. Welch DR, Foster C, Rigoutsos I. Roles of mitochondrial genetics in cancer metastasis. Trends Cancer. 2022 Dec;8(12):1002–18. http://dx.doi.org/10.1016/j.trecan.2022.07.004
185. Schmidt DR, Patel R, Kirsch DG, Lewis CA, Vander Heiden MG, Locasale JW. Metabolomics in cancer research and emerging applications in clinical oncology. CA Cancer J Clin. 2021 Jul;71(4):333–58. http://dx.doi.org/10.3322/caac.21670

186. Bano D, Prehn JHM. Apoptosis-inducing factor (AIF) in physiology and disease: The tale of a repented natural born killer. EBioMedicine. 2018 Apr;30:29–37. https://doi.org/10.1016/j.ebiom.2018.03.016
187. Smith SJ, Long A, Barrow JH, Macarthur DC, Coyle B, Grundy RG, et al. Pediatric high-grade glioma: Identification of poly(ADP-ribose) polymerase as a potential therapeutic target. Neuro Oncol. 2011 Nov;13(11):1171–7. https://doi.org/10.1093/neuonc/nor115
188. Arif T, Krelin Y, Nakdimon I, Benharroch D, Paul A, Dadon-Klein D, et al. VDAC1 is a molecular target in glioblastoma, with its depletion leading to reprogrammed metabolism and reversed oncogenic properties. Neuro Oncol. 2017 Jul 1;19(7):951–64. http://dx.doi.org/10.1093/neuonc/now297
189. Falabella M, Vernon HJ, Hanna MG, Claypool SM, Pitceathly RDS. Cardiolipin, mitochondria, and neurological disease. Trends Endocrinol Metab. 2021 Apr;32(4):224–37. http://dx.doi.org/10.1016/j.tem.2021.01.006
190. Gaitsch H, Franklin RJM, Reich DS. Cell-free DNA-based liquid biopsies in neurology. Brain. 2023 May 2;146(5):1758–74. http://dx.doi.org/10.1093/brain/awac438
191. Peng F, Wang S, Feng Z, Zhou K, Zhang H, Guo X, et al. Circulating cell-free mtDNA as a new biomarker for cancer detection and management. Cancer Biol Med. 2023 Oct 12;21(2). http://dx.doi.org/10.20892/j.issn.2095-3941.2023.0280
192. Jones JJ, Jones KL, Wong SQ, Whittle J, Goode D, Nguyen H, et al. Plasma ctDNA enables early detection of temozolomide resistance mutations in glioma. Neurooncol Adv. 2024 Jan;6(1):vdae041. http://dx.doi.org/10.1093/noajnl/vdae041
193. Panda SS, Sahoo RK, Patra SK, Biswal S, Biswal BK. Molecular insights to therapeutic in cancer: Role of exosomes in tumor microenvironment, metastatic progression and drug resistance. Drug Discov Today. 2024 Aug;29(8):104061. https://doi.org/10.1016/j.drudis.2024.104061
194. Felipe Perez R, Mochi G, Khan A, Woodford M. Mitochondrial Chaperone Code: Just warming up. Cell Stress Chaperones. 2024 Jun;29(3):483–96. http://dx.doi.org/10.1016/j.cstres.2024.05.002
195. Xie S, Wang X, Gan S, Tang X, Kang X, Zhu S. The mitochondrial chaperone TRAP1 as a candidate target of oncotherapy. Front Oncol. 2020;10:585047. http://dx.doi.org/10.3389/fonc.2020.585047
196. Zhang Y, Qu Y, Gao K, Yang Q, Shi B, Hou P, et al. High copy number of mitochondrial DNA (mtDNA) predicts good prognosis in glioma patients. Am J Cancer Res. 2015 Feb 15;5(3):1207–16. https://www.ncbi.nlm.nih.gov/pubmed/26045999
197. Chen N, Wen S, Sun X, Fang Q, Huang L, Liu S, et al. Elevated mitochondrial DNA copy number in peripheral blood and tissue predict the opposite outcome of cancer: A meta-analysis. Sci Rep. 2016 Nov 18;6:37404. https://doi.org/10.1038/srep37404
198. Meyer N, Zielke S, Michaelis JB, Linder B, Warnsmann V, Rakel S, et al. AT 101 induces early mitochondrial dysfunction and HMOX1 (heme oxygenase 1) to trigger mitophagic cell death in glioma cells. Autophagy. 2018 Jul 21;14(10):1693–709. http://dx.doi.org/10.1080/15548627.2018.1476812
199. Rio M, Lebre AS, de Lonlay P, Valayannopoulos V, Desguerre I, Dufier JL, et al. Mitochondrial ND5 mutations mimicking brainstem tectal glioma. Neurology. 2010 Jul 6;75(1):93. http://dx.doi.org/10.1212/WNL.0b013e3181e6214a
200. Oliva CR, Markert T, Gillespie GY, Griguer CE. Nuclear-encoded cytochrome c oxidase subunit 4 regulates BMI1 expression and determines proliferative capacity of high-grade gliomas. Oncotarget. 2015 Feb 28;6(6):4330–44. https://doi.org/10.18632/oncotarget.3015
201. Ma D, Lu B, Feng C, Wang C, Wang Y, Luo T, et al. Deoxypodophyllotoxin triggers parthanatos in glioma cells via induction of excessive ROS. Cancer Lett. 2016 Feb 28;371(2):194–204. http://dx.doi.org/10.1016/j.canlet.2015.11.044
202. Sevrioukova IF. Apoptosis-inducing factor: Structure, function, and redox regulation. Antioxid Redox Signal. 2011 Jun 15;14(12):2545–79. http://dx.doi.org/10.1089/ars.2010.3445
203. Shteinfer-Kuzmine A, Arif T, Krelin Y, Tripathi SS, Paul A, Shoshan-Barmatz V. Mitochondrial VDAC1-based peptides: Attacking oncogenic properties in glioblastoma. Oncotarget. 2017 May 9;8(19):31329–46. http://dx.doi.org/10.18632/oncotarget.15455
204. Arif T, Krelin Y, Shoshan-Barmatz V. Reducing VDAC1 expression induces a non-apoptotic role for pro-apoptotic proteins in cancer cell differentiation. Biochim Biophys Acta. 2016 Aug;1857(8):1228–42. http://dx.doi.org/10.1016/j.bbabio.2016.04.005
205. Park HK, Hong JH, Oh YT, Kim SS, Yin J, Lee AJ, et al. Interplay between TRAP1 and sirtuin-3 modulates mitochondrial respiration and oxidative stress to maintain stemness of glioma stem cells. Cancer Res. 2019 Apr 1;79(7):1369–82. http://dx.doi.org/10.1158/0008-5472.CAN-18-2558

206. Wang N, Zhu P, Huang R, Sun L, Dong D, Gao Y. Suppressing TRAP1 sensitizes glioblastoma multiforme cells to temozolomide. Exp Ther Med. 2021 Nov;22(5):1246. http://dx.doi.org/10.3892/etm.2021.10681
207. Kosti A, Chiou J, Guardia GDA, Lei X, Balinda H, Landry T, et al. ELF4 is a critical component of a miRNA-transcription factor network and is a bridge regulator of glioblastoma receptor signaling and lipid dynamics. Neuro Oncol. 2023 Mar 14;25(3):459–70. http://dx.doi.org/10.1093/neuonc/noac179
208. Jagirdar G, Elsner M, Scharf C, Simm S, Borucki K, Peter D, et al. Re-expression of tafazzin isoforms in TAZ-deficient C6 glioma cells restores cardiolipin composition but not proliferation rate and alterations in gene expression. Front Genet. 2022 Jul 25;13:931017. http://dx.doi.org/10.3389/fgene.2022.931017
209. Mair R, Mouliere F, Smith CG, Chandrananda D, Gale D, Marass F, et al. Measurement of plasma cell-free mitochondrial tumor DNA improves detection of glioblastoma in patient-derived orthotopic xenograft models. Cancer Res. 2019 Jan 1;79(1):220–30. http://dx.doi.org/10.1158/0008-5472.CAN-18-0074
210. Gatto L, Di Nunno V, Ghelardini A, Tosoni A, Bartolini S, Asioli S, et al. Targeting mitochondria in glioma: New hopes for a cure. Biomedicines. 2024 Nov 28;12(12). https://doi.org/10.3390/biomedicines12122730
211. Zielonka J, Joseph J, Sikora A, Hardy M, Ouari O, Vasquez-Vivar J, et al. Mitochondria-targeted triphenylphosphonium-based compounds: Syntheses, mechanisms of action, and therapeutic and diagnostic applications. Chem Rev. 2017 Aug 9;117(15):10043–120. http://dx.doi.org/10.1021/acs.chemrev.7b00042
212. Inigo JR, Kumar R, Chandra D. Targeting the mitochondrial unfolded protein response in cancer: Opportunities and challenges. Trends Cancer. 2021 Dec;7(12):1050–3. http://dx.doi.org/10.1016/j.trecan.2021.08.008
213. Chang X, Huang Y, Qu Y, Guo Y, Fan W, Zhen H. Integrative analysis of mitochondrial-related gene profiling identifies prognostic clusters and drug resistance mechanisms in low-grade glioma. Discov Oncol. 2025 Apr 5;16(1):465. http://dx.doi.org/10.1007/s12672-025-02201-2

11 Plastic Pollution and Cancer

The Emerging Role of Microplastics in Oncology

Niketha Manoj and Shabina Ashraf
National Institute of Technology Calicut, Kozhikode, Kerala, India

11.1 FROM PLASTIC TO MPs

For much of human history, the inherent limitations of materials such as wood, stone, and metal constrained the scope of material aspirations to traditional uses. This paradigm shifted dramatically in the twentieth century with advancements in chemistry that enabled the synthesis and customization of entirely new substances. A key transformation happened with the invention of Bakelite, the first synthetic plastic, by Leo Baekeland in 1907. Marketed as "the material of a thousand uses", Bakelite symbolized boundless possibilities, even adopting the infinity symbol as its trademark. Today, plastics dominate everyday life, shaping objects through processes like molding, extrusion, and vacuum-forming. The ubiquity of plastic-based items including machines, appliances, and furnishings has altered perceptions of materiality to such an extent that these synthetic materials are now regarded as commonplace and naturalized [1]. The development of Bakelite marked a significant milestone paving the way for the creation of numerous other plastics in the following decades. In their book *Plastics* (first published in 1941), Yarsley and Couzens highlighted the vast potential applications of plastics, describing them as "almost inexhaustible". At that time, global plastic production remained below 1 million tons per year, yet plastics were already being utilized in a wide range of products, from household items like cups and saucers to components for automobiles and aircraft [2]. Plastics have become ubiquitous and serve as a foundational material in modern society due to their exceptional versatility in design, low cost, ease of formability, lightweight nature, and bioinert properties [1]. These characteristics have established plastics as the preferred material across diverse applications, including smartphones, food packaging, and 3D printing. Furthermore, plastics contribute to sustainability efforts by protecting food and reducing waste, facilitating the production of lighter vehicles, and insulating electrical cables to enhance energy efficiency. However, these benefits are counterbalanced by significant environmental challenges. Reports frequently highlight remote beaches littered with plastic debris, while social media is replete with images and videos of marine animals such as seabirds, dolphins, and turtles entangled in or fatally impacted by plastic waste [3]. Plastic pollution has permeated virtually every part of the planet, including oceans, soil, drinking water, human and animal bodies, and even the atmosphere (**Figure 11.1**). With global plastic production projected to double within the next two decades, current waste management and recycling systems are expected to be insufficient to address the escalating environmental impacts [4].

The rapid growth of plastic production has led to severe environmental pollution, with global production exceeding 300 million tons per year [5, 6]. Plastics are highly resistant to degradation, persisting for centuries and breaking down into microplastics (MPs) that harm ecosystems. Driven by UV radiation, photodegradation alters plastic properties, causing fragmentation and structural defects.

 DOI: 10.1201/9781003644309-11

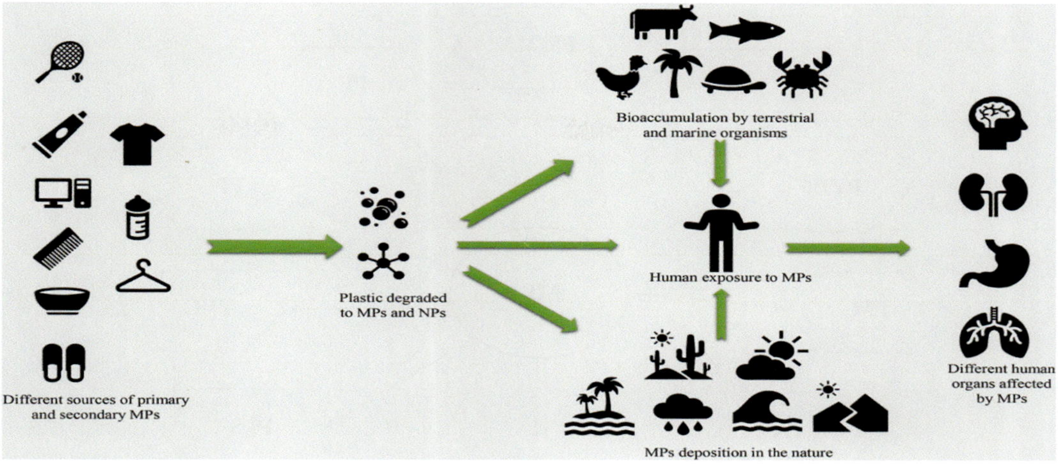

FIGURE 11.1 Generation of MPs, NPs and their effect on the environment.

This process contributes to the accumulation of MPs in marine ecosystems, posing a significant environmental challenge [6].

11.2 MPs TYPES AND SOURCES

Primary MPs are intentionally manufactured plastic particles released into the environment in their original small size, typically smaller than 5 mm. These MPs serve various applications, including as scrubbing agents in personal care products such as shower gels and facial scrubs, plastic pellets used in industrial manufacturing, and synthetic fibers shed during the laundering of textiles like nylon [7]. They can also originate from the abrasion of larger plastic objects during use or maintenance, such as tire erosion while driving or the shedding of synthetic textile fibers during washing [8]. Common types of primary MPs are the following: polypropylene (PP), polyethylene (PE), polymethyl methacrylate (PMMA), polyurethane (PU), polyethylene terephthalate (PET), polystyrene (PS), polyester (PES), polyamide (PA), polycarbonate (PC), polyvinyl chloride (PVC), high-density polyethylene (HDPE), polyvinylidene fluoride (PVDF), and polyoxymethylene (PM) [9]. These MPs contribute significantly to environmental pollution, entering ecosystems through wastewater systems, industrial spills, and other pathways (**Figure 11.2**).

Secondary MPs are formed through the degradation of larger plastic debris into smaller fragments once exposed to environmental conditions, particularly in marine ecosystems [10]. This degradation occurs via processes such as photodegradation, mechanical abrasion, and biological activity. Photodegradation, driven by UV radiation, leads to oxidative reactions that weaken polymer structures and cause fragmentation. Mechanical forces, such as wave action and sediment friction, further break down macro-plastics into MPs, while microbial activity contributes to degradation by secreting enzymes and producing localized acids [11]. Common sources of secondary MPs include mismanaged waste such as discarded plastic bags, bottles, and fishing nets. However, accurately quantifying secondary MPs is challenging due to their diffuse origins, varied polymer types, continuous fragmentation into nanoscale particles, and dynamic distribution in the environment. Their widespread presence in marine ecosystems makes source attribution difficult, as well as assessing how much macro-plastic has converted into MPs over time (**Figure 11.3**). Consequently, research efforts often focus on primary MPs, which are easier to trace and quantify using existing datasets. Addressing secondary MPs pollution requires improved waste management systems and strategies to reduce macro-plastic inputs into the environment [12].

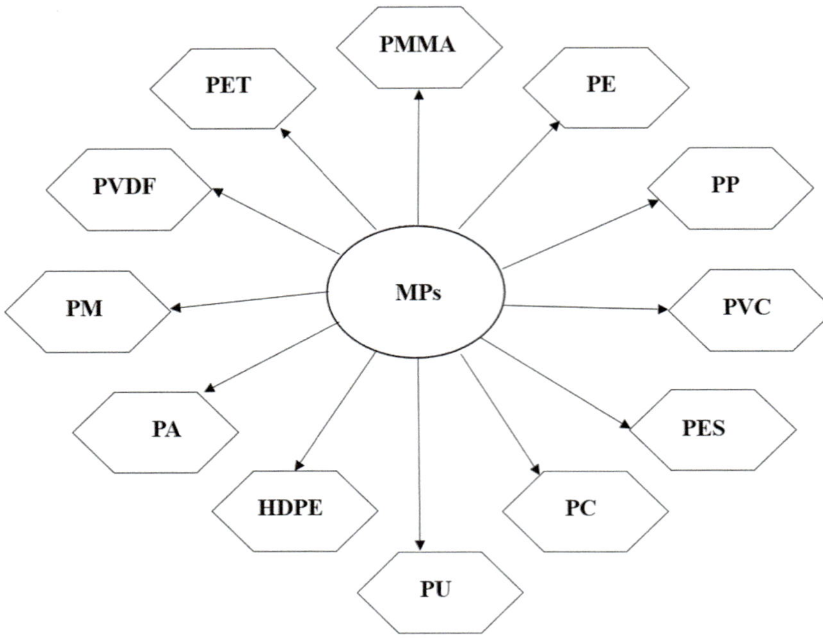

FIGURE 11.2 Different types of MPs.

The International Union for the Conservation of Nature (IUCN) identified various human activities that release MPs into the environment, including washing synthetic clothes, tire wear, furniture abrasion, plastic processing and transportation, and personal care products like exfoliating scrubs. These everyday activities and industrial processes contribute significantly to MPs pollution [12,13]. The World Health Organization (WHO) has reported that plastic particles can travel through various pathways, including the discharge of effluents from wastewater treatment plants and the deposition

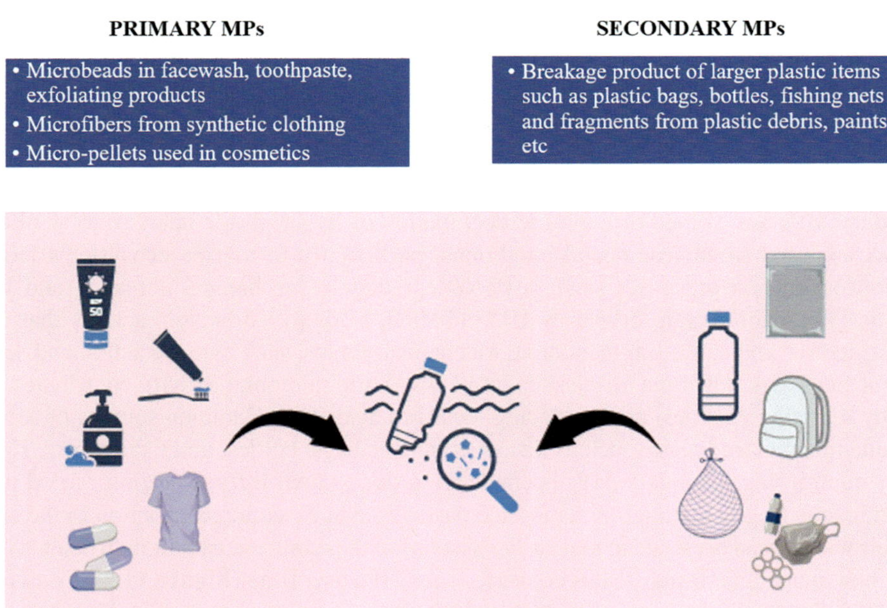

FIGURE 11.3 Primary and Secondary sources of MPs in daily life.

of MPs onto the ground through processes such as surface runoff. These pathways enable MPs to enter aquatic systems, including groundwater and rivers, highlighting their widespread environmental dispersion and potential impact on ecosystems and human health [14]. Additionally, wind can transport primary MPs generated through processes such as natural degradation or mechanical abrasion, dispersing them into the air and facilitating their widespread distribution across different environments [15].

11.3 HUMAN EXPOSURE TO MPs

MPs exposure to humans include ingestion, inhalation, and dermal penetration. Ingestion of MPs was regarded as the primary route of entry into humans [16]. Once MPs are ingested, they undergo several processes and travel through various organs of the body. These MPs are capable of penetrating through the gastrointestinal tract and can get integrated into the circulatory system via lymphatic system or through the intestinal epithelium. MPs smaller than 150 μm, are likely to cross the intestinal barrier and pose potential risk of entering the bloodstream [17]. Due to the immense presence of MPs in the ocean, they often contaminate the aquatic life by ingestion and easily enter the food web by trophic transfer [18]. The sea surface environment of pacific oceanic region is now dominated by PE and PP pieces, including other artificial and natural floating debris with ~6.4 k metric tons of MPs [19]. The assimilation of MPs in humans through food could be understood by the fact that the ingested food sources are often contaminated by plastics particulates. Recently, the samples of table salt have been found to be contaminated by MPs. The MPs in sea salt, lake salt, and rock/well salt were found to be more than 550, 43, and 7 items/kg, respectively [20]. This suggests the widespread contamination of plastic particulates in food which accumulate across different trophic levels of food chains.

Often, the growth of crops includes agricultural practices that use contaminated water. It is known that plastics are constantly being degraded by microorganisms in the soils, which can be taken up by crops during cultivation [21]. Food sources including crops, dairy products derived from animals, and drinking water resources pave a mechanism for the inclusion of MPs in consumption products, thereby resulting in the ingestion by humans [22].

Another potential mode of plastic particulates' entry in humans is through inhalation with daily intake levels fluctuating considerably based on air quality and environmental condition The use of medical devices made up of plastics, such as an inhaler, nebulizers, and other respiratory aides and therapeutic agents, can also contribute to MPs/NNPs' release to the lungs [23]. Humans face significant secondary exposure to MPs and nanoplastics (NPs) through plastic particulates suspended in air and dust. These particles originate from the shedding of synthetic textile fibers as well as fragments from plastic furniture and building materials [24]. Inhalation causes the accumulation of plastic particulates into the respiratory system, with the MPs/NPs depositing in the lung tissues [25]. Additionally, the other modes of MP internalization in humans are also via the transdermal pathways. Human skin has a surface area of about 1.5–2 m^2 and provides a large interface for the MPs in the surrounding environment to interact with humans. The plastic particulates transmit through the sublayers of epidermis and then they will be assimilated into the microcirculation in the dermis. Following this, they gain entry to the human circulation system from where they make their way to various organs of the body. However, the transdermal route is not the most preferred pathway of MPs entry and hence has received lesser attention, as the dermal barrier inhibits the MPs' absorption [26]. Specifically, it was found that plastic particulates less than 100 nm can only gain entry through the transdermal pathways, which breach the dermal barrier. Direct contact of water contaminated with MPs/NPs with skin occurs during daily activities like washing or by using facial/body scrubs containing plastic particulates [27].

Over time, MPs may build up in the body and may have long-term negative consequences on human health. This is especially problematic for heavy metals and persistent organic pollutants (POPs) that could be adsorbed onto MPs, which can bioaccumulate within the body and have harmful effects. Once MPs enter the human body, they translocate to other body organs like the kidney and liver. The liver is a primary site for MPs accumulation as the toxins are filtered from the blood by the liver where the ingested MPs will get deposited. The functioning of the kidneys is to excrete waste from the body which may end up accumulating MPs that do not leave the body. MPs that evade the filtration and excretion processes can get deposited in other organs through recirculation causing severe health issues over prolonged periods [28].

11.4 MECHANISMS OF CARCINOGENESIS

MPs and NPs play a vital role in human health and are strongly linked to cancers of the respiratory and digestive systems, and the skin. Cellular damage by irregularly shaped plastic particulates and their subsequent influence on DNA mutations through multiple pathways could potentially lead to cancer development (**Figure 11.4**). The penetration of MPs/NPs into cellular membranes causes mechanical stress in the cells, which causes tissue inflammation, an elevated release of reactive oxygen species (ROS), often leading to apoptosis or necrosis [29]. In addition, ROS is also responsible in damaging cellular components like lipids, DNA, and proteins, which promote carcinogenesis [30]. An imbalance between the regulated and dysregulated cell death is another potential cause for cancer, which is triggered by plastic particulate-induced programmed cell death pathways [31]. MPs often act as vectors in carrying heavy metals, harmful chemicals, and persistent organic pollutants (POPs). They also interact with immune cells like the macrophages which results in chronic inflammation by frustrated phagocytosis, thus providing a microenvironment for cellular proliferation and mutagenesis. Human hormonal disturbance is related to carcinogenesis and MPs function as endocrine-disrupting chemicals (EDC) perturbates the hormonal regulation, indicating the indirect association of MPs with hormone-related cancers. The modifications at the genetic level like changes in the DNA methylation patterns, histone modifications, and non-coding RNA regulation can all have profound effects on cellular function and in inducing inflammation, potentially leading to the initiation and progression of cancer [32–34].

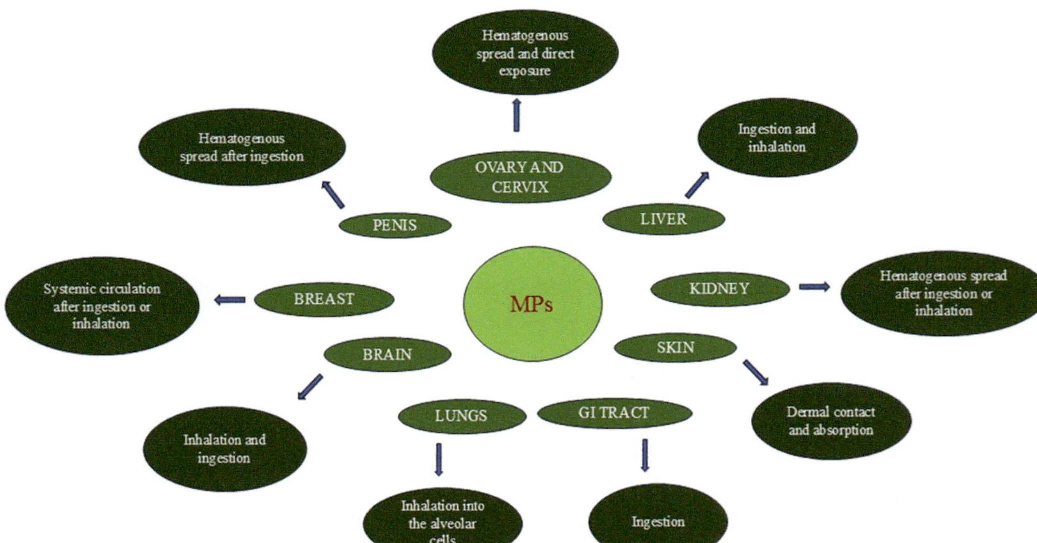

FIGURE 11.4 Various cancer in humans due to MPs and its potential exposure routes.

11.5 MPs AFFECT ON BODY ORGANS LUNGS

The deposition of plastic particulates in lungs is primarily by inhalation, as previously discussed. It was observed that particles less than 10μm can penetrate into the alveolar cells [35]. The particulates reaching the termini of alveoli accumulate over a lifetime, thus altering the cellular metabolic processes and causing a compromise in the lung tissue integrity [25, 36]. A wide range of inflammatory responses were observed upon the exposure of MPs to human bronchial cells, which indicate the potential risks due to MPs inhalation. A normal human bronchial cell line was exposed to plastic particulates of 2 μm polystyrene microplastics (PS-MPs), and the cell line exhibited an elevated level of inflammatory proteins, and higher ROS level at higher concentrations of MPs [35]. When the alveolar lung cell line A549 was exposed to 70 nm PS-NPs, the S-phase of the cell cycle was blocked, thus resulting in the associated changes in expression and proliferation of specific genes Ki67 and cyclin D [36]. This is also associated with an elevated expression of nuclear factor kappa B (NF-κB) and pro-inflammatory cytokines [37].

MPs are known to induce senescence in two lung-related cell lines, as shown by increased SA-β-gal positive cells, higher expression of p16 and p21 proteins, and elevated secretion of senescence-associated secretory phenotype (SASP) factors, while PVC exposure impaired physical function, caused tissue injury, and led to the accumulation of senescent cells. Researchers have found that exposure to PVC induces cellular senescence in A549 cells by increasing intracellular ROS levels and causing mitochondrial dysfunction [38]. The process can be reversed by antioxidant treatment, establishing a relationship between ROS signaling and PVC-induced cellular senescence. Proteomic analysis reveals changes in mitochondrial-related protein expression, supporting the role of mitochondrial dysfunction in increased ROS production. These observations provide prominent insights into the molecular mechanisms, underlying PVC-induced cellular senescence, and highlight the potential health risks associated with PVC exposure [38]. MPs, specifically PS, play a significant role in disrupting the biophysical function of pulmonary surfactants in the lungs. By adsorbing phospholipid components and altering the ultrastructure and mobility of pulmonary surfactants, MPs can cause the collapse of the surfactant film, leading to increased surface tension and potentially impairing respiratory function. Furthermore, MPs can generate ROS, such as hydrogen peroxide and hydroxyl radicals, which can damage lung tissue and contribute to cancer initiation and further progression. The disruption of pulmonary surfactant function and the resulting oxidative stress can create a microenvironment that fosters tumor growth and metastasis, highlighting the potential role of MPs in cancer progression [38, 39].

MPs promote inflammation and create a tumor-promoting microenvironment by inducing the production of cytokines, including transforming growth factor-beta (TGF-β). Excessive production of TGF-β can result in enhanced tumor growth and metastasis. UV-induced degradation of MPs, such as PS particles, have enhanced their toxicity, leading to elevated levels of oxidative stress, membrane damage, and mitochondrial dysfunction in A549 cells. Transcriptome analysis reveals that aged MPs exhibit greater toxicity with more differentially expressed genes and related functional pathways. These findings suggest that MPs exposure contributes to cancer progression in lung tissue by promoting inflammation, DNA damage, and cellular toxicity [40]. MPs exposure can thus contribute to cancer progression in lung cells by inducing oxidative damage to DNA, thus causing the formation of DNA lesions and impairing normal gene function. This can lead to the uncontrolled growth and proliferation of cancerous cells, eventually leading to lung cancer. The interplay between MPs exposure, oxidative stress, and cellular dysfunction highlights the potential role of MPs in promoting lung carcinogenesis [41].

11.6 BRAIN

Exposure to MPs has been found to have a concentration-dependent effect on brain cancer cell viability. Low levels of MPs (2%) can promote cancer cell growth, with a significant increase in cell proliferation (approximately 149.5% compared to the control). However, higher concentrations of MPs (10% and 20%) induce cytotoxic effects, leading to a decrease in live cell count [42]. The mechanisms underlying MP-induced cancer cell growth is thought to involve chemical leaching, where carcinogenic chemicals such as bisphenol A (BPA) and phthalates are released, and physical leaching, where MPs interaction causes physical damage or stress responses in cells and tissues [43]. The geometric factors and surface characteristics of MPs can also influence their biological interactions, potentially leading to enhanced cellular stress, which is known to contribute to cancer progression. These findings highlight the potential role of MPs in promoting brain cancer cell growth and the need for further research into the effects of MPs exposure on human health [29, 42].

11.7 CERVIX AND OVARIES

For the first time, research using micro-Raman spectroscopy has identified and confirmed the presence of MPs in the blood, as well as in cancerous and para-cancerous tissues of human cervical cancer patients [44]. MPs exhibit direct pathophysiological effects on ovarian function through cellular infiltration and molecular dysregulation, potentiating reproductive oncogenesis. MPs infiltrate ovarian granulosa cells via clathrin-mediated endocytosis, inducing follicular hyperplasia with a 37% increase in primordial follicle count while concurrently suppressing anti-Müllerian hormone (AMH) secretion by 62%, thereby disrupting follicular recruitment homeostasis. This cellular intrusion triggers NADPH oxidase 4 (NOX4)-mediated oxidative stress, manifesting as mitochondrial membrane potential collapse (55% $\Delta\Psi m$ reduction) and caspase-3-activated apoptosis (3.2-fold elevation), compounded by genomic instability through 8-hydroxy-2′-deoxyguanosine (8-OHdG) DNA adduct formation. Concurrently, MPs activate the TGF-β1/Smad3 signaling axis, driving fibrotic transformation via 4.1-fold increased collagen I/III deposition and 83% proliferation of α-smooth muscle actin-positive (α-SMA+) myofibroblasts, while tissue inhibitor of metalloproteinases-1 (TIMP-1) overexpression inhibits extracellular matrix (ECM) remodeling [45]. These interconnected mechanisms altered folliculogenesis, oxidative DNA damage, and stromal fibrosis, collectively establish a pro-metastatic niche characterized by compromised tissue architecture and enhanced cellular plasticity, significantly elevating risks of neoplastic transformation and metastatic dissemination in reproductive tissues [46].

The phthalate metabolite mono-ethylhexyl phthalate (MEHP) exhibits estrogen-mimetic oncogenic activity in cervical carcinogenesis through selective activation of the Akt signaling pathway. Experimental studies using HeLa and SiHa cervical cancer cells demonstrate that nanomolar concentrations of MEHP (10–100 nM) induce dose-dependent proliferation (1.7-fold increase vs. controls) via G protein-coupled estrogen receptor (GPER)-mediated phosphorylation of Akt at Ser473, without affecting ERK1/2 or NF-κB pathways [47]. This activation triggers nuclear translocation of phosphorylated Akt, upregulating proliferating cell nuclear antigen (PCNA) expression and promoting cell cycle progression. Pharmacological inhibition of GPER (using G15 inhibitor) or Akt (via MK-2206 or siRNA) completely abolishes MEHP-induced proliferative effects, confirming the specificity of the GPER/Akt axis in this process. The mechanism involves GPER-dependent transactivation of epidermal growth factor receptor (EGFR), which initiates downstream PI3K/Akt signaling cascades that override normal cell cycle checkpoints [48]. These findings position MEHP as an environmental endocrine disruptor that hijacks conserved growth regulatory pathways, potentially exacerbating cervical cancer risk through chronic low-dose exposure [47].

11.8 BREAST

The accumulation of interleukin-17 (IL-17) in breast cancer (BC) cells plays a pivotal role in regulating MP-induced mitophagy, a process that significantly impacts mitochondrial function and quality control [49]. Elevated IL-17 levels have been shown to enhance MP-induced mitochondrial dysfunction by promoting the upregulation of mitophagy-related proteins such as BNIP3L/NIX and stabilizing PINK1, which facilitates the selective degradation of damaged mitochondria. This process disturbs mitochondrial homeostasis, resulting in an impaired autophagic flux and enhanced mitochondrial clearance, ultimately causing the cellular energy metabolism processes to compromise. Furthermore, IL-17-mediated mitophagy is also linked to the activation of oncogenic pathways, including HIF-1α stabilization and metabolic reprogramming toward glycolysis, which supports tumor progression and is also responsible for chemoresistance [50]. Studies demonstrate that IL-17 knockdown can alleviate these effects by restoring mitochondrial biogenesis and decreasing MP-induced cytotoxicity. These findings aid in understanding the critical role of IL-17 in modulating MP-induced mitophagy and also emphasize its role as a therapeutic target in BC progression influenced by the exposure to environmental MPs [51].

MP infiltration in tumor microenvironment (TME) exhibits material-specific biodistribution patterns and pathophysiological interactions that potentiate BC progression [49]. PS-MPs specifically activate NLRP3 inflammasomes in BC cells, generating mitochondrial ROS (2.8 × baseline) that stabilize HIF-1α under normoxia, resulting in glycolytic metabolic reprogramming [52]. Immunomodulatory effects include MP-laden BC cells upregulate IL-17 secretion (5.7-fold via NLRP3 activation), which acts in synergy with MP-induced TGF-β, to polarize tumor-associated macrophages (TAMs) toward an immunosuppressive M2 phenotype. [50, 53].

The convergence of MP-induced oxidative stress (8-OHdG DNA lesions) and chronic inflammation creates a self-perpetuating tumor-promoting environment. PS-MPs influence genomic instability through ANXA2-mediated mitophagy inhibition, impairing mitochondrial quality control [49]. These pathophysiological interactions position MPs as novel environmental cofactors in BC progression, with material properties (size, polymer type) and tumor-specific accumulation patterns critically determining the oncogenic potential [54]. In BC cells, it was observed that the exposure to MPs upregulates metastasis-related gene expression and inflammatory cytokine production, thereby aggravating BC metastasis [55].

11.9 PENILE

MPs were identified in human penile cancer samples based on the type and size analysis of plastic particulates, where the frequently found compositions included PE, PVC, and PA particles. Majority of the MPs were between 20 and 50 μm. MPs have been found to accumulate selectively in human penile cancer tissues, with a higher abundance and diversity compared to adjacent normal tissues. The widely observed types of MPs were PE, PA, and PVC having a 20–50 μm size [56]. The distinct types and distribution of MPs in cancerous tissues suggest that they may play a role in carcinogenesis, potentially contributing to cancer progression [54, 57]. These findings raise concerns about the impact of MPs exposure on human health and highlight the need for further research into the relationship between MPs and cancer development [56].

11.10 KIDNEY

A specialized microfluidic platform, kidney-testis microfluidic platform (KTP) that mimic the basic structure and function of the kidney and testis in a laboratory settings, have been developed by researchers wherein this platform allows for controlled experimentation and observation of cellular responses. Using KTP scientist investigated how PS-NPs interact with human kidney (HK-2) and testis (NTE) cells and found that PS-NPs enter the cells through endocytosis and triggers the activation of key signaling pathways associated with cancer development and progression. This includes MAPK signaling pathway which regulates the cell growth, differentiation, stress response, and apoptosis in which the activated protein involved are RTK, RAS, ERK, JNK, P38, NRF2, TNF-α, and TNF-α-R. PI3K- Akt signaling pathway which controls cell survival, growth, and metabolism with activated proteins including PI3K, AKT, MDM2, P53, and BAD is also affected [58].

11.11 SKIN

The penetration of MPs/NPs across the skin is particle size dependent, with particles smaller than 100 nm able to cross the stratum corneum, the outermost layer of the skin. The presence of chemical enhancers, such as oleic acid and ethanol, can increase the transdermal transport of MPs/NPs by enhancing the intercellular lipid fluidity or by removing lipids from the stratum corneum, further exacerbating their potential harm. Notably, human exposure studies have found significant amounts of MPs in hair, facial skin, and hand skin samples, with the highest concentration found in hair samples (>7000 MPs particles). The accumulation of MPs/NPs in human tissues may lead to chronic inflammation, oxidative stress, and DNA damage, ultimately contributing to the development of cancer [26, 59].

Exposure to MPs/NPs has been shown to induce oxidative stress, leading to the restriction of cell growth, autophagy, and premature aging [41]. Studies have demonstrated that MPs/NPs can increase the levels of ROS in a size-dependent manner, triggering a defense response that activates antioxidant-related enzymes, which include the following: superoxide dismutase, glutathione s-transferases, glutathione reductase, and glutathione peroxidase. The chronic activation of antioxidant defenses can lead to an imbalance in the redox state, resulting in oxidative stress-mediated damage to cellular components, including DNA, lipids, and proteins [60]. This can contribute to the development of oncogenesis by promoting genetic mutations, epigenetic alterations, and the activation of oncogenic pathways. The accumulation of ROS can also lead to the dysregulation of cellular signaling pathways, including those involved in cell cycle regulation, apoptosis, and DNA repair, ultimately increasing the risk of cancer development [61].

The infiltration of MPs/NPs into cells can occur through various endocytic mechanisms, including channels, transport proteins, phagocytosis, macropinocytosis, clathrin-mediated endocytosis, and caveolae-mediated endocytosis [59]. Once internalized, MPs/NPs can accumulate in the cytoplasm and within lysosomes, leading to direct cellular damage. This damage is attributed to the induction of inflammation and oxidative stress, which can contribute to the development of cancer. The accumulation of MPs/NPs within cells can disrupt normal cellular function, leading to genetic mutations, epigenetic alterations, and the activation of oncogenic pathways. The resulting chronic inflammation and oxidative stress can further exacerbate the carcinogenic process, ultimately contributing to the genesis of cancer [62].

The interaction between MPs/NPs and skin triggers an immune response, which is initiated by the recognition of pathogen-associated molecular patterns (PAMPs) and damage-associated molecular patterns (DAMPs) by cellular receptors on various skin cells, including keratinocytes, Langerhans cells, dendritic cells, melanocytes, macrophages, and T cells [63]. This recognition leads to the activation of immune cells and the secretion of pro-inflammatory molecules, such as ILs (IL-1, IL-6, IL-10, IL-17, IL-18, and IL-22) and tumor necrosis factor (TNF), which compromise the skin's barrier integrity. The immune response also involves the upregulation of pro-apoptotic proteins, including BAX, caspase-3, caspase-8, caspase-9, DR5, and the activation of the mitochondrial apoptotic pathway, ultimately contributing to the disruption of skin homeostasis [64, 65].

MPs can bind to proteins, altering their structure and function by changing protein folding and forming dysfunctional proteins [66]. This interaction can lead to the formation of a "protein corona" on the surface of plastic particles, modifying the biological response and potentially contributing to carcinogenesis. The presence of a protein corona on MPs can alter their interaction with cells, disrupting normal cellular processes and progressively leading to cancer development by affecting DNA repair, cell cycle regulation, and apoptosis [66, 67].

Exposure to NPs from commercial face scrubs can adhere to and be internalized by human skin cells, causing harmful effects that depend on the concentration [65]. The attachment of NPs to the keratin layer facilitates protein-corona formation, which triggers macropinocytosis and subsequent macropinolysosomal processes. The internalized NPs induce oxidative stress, leading to the downregulation of cell growth and proliferation inhibition. Chronic exposure to NPs results in autophagic structures and premature aging, indicating a potential link to oncogenesis [7]. Small plastic particulates get internalized in skin cells, and the process of internalization is time- and concentration-dependent. This triggers mitochondrial oxidative stress, membrane depolarization, and GSDMD (Gasdermin-D) recruitment, which releases mtDNA into the cytoplasm. This activates the AIM2 inflammasome, upregulating pro-inflammatory cytokines (IL-1β, IL-18) and inducing cellular senescence via p16/p21 overexpression [68]. Chronic exposure impairs skin regeneration, amplifies inflammation, and disrupts homeostasis, promoting genetic mutations, epigenetic alterations, and oncogenic pathways linked to skin cancer initiation and progression [43].

11.12 GASTROINTESTINAL

Mucus is the primary interaction layer in the gastrointestinal tract, which interacts with the foreign particles. This mucus layer serves as the first interface between the host and external particles, with its functionality strongly related to the gut microbiome [69]. Dysbiosis and foreign particles like MPs/NPs can disrupt this balance, leading to pathological consequences. MNPs interact directly with the mucus layer, adhering to intestinal epithelial cells and inducing local inflammation [70]. Exposure to MNPs reduces *MUC2* expression in some studies, thinning the mucus layer, while others report increased mucin secretion as a compensatory response. This structural compromise allows pathogens and MNPs to penetrate the epithelium, triggering oxidative damage, immune activation, and "leaky gut" syndrome [71]. MNPs also act as vectors for biofilm-associated pathogens (e.g., antibiotic-resistant *Escherichia coli*) and horizontal gene transfer, amplifying antimicrobial resistance [72]. The uptake of MPs in the intestines occurs through diverse mechanistic pathways which include macropinocytosis, caveolae-mediated endocytosis, clathrin-mediated endocytosis, and membrane disruption [73].

MPs, upon oral exposure, are translocated by M cells in the gut mucosa into the bloodstream, potentially accumulating in organs and crossing biological barriers [70]. Their small size and hydrophobic properties enable them to reach the gastrointestinal tract, where chronic exposure may lead to inflammation, oxidative stress causing ROS generation, and DNA damage, potentially contributing to gastrointestinal oncogenesis. The interaction between MPs and the gut microenvironment may disrupt cellular homeostasis, promoting epigenetic alterations and genetic mutations that can result in the initiation and progression of gastrointestinal cancer [17, 69, 74].

The gut-associated lymphoid tissues, specifically Peyer's patches in the ileum, play a crucial role in immune homeostasis by sampling and transporting particles from the intestinal lumen. M cells in Peyer's patches can take up MPs and NPs, potentially leading to their accumulation in the subepithelial dome [70]. This accumulation may compromise local immunity, disrupt immune-sensing, and surveillance, potentially leading to chronic inflammation and increased cancer risk in the gastrointestinal tract. The hijacking of this route by MPs could contribute to the development of gastrointestinal cancer by promoting genetic mutations, epigenetic alterations, and disrupting cellular homeostasis [17].

The translocation of MPs, such as PVC particles, across the gastrointestinal epithelium occurs through paracellular pathways, particularly in areas of desquamation and between villi. Particles are transported through the body via two primary routes. They travel through the lymphatic route via the chyle of underlying lymph vessels. They also travel through the portal circulation route where they are detected in the mesenteric veins [75, 76]. The rapid appearance of MPs in the bloodstream, bile, urine, and cerebrospinal fluid suggests systemic distribution [77]. Larger particles tend to accumulate in tissues and organs, such as the liver. Chronic exposure may lead to epigenetic alterations, DNA damage, and disruption of cellular homeostasis, thereby contributing to gastrointestinal carcinogenesis through mechanisms involving persistent inflammatory responses, altered cellular signaling pathways, and compromised immune surveillance [76].

Exposure to PS particles disrupts liver function by altering energy metabolism, lipid metabolism, and inducing oxidative stress [78]. Notably, PS-MPs decrease ATP levels, increase LDH activity, and reduce total cholesterol and triglyceride levels. The MPs also induce oxidative stress, as evidenced by changes in antioxidant enzyme activities, including increased GSH-Px and SOD, and decreased CAT. Furthermore, PS-MPs exhibit neurotoxic potential by inhibiting AChE activity. These alterations may contribute to gastrointestinal cancer development by promoting chronic inflammation, oxidative damage, and disrupting cellular homeostasis. The size-dependent effects of MPs on liver's functioning suggest that smaller particles may have a greater impact on certain biomarkers, potentially exacerbating cancer risk [79].

The unique physicochemical properties of MPs, including their small size and high surface area-to-volume ratio, facilitate the adsorption and concentration of environmental carcinogens, such as PAHs and heavy metals [80]. Upon ingestion, these MPs-bound pollutants can be released, exposing gastrointestinal tissues to carcinogenic agents and potentially inducing malignant transformations. The prolonged retention of MPs in the gastrointestinal tract may amplify the adverse effects of these adsorbed pollutants, contributing to the development of gastrointestinal cancer through mechanisms involving chronic inflammation, DNA damage, and epigenetic alterations [80, 81].

11.13 POTENTIAL THERAPEUTIC INTERVENTIONS FOR MPs-INDUCED CANCER

Current strategies focus on pharmacological agents, pathway inhibition, and novel technologies to counteract MP-driven carcinogenesis (**Figure 11.5**).

11.14 PHARMACOLOGICAL APPROACHES

Existing Anticancer Drugs: Taxanes and targeted therapies including paclitaxel, sorafenib, and vemurafenib show efficacy against MP-affected cancers by targeting proliferation and metastasis pathways [82]. Paclitaxel is widely used for breast, ovarian, and other solid tumors. It induces cell cycle arrest during the G2/M phase and also promotes apoptosis. It stabilizes microtubules, preventing their disassembly during mitosis. Additionally, it modulates microRNA expression and immune responses, enhancing tumor suppression. Often combined with other agents like doxorubicin or bevacizumab to improve progression-free survival and reduce recurrence rates [83]. Sorafenib is

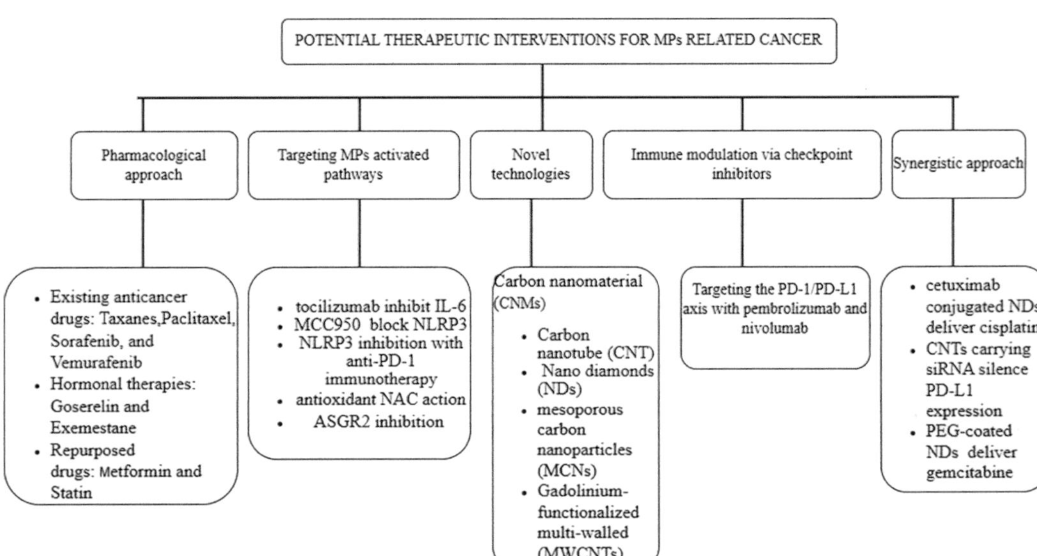

FIGURE 11.5 Emerging therapeutic strategies for mitigating MPs related carcinogenesis.

a first-line treatment for advanced hepatocellular carcinoma (HCC), targeting proliferation and angiogenesis pathways. However, resistance develops in many patients within six months. It inhibits multiple kinases in the RAF/MEK/ERK pathway and blocks VEGFR and PDGFR to reduce tumor growth and vascularization. Sorafenib is often combined with other agents like disulfiram to overcome resistance and enhance efficacy by targeting cancer stem cells [84]. Vemurafenib inhibits mutated BRAF kinase, suppressing ERK signaling and tumor proliferation. Standard care for BRAF-mutated melanoma resistance remains a challenge requiring combination strategies [85].

Hormonal Therapies: Goserelin and exemestane are highlighted for their potential in MP-associated breast and ovarian cancers [43]. Goserelin improves disease-free survival in women during the premenopausal stage, with hormone-receptor-positive BC. It also preserves ovarian function during chemotherapy. As a gonadotropin-releasing hormone agonist, it suppresses ovarian estrogen production, reducing hormone-driven tumor growth, and is administered as adjuvant therapy with endocrine agents like tamoxifen or aromatase inhibitors for BC management [86, 87]. Exemestane significantly reduces recurrence rates in hormone-receptor-positive BC when combined with ovarian suppression therapies. It inhibits aromatase enzyme activity, lowering estrogen levels to prevent tumor progression. This is used alongside ovarian suppression agents like goserelin for enhanced therapeutic outcomes in premenopausal women [88]. These drugs demonstrate significant efficacy against MP-associated cancers by targeting proliferation, metastasis pathways, or hormone dependence. Combination approaches are increasingly utilized to enhance outcomes and address drug resistance.

Repurposed Drugs: There are drugs like metformin and statin that are used to mitigate MP-induced oxidative stress, inflammation and to disrupt cancer-promoting pathways. Metformin mitigate MP-induced oxidative stress and inflammation, which are critical in TME modulation. Metformin and statins show promise in cancer treatment by targeting the TME through multiple mechanisms [89]. The former reduces oxidative stress and tumor growth by activating AMPK and inhibiting mTOR signaling. It also boosts antitumor immunity by enhancing CD8+ T cell and NK cell activity while suppressing immunosuppressive cells. When combined with chemotherapy or radiation, metformin can sensitize cancer cells and improve treatment outcomes by normalizing TME hypoxia and inflammation. This highlights the potential for repurposing these drugs to enhance cancer therapy [43].

Inhibiting the cholesterol pathway with statins can disrupt cancer-promoting signaling and reduce metastasis by lowering membrane cholesterol and suppressing pro-inflammatory pathways [90]. Statins also prevent metastasis by downregulating invasion-related genes. When combined with metformin, statins show promise in preclinical models, jointly targeting multiple pathways to induce cancer cell death and senescence, highlighting the potential for improved cancer treatment outcomes through combination therapy. These repurposed drugs offer a multifaceted approach to counteract MP-induced oxidative stress and inflammation, highlighting their utility in adjuvant cancer therapy [89].

11.15 TARGETING MP-ACTIVATED PATHWAYS

PS-MPs promote therapy resistance in gastric cancer by upregulating the ASGR2 receptor, which enhances stemness and multidrug resistance through PD-L1. Targeting ASGR2 via knockdown or inhibition may restore sensitivity to chemotherapy and monoclonal antibodies. Studies have shown that silencing ASGR2 significantly reduces gastric cancer cell proliferation, migration, and invasion, while also reversing resistance to paclitaxel, trastuzumab, and bortezomib, thereby enhancing treatment efficacy. This approach highlights the potential for ASGR2 inhibition as a therapeutic strategy to mitigate MP-induced therapy resistance in gastric cancer [91] (**Figure 11.5**).

MPs exposure can lead to increased IL-6 levels and NLRP3 inflammasome activation, contributing to inflammation and metastasis. Potential therapeutic strategies to counteract these effects include using tocilizumab to inhibit IL-6 and MCC950 to block NLRP3, which may help mitigate the pro-inflammatory and pro-metastatic consequences of MPs exposure [92]. Tocilizumab, a monoclonal antibody that targets IL-6 receptors, has shown promise in preclinical studies for reducing inflammation and tumor growth driven by MPs-induced IL-6 elevation. By blocking IL-6 signaling, tocilizumab may mitigate the pro-tumorigenic effects of MPs exposure, offering a potential therapeutic strategy [93].

Inhibiting the NLRP3 inflammasome can suppress tumor-promoting inflammation and enhance anti-tumor immunity by reducing myeloid-derived suppressor cells (MDSCs) and boosting CD8+ T cell activity. Notably, combining NLRP3 inhibition with anti-PD-1 immunotherapy, such as with MCC950, can synergistically enhance anti-tumor effects, leading to greater tumor volume reduction than either therapy alone, highlighting the potential for improved cancer treatment outcomes [94]. The antioxidant N-acetylcysteine (NAC) can mitigate MPs-induced oxidative stress by scavenging mitochondrial ROS, thereby preventing DNA damage and alterations in the TME. NAC has been shown to reduce oxidative DNA damage and suppress PI3K/Akt pathway activation [95]. NAC serves as a chemotherapy adjuvant by reducing oxidative stress, as evidenced by a 40% decrease in malondialdehyde (MDA) levels and enhanced glutathione peroxidase activity. This leads to reduced hepatotoxicity and hematological complications in acute lymphoblastic leukemia (ALL) patients. Additionally, NAC synergizes with cisplatin in triple-negative breast cancer (TNBC) by normalizing hypoxia and increasing treatment [96].

11.16 NOVEL TECHNOLOGIES

Carbon nanomaterials (CNMs) have emerged as promising tools for targeted cancer therapy, enabling precise drug delivery to tumor cells while minimizing off-target effects. By leveraging covalent modifications, pH-sensitive release mechanisms, and dual functionality, CNMs such as carbon nanotubes (CNTs) and nanodiamonds (NDs) can enhance therapeutic efficacy and reduce systemic toxicity. For instance, CNTs can be engineered to release drugs in response to acidic TME while NDs can target mitochondria in cancer cells to overcome drug resistance. Additionally, mesoporous carbon nanoparticles (MCNs) can be designed with gatekeeper systems that allow for spatiotemporal control of drug release, highlighting the potential of CNMs to improve cancer treatment outcomes [97]. pH-sensitive CNTs release drugs in acidic TME conditions, improving efficacy in gastric and BCs. Gadolinium-functionalized multi-walled CNTs (MWCNTs) serve dual roles in drug delivery and MRI contrast enhancement, with stability in biological fluids [98, 99]. NDs and MCNs offer targeted cancer therapy approaches. NDs deliver cisplatin to mitochondria, overcoming drug resistance in HCC. MCNs release drugs in response to pH changes or near-infrared light, enabling spatiotemporal control in colorectal cancer [97].

11.17 IMMUNE MODULATION VIA CHECKPOINT INHIBITORS

By using checkpoint inhibitors to targeting the PD-1/PD-L1 axis, such as pembrolizumab and nivolumab, one can counteract TME suppression mediated by MPs. By blocking PD-1/PD-L1 interactions, these therapies restore cytotoxic T cell activity and promote anti-tumor immunity. Notably, nivolumab has shown significant clinical benefit, improving five-year survival rates in advanced melanoma. To overcome resistance, combining anti-PD-1 therapies with NLRP3 inhibitors, such as MCC950, may enhance CD8+ T cell responses by reducing MDSC infiltration, thereby augmenting the efficacy of immunotherapy [100].

Remodeling the TME through macrophage repolarization involves shifting TAMs from an immunosuppressive phenotype to a pro-inflammatory M1 phenotype, characterized by increased secretion of TNF-α and IL-6. This repolarization enhances the penetration of anti-PD-1 antibodies by degrading the collagen-rich ECM, ultimately facilitating CD8+ T cell infiltration and augmenting the efficacy of immunotherapy [101].

11.18 SYNERGISTIC APPROACHES

CNM-immunotherapy combinations show promise, such as cetuximab-conjugated NDs that deliver cisplatin while targeting EGFR, resulting in significant reduction of HepG2 cell viability. Additionally, CNTs carrying siRNA can silence PD-L1 expression in TAMs, synergizing with anti-CTLA-4 therapy to delay melanoma progression, highlighting the potential of CNMs in enhancing cancer immunotherapy [99].

PEG-coated NDs have shown promise in delivering gemcitabine for pancreatic cancer treatment by enabling sustained release and maintaining stable plasma concentrations. By either physically absorbing or chemically conjugating gemcitabine to NDs, these systems facilitate controlled drug release, enhance stability, and promote intracellular delivery in pancreatic cancer cells, potentially improving therapeutic outcomes [97, 102]. PEGylation of ND systems can reduce opsonization and extend circulation time, similar to PEGylated micellar systems, which have shown enhanced tumor accumulation of gemcitabine. While PEG-NDs stabilize plasma levels, incorporating targeting ligands may further improve tumor-specific delivery and efficacy. The complexity of cancer treatment suggests that combining ND-based delivery systems with other therapies, such as checkpoint inhibitors or metabolic modulators, may be necessary to achieve optimal outcomes, highlighting the need for multifaceted approaches to cancer treatment [102]. Researchers are investigating checkpoint inhibitors, such as anti-PD-1 therapies, to potentially overcome the immunosuppressive effects of MPs in the TME, thereby increasing the body's natural ability toward anti-tumor immune responses [43].

11.19 FUTURE PERSPECTIVE

Emerging evidence implicates MPs in carcinogenesis, necessitating further research to elucidate underlying mechanisms. Key priorities include investigating MP-induced epigenetic changes, immune modulation, and hormonal disruptions. Standardized assessment models, biomonitoring, and epidemiological studies are crucial to establish causal links between MP exposure and cancer incidence. Regulatory frameworks, therapeutic innovations, and public awareness campaigns are essential for mitigating MP-related health risks. Interdisciplinary collaboration is vital to address the complex interactions between MPs, human health, and the environment, ultimately informing evidence-based policies and interventions to reduce MP exposure and associated health impacts.

ABBREVIATIONS

BC: breast cancer
MP: microplastic
NAC: N-acetylcysteine
NP: nanoplastic
PS-MP: polystyrene microplastics
ROS: reactive oxygen species
TME: tumor microenvironment

REFERENCES

1. Meikle, Jeffrey L. 1997. "Material Doubts: The Consequences of Plastic." *Environmental History* 2 (3): 278–300. https://doi.org/10.2307/3985351.
2. Thompson, Richard C., Shanna H. Swan, Charles J. Moore, and Frederick S. vom Saal. 2009. "Our Plastic Age." *Philosophical Transactions of the Royal Society B: Biological Sciences* 364 (1526): 1973–76. https://doi.org/10.1098/rstb.2009.0054.

3. Valliant, Melissa, and Dustin Cranor. 2020. *Oceana Finds Plastic Entangling, Choking 1,800 Marine Animals in U.S. Waters*. Washington, DC: Oceana USA.
4. Nielsen, Tobias D., Jacob Hasselbalch, Karl Holmberg, and Johannes Stripple. 2020. "Politics and the Plastic Crisis: A Review throughout the Plastic Life Cycle." *Wiley Interdisciplinary Reviews: Energy and Environment* 9 (1): e360. https://doi.org/10.1002/wene.360.
5. Le Guern, Claire. 2019. "When the Mermaids Cry: The Great Plastic Tide." *Coastal Care* 10 (2).
6. Bajt, Oliver. 2021. "From Plastics to Microplastics and Organisms." *FEBS Open Bio* 11 (4): 954–66. https://doi.org/10.1002/2211-5463.13120.
7. Gopinath, Ponnusamy Manogaran, Krishna Sundar Twayana, Palaniyandi Ravanan, John Thomas, Amitava Mukherjee, David F. Jenkins, and Natarajan Chandrasekaran. 2021. "Prospects on the Nano-Plastic Particles Internalization and Induction of Cellular Response in Human Keratinocytes." *Particle and Fibre Toxicology* 18 (1): 35. https://doi.org/10.1186/s12989-021-00428-9.
8. Rahim, Nur Anis Sofia M., Farida Islahudin, Nurfaiza Abu Tahrim, and Malina Jasamai. 2022. "Microplastics in Cosmetics and Personal Care Products: Impacts on Aquatic Life and Rodents with Potential Alternatives." *Sains Malaysiana* 51 (3). http://doi.org/10.17576/jsm-2022-5108-12.
9. Osman, Ahmed I., Mohamed Hosny, Abdelazeem S. Eltaweil, Sara Omar, Ahmed M. Elgarahy, Mohamed Farghali, Pow-Seng Yap, et al. 2023. "Microplastic Sources, Formation, Toxicity and Remediation: A Review." *Environmental Chemistry Letters* 21 (4): 2129–69. https://doi.org/10.1007/s10311-023-01593-3.
10. Yang, Yulu, Mohammed Jalalah, Saeed A. Alsareii, Farid A. Harraz, Nandini Thakur, Yuanzhang Zheng, Yeojoon Yoon, and El-Sayed Salama. 2024. "Plastic Wastes (PWs) and Microplastics (MPs) Formation: Management, Migration, and Environmental Impact." *Journal of Environmental Chemical Engineering* 12 (3): 112926. https://doi.org/10.1016/j.jece.2024.112926.
11. Zhang, Kai, Amir Hossein Hamidian, Aleksandra Tubić, Yu Zhang, James K. H. Fang, Chenxi Wu, and Paul K. S. Lam. 2021. "Understanding Plastic Degradation and Microplastic Formation in the Environment: A Review." *Environmental Pollution* 274: 116554. https://doi.org/10.1016/j.envpol.2021.116554.
12. Boucher, Julien, and Damien Friot. 2017. *Primary Microplastics in the Ocean: A Global Evaluation of Sources*. Gland, Switzerland: International Union for Conservation of Nature. http://dx.doi.org/10.2305/IUCN.CH.2017.01.en
13. Wright, Stephanie L., Jessica Ulke, Anna Font, K. L. Andrew Chan, and Frank J. Kelly. 2020. "Atmospheric Microplastic Deposition in an Urban Environment and an Evaluation of Transport." *Environment International* 136: 105411. https://doi.org/10.1016/j.envint.2019.105411.
14. World Health Organization. 2022. *Dietary and Inhalation Exposure to Nano- and Microplastic Particles and Potential Implications for Human Health*. Geneva: World Health Organization.
15. Cai, Liqi, Jundong Wang, Jinping Peng, Zhi Tan, Zhiwei Zhan, Xiangling Tan, and Qiuqiang Chen. 2017. "Characteristic of Microplastics in the Atmospheric Fallout from Dongguan City, China: Preliminary Research and First Evidence." *Environmental Science and Pollution Research* 24 (32): 24928–35. https://doi.org/10.1007/s11356-017-0116-x.
16. Prata, Joana Correia, João P. da Costa, Isabel Lopes, Armando C. Duarte, and Teresa Rocha-Santos. 2020. "Environmental Exposure to Microplastics: An Overview on Possible Human Health Effects." *Science of the Total Environment* 702: 134455. https://doi.org/10.1016/j.scitotenv.2019.134455.
17. Wright, Stephanie L., and Frank J. Kelly. 2017. "Plastic and Human Health: A Micro Issue?" *Environmental Science & Technology* 51 (12): 6634–47. https://doi.org/10.1021/acs.est.7b00423.
18. Lindeque, Penelope K., Matthew Cole, Rachel L. Coppock, Ceri N. Lewis, Rachael Z. Miller, Andrew J. R. Watts, Alice Wilson-McNeal, Stephanie L. Wright, and Tamara S. Galloway. 2020. "Are We Underestimating Microplastic Abundance in the Marine Environment? A Comparison of Microplastic Capture with Nets of Different Mesh-Size." *Environmental Pollution* 265: 114721. https://doi.org/10.1016/j.envpol.2020.114721.
19. Lebreton, Laurent, Boyan Slat, Francesco Ferrari, Bruno Sainte-Rose, James Aitken, Robin Marthouse, Sarah Hajbane, et al. 2018. "Evidence That the Great Pacific Garbage Patch Is Rapidly Accumulating Plastic." *Scientific Reports* 8 (1): 4666. https://doi.org/10.1038/s41598-018-22939-w.
20. Yang, Dongqi, Huahong Shi, Lan Li, Jiana Li, Khalida Jabeen, and Prabhu Kolandhasamy. 2015. "Microplastic Pollution in Table Salts from China." *Environmental Science & Technology* 49 (22): 13622–27. https://doi.org/10.1021/acs.est.5b03163.
21. Corradini, Fabio, Pablo Meza, Raúl Eguiluz, Francisco Casado, Esperanza Huerta-Lwanga, and Violette Geissen. 2019. "Evidence of Microplastic Accumulation in Agricultural Soils from Sewage Sludge Disposal." *Science of the Total Environment* 671: 411–20. https://doi.org/10.1016/j.scitotenv.2019.03.368.

22. Wu, Panfeng, Jinsheng Huang, Yuling Zheng, Yicheng Yang, Yue Zhang, Feng He, Hao Chen, et al. 2019. "Environmental Occurrences, Fate, and Impacts of Microplastics." *Ecotoxicology and Environmental Safety* 184: 109612. https://doi.org/10.1016/j.ecoenv.2019.109612.
23. Krishnan, Kannabiran. 2023. "A Systematic Review on the Impact of Micro-Nanoplastics Exposure on Human Health and Diseases." *Biointerface Research in Applied Chemistry* 13 (4): 1–12. https://doi.org/10.33263/BRIAC134.381.
24. Prata, Joana Correia. 2018. "Airborne Microplastics: Consequences to Human Health?" *Environmental Pollution* 234: 115–26. https://doi.org/10.1016/j.envpol.2017.11.043.
25. Dris, Rachid, Johnny Gasperi, Cécile Mirande, Corinne Mandin, Mohamed Guerrouache, Valérie Langlois, and Bruno Tassin. 2017. "A First Overview of Textile Fibers, Including Microplastics, in Indoor and Outdoor Environments." *Environmental Pollution* 221: 453–58. https://doi.org/10.1016/j.envpol.2016.12.013.
26. Menichetti, Arianna, Dario Mordini, and Marco Montalti. 2024. "Penetration of Microplastics and Nanoparticles through Skin: Effects of Size, Shape, and Surface Chemistry." *Journal of Xenobiotics* 15 (1): 6. https://doi.org/10.3390/jox15010006.
27. Hernandez, Laura M., Nariman Yousefi, and Nathalie Tufenkji. 2017. "Are There Nanoplastics in Your Personal Care Products?" *Environmental Science and Technology Letters* 4 (7): 280–85. http://dx.doi.org/10.1021/acs.estlett.7b00187.
28. Bhuyan, Md. Simul. 2022. "Effects of Microplastics on Fish and in Human Health." *Frontiers in Environmental Science* 10: 827289. https://doi.org/10.3389/fenvs.2022.827289.
29. Kumar, Naveen, Mridul Lamba, Ashok Kumar Pachar, Sonal Yadav, and Arbind Acharya. 2024. "Microplastics – A Growing Concern as Carcinogens in Cancer Etiology: Emphasis on Biochemical and Molecular Mechanisms." *Cell Biochemistry and Biophysics* 82 (4): 3109–21. https://doi.org/10.1007/s12013-024-01436-0.
30. Płuciennik, Kamil, Paulina Sicińska, and Weronika Misztal. 2024. "Important Factors Affecting Induction of Cell Death, Oxidative Stress and DNA Damage by Nano- and Microplastic Particles in Vitro." *Cells* 13 (9): 768. https://doi.org/10.3390/cells13090768.
31. Xuan, Lihui, Liang Xiao, and Ruixue Huang. 2023. "The Geno-toxicological Impacts of Microplastic (MP) Exposure on Health: Mechanistic Pathways and Research Trends from a Chinese perspective." *Environmental Science: Processes and Impacts* 25 (1): 26–36. https://doi.org/10.1039/d2em00301e.
32. Blackburn, Kirsty, and Dannielle Green. 2022. "The Potential Effects of Microplastics on Human Health: What Is Known and What Is Unknown." *Ambio* 51 (3): 518–30. https://doi.org/10.1007/s13280-021-01589-9.
33. Wade, Miranda J., Kennedy Bucci, Chelsea M. Rochman, and Mariah H. Meek. 2025. "Microplastic Exposure Is Associated with Epigenomic Effects in the Model Organism *Pimephales promelas* (Fathead Minnow)." *Journal of Heredity* 116 (2): 113–25. https://doi.org/10.1093/jhered/esae027.
34. Noventa, Seta, Matthew S. P. Boyles, Andreas Seifert, Simone Belluco, Aracaeli Sánchez Jiménez, Helinor J. Johnston, et al. 2021. "Paradigms to Assess the Human Health Risks of Nano- and Microplastics." *Microplastics and Nanoplastics* 1 (1): 9. https://doi.org/10.1186/s43591-021-00011-1.
35. Vasse, Gwenda F., and Barbro N. Melgert. 2024. "Microplastic and Plastic Pollution: Impact on Respiratory Disease and Health." *European Respiratory Review* 33 (172). https://doi.org/10.1183/16000617.0226-2023.
36. Goodman, Kerestin E., Joan T. Hare, Zahraa I. Khamis, Timothy Hua, and Qing-Xiang Amy Sang. 2021. "Exposure of Human Lung Cells to Polystyrene Microplastics Significantly Retards Cell Proliferation and Triggers Morphological Changes." *Chemical Research in Toxicology* 34 (4): 1069–81. https://doi.org/10.1021/acs.chemrestox.0c00486.
37. Cao, Jingwen, Ran Xu, Yuan Geng, Shiwen Xu, and Mengyao Guo. 2023. "Exposure to Polystyrene Microplastics Triggers Lung Injury via Targeting Toll-Like Receptor 2 and Activation of the NF-κB Signal in Mice." *Environmental Pollution* 320: 121068. https://doi.org/10.1016/j.envpol.2023.121068.
38. Jin, Wenhua, Weibo Zhang, Hejing Tang, Pengjie Wang, Yan Zhang, Siyuan Liu, et al. 2024. "Microplastics Exposure Causes the Senescence of Human Lung Epithelial Cells and Mouse Lungs by Inducing ROS Signaling." *Environment International* 185: 108489. https://doi.org/10.1016/j.envint.2024.108489.
39. Lu, Kuo, Danting Zhan, Yingying Fang, Lei Li, Guobin Chen, Shanze Chen, and Lingwei Wang. 2022. "Microplastics, Potential Threat to Patients with Lung Diseases." *Frontiers in Toxicology* 4: 958414. https://doi.org/10.3389/ftox.2022.958414.

40. Shi, Qingying, Jingchun Tang, Xiaomei Liu, and Rutao Liu. 2021. "Ultraviolet-Induced Photodegradation Elevated the Toxicity of Polystyrene Nanoplastics on Human Lung Epithelial A549 Cells." *Environmental Science: Nano* 8 (9): 2660–75. https://doi.org/10.1039/D1EN00465D.
41. Kadac-Czapska, Kornelia, Justyna Ośko, Eliza Knez, and Małgorzata Grembecka. 2024. "Microplastics and Oxidative Stress—Current Problems and Prospects." *Antioxidants* 13 (5): 579. https://doi.org/10.3390/antiox13050579.
42. Lee, Hanjun. 2024. "From Bottles to Brains: The Role of Microplastics in Enhancing." *International Journal of High School Research* 6 (11). https://doi.org/10.36838/v6i11.9.
43. Chen, Yunjie, Zihang Zhang, Kangming Ji, Qiuchen Zhang, Lijun Qian, and Chuang Yang. 2025. "Role of Microplastics in the Tumor Microenvironment (Review)." *Oncology Letters* 29 (4): 193. https://doi.org/10.3892/ol.2025.14939.
44. Xu, Hongwen, Chunlin Dong, Zhilong Yu, Yukihiro Ozaki, and Zhenyang Hua. 2024. "Detection and Analysis of Microplastics in Tissues and Blood of Human Cervical Cancer Patients." *Environmental Research* 259: 119498. https://doi.org/10.1016/j.envres.2024.119498.
45. Hou, Junyu, Zhimin Lei, Linlu Cui, Yun Hou, Long Yang, Ru An, et al. 2021. "Polystyrene Microplastics Lead to Pyroptosis and Apoptosis of Ovarian Granulosa Cells via NLRP3/Caspase-1 Signaling Pathway in Rats." *Ecotoxicology and Environmental Safety* 212: 112012. https://doi.org/10.1016/j.ecoenv.2021.112012.
46. An, Ru, Xiaoqing Wang, Long Yang, Junyu Zhang, Ning Wang, Feng Xu, Yun Hou, Hongqin Zhang, and Lianshuang Zhang. 2021. "Polystyrene Microplastics Cause Granulosa Cells Apoptosis and Fibrosis in Ovary through Oxidative Stress in Rats." *Toxicology* 449: 152665. https://doi.org/10.1016/j.tox.2020.152665.
47. Yang, Weili, Wen Tan, Jingfei Zheng, Biyan Zhang, Hongfeng Li, and Xuehe Li. 2018. "MEHP Promotes the Proliferation of Cervical Cancer via GPER Mediated Activation of Akt." *European Journal of Pharmacology* 824: 11–16. https://doi.org/10.1016/j.ejphar.2018.01.040.
48. Silva, Christian David Hernández, Julio César Villegas-Pineda, and Ana Laura Pereira Suárez. 2020. "Expression and Role of the G Protein-Coupled Estrogen Receptor (GPR30/GPER) in the Development and Immune Response in Female Reproductive Cancers." *Frontiers in Endocrinology* 11: 544. https://doi.org/10.3389/fendo.2020.00544.
49. Tian, Ziying, Boni Ding, Yilin Guo, Jieyu Zhou, Su Jiang, Jiaxue Lu, Nan Li, Xiao Zhou, and Wenling Zhang. 2025. "Microplastics Accumulated in Breast Cancer Patients Lead to Mitophagy via ANXA2-Mediated Endocytosis and IL-17 Signaling Pathway." *Environmental Pollution* 364: 125321. https://doi.org/10.1016/j.envpol.2024.125321.
50. Chen, Cong, Aizhai Xiang, Xia Lin, Jufeng Guo, Jian Liu, Shufang Hu, Tao Rui, and Qianwei Ye. 2024. "Mitophagy: Insights into Its Signaling Molecules, Biological Functions, and Therapeutic Potential in Breast Cancer." *Cell Death Discovery* 10 (1): 457. https://doi.org/10.1038/s41420-024-02226-6.
51. Ramakrishnan, Rakhee K., Khuloud Bajbouj, Saba Al Heialy, Bassam Mahboub, Abdul Wahid Ansari, Ibrahim Y. Hachim, Surendra Rawat, et al. 2020. "IL-17 Induced Autophagy Regulates Mitochondrial Dysfunction and Fibrosis in Severe Asthmatic Bronchial Fibroblasts." *Frontiers in Immunology* 11: 1002. https://doi.org/10.3389/fimmu.2020.01002.
52. Nikolaou, Savvas, and Laura M. Machesky. 2020. "The Stressful Tumour Environment Drives Plasticity of Cell Migration Programmes, Contributing to Metastasis." *The Journal of Pathology* 250 (5): 612–23. https://doi.org/10.1002/path.5395.
53. Gorczynski, Reginald M. 2020. "IL-17 Signaling in the Tumor Microenvironment." *Advances in Experimental Medicine and Biology* 1240: 47–58. https://doi.org/10.1007/978-3-030-38315-2_4.
54. Schnee, Maximilian, Mareike Sieler, Jessica Dörnen, and Thomas Dittmar. 2024. "Effects of Polystyrene Nano-and Microplastics on Human Breast Epithelial Cells and Human Breast Cancer Cells." *Heliyon* 10 (20). https://doi.org/10.1016/j.heliyon.2024.e38686.
55. Zhu, Leilei, Peihao Xu, Mingyuan Zhou, Kewei Li, Shasha Tian, Xuemei Fan, Junling Liu, Baodong Ye, Zhishan Ding, and Yingzhi Shen. 2025. "Synergistic Promotion of Triple-Negative Breast Cancer Tumorigenesis and Metastasis by Oral Polystyrene Nanoplastics Exposure via *Alloprevotella*-Derived Glutamate and Platelet Activation." *Advanced Science* 12 (1): e2405612. https://doi.org/10.1002/advs.202508310
56. Wang, Ming, Qiushi Liu, Xueping Zhang, Hui Jiang, and Xiansheng Zhang. 2025. "Identification and Analysis of Microplastics in Human Penile Cancer Tissues." *Science of the Total Environment* 969: 178815. https://doi.org/10.1016/j.scitotenv.2025.178815.
57. Cross, Paul Ian. 2024. "Could Microplastics Found in Penises Affect Fertility and Sperm Count?" *Medical News Today.*

58. Xiao, Mingming, Xinran Li, Xinlian Zhang, Xiaoxiao Duan, Houwei Lin, Sixiu Liu, and Guodong Sui. 2023. "Assessment of Cancer-Related Signaling Pathways in Responses to Polystyrene Nanoplastics via a Kidney-Testis Microfluidic Platform (KTP)." *Science of the Total Environment* 857: 159306. http://dx.doi.org/10.1016/j.scitotenv.2022.159306.
59. Yee, Maxine Swee-Li, Ling-Wei Hii, Chin King Looi, Wei-Meng Lim, Shew-Fung Wong, Yih-Yih Kok, et al. 2021. "Impact of Microplastics and Nanoplastics on Human Health." *Nanomaterials* 11 (2): 496. https://doi.org/10.3390/nano11020496.
60. Jeong, Chang-Bum, Hye-Min Kang, Min-Chul Lee, Duck-Hyun Kim, Jeonghoon Han, Dae-Sik Hwang, Sami Souissi, et al. 2017. "Adverse Effects of Microplastics and Oxidative Stress-Induced MAPK/Nrf2 Pathway-Mediated Defense Mechanisms in the Marine Copepod *Paracyclopina nana*." *Scientific Reports* 7 (1): 41323. https://doi.org/10.1038/srep41323.
61. Jeong, Chang-Bum, Eun-Ji Won, Hye-Min Kang, Min-Chul Lee, Dae-Sik Hwang, Un-Ki Hwang, Bingsheng Zhou, et al. 2016. "Microplastic Size-Dependent Toxicity Oxidative Stress Induction, and p-JNK and p-p38 Activation in the Monogonont Rotifer (*Brachionus koreanus*)." *Environmental Science and Technology* 50 (16): 8849–57. http://dx.doi.org/10.1021/acs.est.6b01441.
62. Mishra, Sarvesh Kumar, Tapojyoti Sanyal, Pritha Kundu, Rupesh Kumar, Dipanjan Ghosh, Gopal Chakrabarti, Nilabja Sikdar, et al. 2025. "Microplastics as Emerging Carcinogens: From Environmental Pollutants to Oncogenic Drivers." *Molecular Cancer* 24 (1): 1–34. https://doi.org/10.1186/s12943-025-02409-4.
63. Li, Danyang, and Minghua Wu. 2021. "Pattern Recognition Receptors in Health and Diseases." *Signal Transduction and Targeted Therapy* 6 (1): 291. https://doi.org/10.1038/s41392-021-00687-0.
64. Wang, Hui, Huinuan Wang, Jiawen Guan, Weijun Guan, and Zheng Liu. 2023. "Lead Induces Mouse Skin Fibroblast Apoptosis by Disrupting Intracellular Homeostasis." *Scientific Reports* 13 (1): 9670. https://doi.org/10.1038/s41598-023-36835-5.
65. Sözener, Zeynep Celebi, Lacin Cevhertas, Kari Nadeau, Mübeccel Akdis, and Cezmi A. Akdis. 2020. "Environmental Factors in Epithelial Barrier Dysfunction." *Journal of Allergy and Clinical Immunology* 145 (6): 1517–28. https://doi.org/10.1016/j.jaci.2020.04.024.
66. Hollóczki, Oldamur, and Sascha Gehrke. 2019. "Nanoplastics Can Change the Secondary Structure of Proteins." *Scientific Reports* 9 (1): 16013. https://doi.org/10.1038/s41598-019-52495-w.
67. Treuel, Lennart, Stefan Brandholt, Pauline Maffre, Sarah Wiegele, Li Shang, and G. Ulrich Nienhaus. 2014. "Impact of Protein Modification on the Protein Corona on Nanoparticles and Nanoparticle-Cell Interactions." *ACS Nano* 8 (1): 503–13. https://doi.org/10.1021/nn405019v.
68. Han, Wang, Jiayue Cui, Gao Sun, Xiao Miao, Zhang Pufang, and Li Nannan. 2024. "Nano-Sized Microplastics Exposure Induces Skin Cell Senescence via Triggering the Mitochondrial Localization of GSDMD." *Environmental Pollution* 349: 123874. https://doi.org/10.1016/j.envpol.2024.123874.
69. Wang, Chia-Ming, Matthew T. Fernez, Benjamin M. Woolston, and Rebecca L. Carrier. 2023. "Native Gastrointestinal mucus: Models and Techniques for Studying Interactions with Drugs, Drug Carriers, and Bacteria." *Advanced Drug Delivery Reviews* 200: 114966. https://doi.org/10.1016/j.addr.2023.114966.
70. Kimura, Shunsuke, Yutaka Nakamura, Nobuhide Kobayashi, Katsuyuki Shiroguchi, Eiryo Kawakami, Mami Mutoh, et al. 2020. "Osteoprotegerin-Dependent M Cell Self-Regulation Balances Gut Infection and Immunity." *Nature Communications* 11 (1): 234. https://doi.org/10.1038/s41467-019-13883-y.
71. Sofield, Charlotte E., Ryan S. Anderton, and Anastazja M. Gorecki. 2024. "Mind over Microplastics: Exploring Microplastic-Induced Gut Disruption and Gut-Brain-Axis Consequences." *Current Issues in Molecular Biology* 46 (5): 4186–202. https://doi.org/10.3390/cimb46050256.
72. Piergiacomo, Federica, Lorenzo Brusetti, and Leonardo Pagani. 2022. "Understanding the Interplay between Antimicrobial Resistance, Microplastics and Xenobiotic Contaminants: A Leap towards One Health?" *International Journal of Environmental Research and Public Health* 20 (1): 42. https://doi.org/10.3390/ijerph20010042.
73. Ding, Ruiyang, Yueyue Chen, Xuemin Shi, Yang Li, Yang Yu, Zhiwei Sun, and Junchao Duan. 2024. "Size-Dependent Toxicity of Polystyrene Microplastics on the Gastrointestinal Tract: Oxidative Stress Related-DNA Damage and Potential Carcinogenicity." *Science of the Total Environment* 912: 169514. https://doi.org/10.1016/j.scitotenv.2023.169514.
74. Smith, Madeleine, David C. Love, Chelsea M. Rochman, and Roni A. Neff. 2018. "Microplastics in Seafood and the Implications for Human Health." *Current Environmental Health Reports* 5 (3): 375–86. https://doi.org/10.1007/s40572-018-0206-z.
75. Zhou, Li, Lidan Ran, Yufen He, and Yaxi Huang. 2025. "Mechanisms of Microplastics on Gastrointestinal Injury and Liver Metabolism Disorder (Review)." *Molecular Medicine Reports* 31 (4): 98. https://doi.org/10.3892/mmr.2025.13463.

76. Volkheimer, Gerhard. 1975. "Hematogenous Dissemination of Ingested Polyvinyl Chloride Particle." *Annals of the New York Academy of Sciences* 246: 164–71. https://doi.org/10.1111/j.1749-6632.1975.tb51092.x.
77. Huang, Haipeng, Jiaqi Hou, Mingxiao Li, Fangchao Wei, Yilie Liao, and Beidou Xi. 2025. "Microplastics in the Bloodstream Can Induce Cerebral Thrombosis by Causing Cell Obstruction and lead to Neurobehavioral Abnormalities." *Science Advances* 11 (4): eadr8243. https://doi.org/10.1126/sciadv.adr8243
78. Chiu, Hui-Wen, Chun-Wei Chu, Chih-Chia Huang, Zi-Chun Chia, Yung-Li Wang, and Yu-Hsuan Lee. 2025. "Polystyrene Microplastics Induce Hepatic Lipid Metabolism and Energy Disorder by Upregulating the NR4A1-AMPK Signaling Pathway." *Environmental Pollution* 369: 125850. https://doi.org/10.1016/j.envpol.2025.125850.
79. Deng, Yongfeng, Yan Zhang, Bernardo Lemos, and Hongqiang Ren. 2017. "Tissue Accumulation of Microplastics in Mice and Biomarker Responses Suggest Widespread Health Risks of Exposure." *Scientific Reports* 7 (1): 46687. https://doi.org/10.1038/srep46687.
80. Weis, Judith S., and Juan José Alava. 2025. "Microplastics are Toxic Pollutants." *Toxics* 11 (11):935 https://doi.org/10.3390/toxics11110935.
81. Gruber, Elisabeth S., Vanessa Stadlbauer, Verena Pichler, Katharina Resch-Fauster, Andrea Todorovic, Thomas C. Meisel, Sibylle Trawoeger, et al. 2023. "To Waste or Not to Waste: Questioning Potential Health Risks of Micro- and Nanoplastics with a Focus on Their Ingestion and Potential Carcinogenicity." *Exposure and Health* 15 (1): 33–51. https://doi.org/10.1007/s12403-022-00470-8.
82. Baspakova, Akmaral, Afshin Zare, Roza Suleimenova, Aidar B. Berdygaliev, Bibigul Karimsakova, Kymbat Tussupkaliyeva, Nadiar M. Mussin, et al. 2025. "An Updated Systematic Review about Various Effects of Microplastics on Cancer: A Pharmacological and In-Silico Based Analysis." *Molecular Aspects of Medicine* 101: 101336. https://doi.org/10.1016/j.mam.2024.101336.
83. Liu, Zeng, Yuan-Yuan Zhu, Zhao-Yuan Li, and Si-Qing Ning. 2016. "Evaluation of the Efficacy of Paclitaxel with Curcumin Combination in Ovarian Cancer Cells." *Oncology Letters* 12 (5): 3944–48. https://doi.org/10.3892/ol.2016.5192.
84. Zhang, Gong, Yufeng Wang, Bryan C. Fuchs, Wei Guo, David L. Drum, Derek J. Erstad, Baomin Shi, et al. 2022. "Improving the Therapeutic Efficacy of Sorafenib for Hepatocellular Carcinoma by Repurposing Disulfiram." *Frontiers in Oncology* 12: 913736. https://doi.org/10.3389/fonc.2022.913736
85. Fisher, Rosalie, and James Larkin. 2012. "Vemurafenib: A New Treatment for BRAF-V600 Mutated Advanced Melanoma." *Cancer Management and Research* 4: 243–52. https://doi.org/10.2147/CMAR.S25284.
86. Chen, Nan, Daniella Audi Blotta, Hee Jeong Kim, Salma Sayeed, Joan Cannon, Noran Osman, Rosa Macrito, and Matteo Lambertini. 2025. "Efficacy of Goserelin in Ovarian Function Suppression and Preservation for Pre- and Perimenopausal Breast Cancer Patients: A Systematic Review." *Therapeutic Advances in Medical Oncology* 17: 17588359251319696. https://doi.org/10.1177/17588359251319696.
87. Rody, Achim, Sibylle Loibl, Gunter von Minckwitz, and Manfred Kaufmann. 2005. "Use of Goserelin in the Treatment of Breast Cancer." *Expert Review of Anticancer Therapy* 5 (4): 591–604. https://doi.org/10.1586/14737140.5.4.591.
88. Wang, Jiayu, Binghe Xu, Peng Yuan, Fei Ma, Qing Li, Pin Zhang, Ruigang Cai, et al. 2015. "Phase II Trial of Goserelin and Exemestane Combination Therapy in Premenopausal Women with Locally Advanced or Metastatic Breast Cancer." *Medicine* 94 (26): e1006. http://dx.doi.org/10.1097/MD.0000000000001006.
89. Teper, Yaroslav, Linda Ye, Richard T. Waldron, Aurelia Lugea, Xiaoying Sun, James Sinnett-Smith, Oscar J. Hines, et al. 2023. "Low Dosage Combination Treatment with Metformin and Simvastatin Inhibits Obesity-Promoted Pancreatic Cancer Development in Male KrasG12D Mice." *Scientific Reports* 13 (1): 16144. https://doi.org/10.1038/s41598-023-43498-9.
90. Dorsch, Madeleine, Manuela Kowalczyk, Mélanie Planque, Geronimo Heilmann, Sebastian Urban, Philip Dujardin, Jan Forster, et al. 2021. "Statins Affect Cancer Cell Plasticity with Distinct Consequences for Tumor Progression and Metastasis." *Cell Reports* 37 (8). https://doi.org/10.1016/j.celrep.2021.110056.
91. Kim, Hyeongi, Javeria Zaheer, Eui-Ju Choi, and Jin Su Kim. 2022. "Enhanced ASGR2 by Microplastic Exposure Leads to Resistance to Therapy in Gastric Cancer." *Theranostics* 12 (7): 3217. https://doi.org/10.7150/thno.73226.

92. Park, Jun Hyung, Seungwoo Hong, Ok-Hyeon Kim, Chul-Hong Kim, Jinho Kim, Jung-Woong Kim, Sungguan Hong, and Hyun Jung Lee. 2023. "Polypropylene Microplastics Promote Metastatic Features in Human Breast Cancer." *Scientific Reports* 13 (1): 6252. https://doi.org/10.1038/s41598-023-33393-8.
93. Paniri, Alireza, and Haleh Akhavan-Niaki. 2020. "Emerging Role of IL-6 and NLRP3 Inflammasome as Potential Therapeutic Targets to Combat COVID-19: Role of lncRNAs in Cytokine Storm Modulation." *Life Sciences* 257: 118114. https://doi.org/10.1016/j.lfs.2020.118114.
94. Lu, Yang, Jiamin Gao, Yachen Hou, Han Yang, Dashuai Wang, Ge Zhang, Zhen Qin, et al. 2025. "Targeting the NLRP3 Inflammasome Abrogates Cardiotoxicity of Immune Checkpoint Blockers." *Journal for Immunotherapy of Cancer* 13 (1): e010127. https://doi.org/10.1136/jitc-2024-010127.
95. Xie, Chuan, Jian Yi, Jing Lu, Muwen Nie, Meifang Huang, Jianfang Rong, Zhenhua Zhu, et al. 2018. "N-acetylcysteine Reduces ROS-Mediated Oxidative DNA Damage and PI3K/Akt Pathway Activation Induced by *Helicobacter pylori* Infection." *Oxidative Medicine and Cellular Longevity* 2018: 1874985. https://doi.org/10.1155/2018/1874985.
96. Delneste, Yves, Pascale Jeannin, Laurent Potier, Pedro Romero, and Jean-Yves Bonnefoy. 1997. "N-acetyl-L-cysteine Exhibits Antitumoral Activity by Increasing Tumor Necrosis Factor α-Dependent T-cell Cytotoxicity." *Blood* 90 (3): 1124–32. https://doi.org/10.1182/blood.V90.3.1124.
97. Debnath, Sujith Kumar, and Rohit Srivastava. 2021. "Drug Delivery with Carbon-Based Nanomaterials as Versatile Nanocarriers: Progress and Prospects." *Frontiers in Nanotechnology* 3: 644564. https://doi.org/10.3389/fnano.2021.644564.
98. Rastogi, Vaibhav, Pragya Yadav, Shiv Sankar Bhattacharya, Arun Kumar Mishra, Navneet Verma, Anurag Verma, and Jayanta Kumar Pandit. 2014. "Carbon Nanotubes: An Emerging Drug Carrier for Targeting Cancer Cells." *Journal of Drug Delivery* 2014: 670815. http://dx.doi.org/10.1155/2014/670815.
99. Saleem, Jabran, Liming Wang, and Chunying Chen. 2018. "Carbon-Based Nanomaterials for Cancer Therapy via Targeting Tumor Microenvironment." *Advanced Healthcare Materials* 7 (20): 1800525. https://doi.org/10.1002/adhm.201800525.
100. Singh, Sidhartha, Navneet Singh, Manoj Baranwal, Siddharth Sharma, S. S. Kirthiga Devi, and Sandeep Kumar. 2023. "Understanding Immune Checkpoints and PD-1/PD-L1-Mediated Immune Resistance towards Tumour Immunotherapy." *3 Biotech* 13 (12): 411. https://doi.org/10.1007/s13205-023-03826-2.
101. Wei, Zhaohan, Xiaoqiong Zhang, Tuying Yong, Nana Bie, Guiting Zhan, Xin Li, Qingle Liang, et al. 2021. "Boosting Anti-PD-1 Therapy with Metformin-Loaded Macrophage-Derived Microparticles." *Nature Communications* 12 (1): 440. https://doi.org/10.1038/s41467-020-20723-x.
102. Han, Haijie, Su Li, Yueyang Zhong, Yue Huang, Kai Wang, Qiao Jin, Jian Ji, and Ke Yao. 2022. "Emerging Pro-drug and Nano-drug Strategies for Gemcitabine-Based Cancer Therapy." *Asian Journal of Pharmaceutical Sciences* 17 (1): 35–52. https://doi.org/10.1016/j.ajps.2021.06.001.

12 Bioactive Compounds in Colorectal Cancer Therapy

Emerging Challenges and Future Directions

Ashiq Shibili P[#], *Sneha Pallatt*[#], *Antara Banerjee, and Surajit Pathak*
Chettinad Academy of Research and Education (CARE), Chettinad Hospital and Research Institute (CHRI), Chennai, Tamil Nadu, India

12.1 INTRODUCTION

Colorectal cancer (CRC) continues to be one of the most prevalent and deadly cancers worldwide, representing nearly 10% of all cancer cases [1]. As of 2022, it was estimated that over 1.9 million new cases of CRC were diagnosed, leading to more than 930,000 deaths globally. This extremely high rate of mortality is also projected to rise, with an estimated increase in deaths of 60% by the year 2035 [2]. CRC usually begins in the glandular epithelial cells that are part of the large intestine, primarily caused by a combination of epigenetic and genetic variations that impact multiple signaling pathways [3]. Red meat intake, obesity, sedentary lifestyles, alcohol use, and tobacco use are the main causes of the rise in CRC. Moreover, the two primary risk factors for CRC are a diet heavy in carbohydrates and lipids and insufficient physical exercise, which induces an inflammatory response that elevates reactive oxygen species (ROS) levels and produces pro-inflammatory cytokines in the gut lining [4]. As a result, early detection and diagnosis are crucial for preventing CRC. Although progress has been made in surgical and multimodal therapy, as well as the availability of advanced techniques for early CRC screening, the poor prognosis and late detection of CRC still remain significant [5]. The current conventional treatment for CRC includes surgery, radiotherapy, chemotherapy, and immunotherapy [6]. Although significant advances have been made in the development of these therapies, they often come with limitations, including significant side effects, risk of recurrence, and reduced efficacy, especially in advanced stages of the disease [7]. For instance, chemotherapy may harm healthy cells as well as cancerous cells, and cause side effects such as fatigue, nausea, and immunosuppression [8]. Additionally, resistance to chemotherapeutic drugs continues to pose a significant issue in the treatment of CRC, especially in those with metastatic disease [8]. Radiation therapy, although effective for localized tumors, can also cause long-term damage to surrounding healthy tissues [9]. Hence, the dependence on such traditional therapies supports the necessity of developing alternative therapeutic options that are more precise and have fewer side effects. In this regard, advances in CRC management increasingly emphasize tailoring therapeutic strategies based on tumor-specific features, including genetic alterations, molecular

[#] Equal Contributing Authors

 DOI: 10.1201/9781003644309-12

characteristics, and clinically relevant biomarkers, to improve treatment efficacy and patient outcomes [10]. By focusing on the distinctive biological and molecular features of cancer, this approach aims to improve treatment effectiveness, reduce unnecessary adverse effects, and avoid the use of ineffective therapies [10, 11]. This approach also has the potential to overcome the limitations of conventional treatments by targeting the specific molecular drivers of CRC [11]. For instance, targeted therapies and immunotherapies, based on the molecular characterization of tumors, have demonstrated promising outcomes in certain CRC patients, yet challenges remain in identifying the most effective targets and ensuring long-term efficacy [12, 13]. One promising therapeutic strategy involves the use of bioactive compounds derived from natural sources. Bioactive compounds, including polyphenols, flavonoids, carotenoids, glucosinolates, and terpenoids, are abundantly present in commonly consumed foods such as fruits, vegetables, nuts, seeds, and herbs [14]. These compounds have diverse biological activities, such as antioxidant, anti-inflammatory, apoptotic, and anticancer properties [15]. They have been found to regulate significant signaling pathways related to CRC, like those controlling cell cycle progression, apoptosis, DNA repair, inflammation, and angiogenesis, such as Wnt/β-catenin, PI3K/Akt, MAPK, NF-κB, and VEGF signaling pathways [16, 17]. Additionally, bioactive compounds can also influence the tumor microenvironment by enhancing immune responses, supporting DNA repair, and regulating cell growth and differentiation [18]. However, integrating bioactive compounds into clinical CRC therapy faces key challenges, including poor bioavailability, lack of dosage standardization, and variability in patient response due to tumor heterogeneity [16, 17]. Also, as the molecular targets for bioactive compounds in cancer treatment are understood, there is a need for further clinical trials to determine appropriate dosages, treatment schedules, and long-term safety profiles for their application in patients [19]. This chapter summarizes the therapeutic potential of bioactive compounds in CRC management, highlighting their underlying mechanisms of action and clinical benefits. It also discusses the key challenges associated with their use and outlines future strategies to enhance their effective clinical application.

12.2 KEY BIOACTIVE COMPOUNDS IN CRC THERAPY AND THEIR SOURCES

Bioactive compounds are phytochemicals present naturally in foods like fruits, vegetables, herbs, and whole grains. They offer a variety of health benefits through the modulation of biological processes, suppression of inflammation, and the prevention of chronic diseases, like CRC. They exhibit antioxidant, anti-inflammatory, antimicrobial, and anticancer properties, and thus are valuable in both preventive and therapeutic strategies. The following are key bioactive compounds used in CRC therapy.

12.2.1 Polyphenols

Polyphenols are natural compounds with several phenol units that are obtained from vegetables, fruits, beverages, and cereals. Depending on the fruit, there might be 200–300 mg of polyphenols per 100 g of fresh weight [20]. Studies have shown that polyphenols are excellent antioxidants and may neutralize reactive oxygen or nitrogen species produced as the byproducts of the body's metabolic activities. According to epidemiological research, polyphenols significantly reduce the risk of developing several chronic illnesses, including cancer, asthma, diabetes, heart disease, infections, and aging [21]. Studies show that resveratrol, a polyphenol found in grapes, berries, red wine, and peanuts, reduces pro-inflammatory enzymes such as COX-2 and iNOS, mediators like tumor necrosis factor-α (TNF-α) and interleukin-1β (IL-1β), and signaling pathways including CamKKB/AMPK, talin-FAK, Sirt1, NF-κB, and Mtor [20, 22]. Similarly, epigallocatechin gallate (EGCG) of green tea has shown chemopreventive properties via the downregulation of various tumor-related molecules and signaling pathways, including mTOR, STAT-3, MAPK/ERK,

PI3K/Akt, and NF-κB, to inhibit angiogenesis, proliferation, invasion, and migration of CRC [23]. Curcumin, another polyphenol obtained from turmeric, can decrease cell growth in the human CRC cell line HCT-116 by cell cycle arrest in the G2/M phase and partially at the G1 phase [24]. It also had an impact on the expression of several genes in CRC, including p21, p27, and Cyclin A, which are involved in the development of the cell cycle and are controlled in an E2F4-dependent manner [25].

12.2.2 Flavonoids

Flavonoids are a type of polyphenolic compound that are abundantly present in apples, berries, tea, wine, onion, celery, etc. [26]. Variations in the degree of hydroxylation and glycosylation distinguish the various flavonoid classes, including flavones, isoflavones, flavonols, flavan-3-ols, and anthocyanidins [27]. Many dietary flavonoids have diverse biological modes of action that minimize alterations in colon epithelia, inhibit tumor growth, and function as chemopreventive suppressor agents [28]. A flavonoid, quercetin, present in apples, onions, and berries, can induce apoptosis via downregulation of the Wnt/β-catenin pathway and correlated genes like *cyclin D1* [29]. Quercetin can inhibit CRC cells by regulating signaling pathways like Wnt, P13K/AKT, caspase-3, MAPK, and NF-κB [22]. An *in vitro* study reveals that apigenin found in chamomile, celery, and parsley has cytostatic and chemopreventive properties, which lower angiogenesis and inhibit apoptosis, cell proliferation, and cell cycle arrest [30]. Apigenin can also promote the production of proapoptotic proteins such as p53, NAG-1, and the cell cycle inhibitor p21 in colorectal cells [30]. Likewise, kaempferol is a flavanol found in broccoli, beans, tea, apples, and strawberries and can regulate signaling pathways like mTOR, JMJD2C/β-catenin, Erk/MAPK, and PI3/Akt through inhibitory effects on survival, angiogenesis, proliferation of cells, metastasis, and migration [31]. Kaempferol triggers apoptosis and p53-dependent growth inhibition in CRC cells by activating caspase-3-3 cleavage and releasing cytochrome c from the mitochondria. Kaempferol can also induce G1 and G2/M cell cycle arrest by inhibiting the activities of Cdc2, CDK4, and CDK2 [32, 33].

12.2.3 Carotenoids

Carotenoids are naturally occurring pigments that give many fruits and vegetables their yellow, orange, and red colors. Carrots, spinach, squash, sweet potatoes, broccoli, papayas, and apricots are good sources of carotenoids [34]. Carotenoids are good antioxidants; moreover, they can inhibit the growth of cancerous tumors and trigger programmed cell death [35]. Studies show that lycopene, a well-known red carotenoid found in tomatoes, guava, papaya, watermelon, and other fruits, can prevent the proliferation and survival of cancerous cells by disrupting the insulin-like growth factor (IGF) signaling pathway, P1K3/AKT pathway, and blocking mTOR activity [36]. In CRC treatment, lycopene helps to minimize the side effects by reducing the oxidative stress caused by two chemotherapy drugs, oxaliplatin and 5-FU [37]. Lycopene inhibited the development of HT-29 cells with an IC (50) value of 10 μM. Consequently, this therapy decreased non-phosphorylated beta-catenin protein levels and decreased Akt activation [38]. Likewise, astaxanthin, seen in marine organisms like salmon, shrimp, krill, trout, and crayfish, can suppress the expression of the mesenchymal markers cortactin and vimentin while increasing the expression of the epithelial marker E-cadherin [39]. Astaxanthin inhibits the PI3K/Akt and Erk/MAPK signaling pathways, which causes apoptosis and inhibits cancer. Additionally, it raises the expression of miR-200a and miR-29a-3p, which reduces matrix metalloproteinase-2 (MMP2) and limits the ability of CRC to spread [40]. A derivative of fucoxanthin, fucoxanthinol, found in the chloroplasts of seaweeds and diatoms, can reduce the cell growth in human CRC cells by downregulating pAkt, PPARβ/δ, and PPARγ [41]. By downregulating *BCL-2,* fucoxanthin and fucoxanthinol cause apoptosis in the CRC cell line Caco-2. Additionally, it has been shown that fucoxanthin causes cytostasis in WiDr cells by stopping their cell cycle [41].

12.2.4 Terpenoids

Terpenoids are a group of bioactive compounds obtained from fruits, vegetables, teas, spices, and medicinal plants. They have properties like exhibiting apoptotic, anti-angiogenic, anti-proliferative, and anti-metastatic effects [42]. Terpenoids can trigger autophagy through multiple signaling pathways, including MAPK/ERK/JNK, NF-kB, AMPK, and PI3K/AKT/mTOR [43]. A cyclic monoterpene, D-limonene, is a main component of the essential oils, grapefruit, orange, lemon, mandarin, and lime. According to Jia *et al.*, D-limonene causes dose-dependent inhibition of the LS174T human CRC cells' viability and triggers apoptosis, which is partially mediated by the mitochondrial route. It can also inhibit the PI3K/Akt pathway [44]. Similarly, monoterpene geraniol found in apples, coriander, grapes, ginger, and nutmeg can control many signaling pathways, such as PI3K/AKT/mTOR, NF-κB, and MAPK/ERK1/2. Additionally, it may modify the expression of various molecules, including growth factors, interleukins, CDKs, and cyclins [45]. Geraniol has been shown to induce a cell cycle arrest in the S-phase in the Caco-2 cell line. This reduces the proliferation of cells and may potentially trigger apoptosis in *in vivo* models by decreasing the expression of the anti-apoptotic protein *BCL-2* in tumor tissues [46]. A monoterpene called linalool is present in lavender, rose, and many edible fruits like peaches, plums, guava, and pineapple [47]. Hou *et al.* demonstrated that linalool possesses anticancer properties and induces apoptosis in cancer cells by inhibiting cell division. Cells can be protected from oxidative stress by preventing the activation of NF-κB/p65 and the phosphorylation of ERK1, JNK, and p38. Through the JAK2/STAT3 and Akt/mTOR signaling pathways, linalool promotes apoptosis and suppresses the growth of CRC cells [48].

12.2.5 Glucosinolates

Sulfur-containing bioactive compounds called glucosinolates are mostly present in cruciferous vegetables, which include cabbage, broccoli, sprouts, and kale [49]. Glucosinolates and the products of their hydrolysis have been used in CRC therapy because of their chemopreventive properties, such as antioxidants, anti-inflammation, and apoptosis. Phytochemical sulforaphane, a product of isothiocyanate, is abundant in cabbage, water stress, and broccoli and has anticarcinogenic, anti-inflammatory, antioxidant, and CRC-preventive properties [50]. According to a previous study, sulforaphane may induce human CRC cells to undergo cell-cycle arrest and death as well as enhance UGT1A expression in CRC cells [51]. Various research on CRC cell lines like HT-29, HCT116, SW480, Caco-2, and LoVo have established the antiproliferative properties of sulforaphane through increased ROS, DNA damage, cell cycle arrest, and apoptosis [52]. Another glucosinolate, indole-3-carbinol (I3C), can be found naturally in high concentrations in cauliflower, sprouts, kale, and cabbage. I3C increased ROS levels, caused DNA breakage, apoptosis, and cell cycle arrest, and inhibited growth and migration in LoVo cells of CRC [53]. I3C can alter the PI3K/Akt/mTOR signaling pathway, which has an impact on carcinogenesis and physiological aspects of cell growth and survival [54]. Similarly, phenethyl isothiocyanate (PEITC), derived from broccoli, watercress, and cabbage, triggers apoptosis and demonstrates strong chemopreventive effects against CRC. According to a recent study, PEITC can prevent the Wnt/β-catenin pathway from being activated [55]. According to Liu *et al.*, alterations in a gene-suppressing histone modification mark were linked to the PEITC-induced decrease in NFκB1 expression. This shows that NFκB1's epigenetic regulation may play a role in PEITC's activity and contribute to its anti-inflammatory effects [56]. The key bioactive compounds used in CRC therapy, their sources, and therapeutic roles are summarized in **Table 12.1**.

12.3 MECHANISM OF ACTION OF BIOACTIVE COMPOUNDS IN CRC

Bioactive compounds from natural sources have shown great potential for anticancer activity in CRC treatment. These molecules regulate key cellular pathways that play a role in inflammation,

TABLE 12.1
Key Bioactive Compounds from Natural Sources Used in CRC Therapy: Sources, Mechanism of Actions, and Therapeutic Effects

Compound	Natural Source	Molecular Target	Mechanism of Action	Ref
Resveratrol	Grapes, berries, peanuts	p53, β-catenin, PI3K/Akt	Induces cell cycle arrest and apoptosis, inhibits angiogenesis	[22]
Epigallocatechin gallate	Green tea (*Camellia sinensis*)	EGFR, MAPK, NF-κB	Inhibits tumor growth, angiogenesis, and metastasis	[23]
Curcumin	Turmeric (*Curcuma longa*)	NF-κB, COX-2, STAT3	Inhibits inflammation and cell proliferation, induces apoptosis	[24]
Quercetin	Apples, onions, broccoli	Bcl-2, Bax, p53	Promotes apoptosis, reduces oxidative stress, and inflammation	[29]
Apigenin	Parsley, celery, chamomile	PI3K/Akt, MAPK, NF-κB	Inhibits cancer cell invasion, inflammation, and induces apoptosis	[30]
Kaempferol	Broccoli, beans, tea, apple, strawberries	JMJD2C/β-catenin, PI3/Akt, mTOR, AMPK, Erk/MAPK	Antioxidant, anti-inflammation, inhibit cell proliferation, reduce angiogenesis and metastasis	[31]
Lycopene	Tomatoes, watermelon	IGF-1R, Akt, Cyclin D1	Antioxidant activity, inhibits cell proliferation, and DNA damage	[36]
Astaxanthin	Salmon, trout, shrimp, krill, crayfish	Erk/MAPK, PI3K/Akt, NF-kB, Wnt/β-catenin, Nrf2	Induce apoptosis, inhibit cell growth, reduce oxidative stress, and inflammation	[39]
Fucoxanthin	Seaweed, diatoms	pAkt, PPARβ/δ, PPARγ, PI3K/Akt	Antioxidant, inhibit cell growth, and slow down the cell cycle	[41]
D-limonene	grapefruit, orange, lemon, mandarin, lime	PI3K/Akt/mTOR, Bcl-2, β-catenin, NF-κB	Induces apoptosis, reduces cell proliferation, promotes autophagy, reduces inflammation	[44]
Geraniol	Apple, coriander, grapes, ginger, nutmeg	PI3K/AKT/mTOR, MAPK/ERK1/2, NF-κB	Induce cell cycle arrest, reduce cell proliferation, and induce apoptosis	[45]
Linalool	Peach, plum, guava, pineapple	NF-κB, AKT/mTOR, JAK2/STAT3, p53	Induce apoptosis, autophagy, induce cell cycle arrest	[48]
Sulforaphane	Broccoli, cabbage (*Cruciferous vegetables*)	Nrf2, HDAC, p21	Epigenetic modulation, induces detoxification of enzymes, and apoptosis	[50]
Indole-3-carbinol	Cauliflower, sprouts, kale, broccoli, cabbage	PI3K/Akt/mTOR, Wnt/β-Catenin	Increases ROS level, triggers apoptosis, cell cycle arrest, and prevents angiogenesis.	[53]

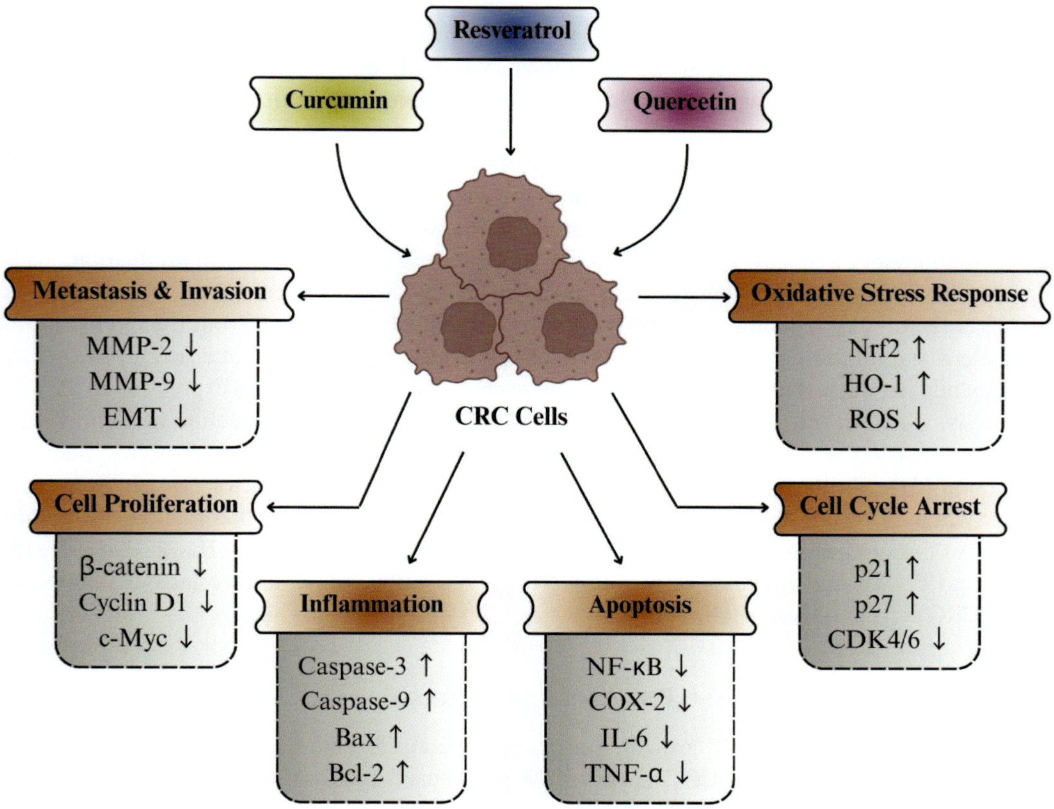

FIGURE 12.1 Schematic representation of the mechanism of action of bioactive compounds in CRC, showing effects on inflammation, apoptosis, and key signaling targets.

oxidative stress, apoptosis, and cell proliferation, thus suppressing tumor growth and development. The following are the major mechanisms through which they exert their effects (**Figure 12.1**).

12.3.1 Antioxidant Effects

Antioxidants are essential for preventing and treating CRC since oxidative stress is a key factor in the origin of cancers. Bioactive compounds have various mechanisms of action that contribute to their anti-cancer properties [57]. ROS can alter DNA, lipids, and proteins, which leads to the development and progression of CRC [58]. By neutralizing ROS, bioactive compounds can decrease the oxidative stress in cancer cells. Onions and apples contain quercetin, which efficiently removes free radicals and protects cells against oxidative damage in CRC. Quercetin works directly as a scavenger of ROS [59]. Superoxide dismutase (SOD) uses glutathione as a hydrogen donor, and quercetin can increase glutathione synthesis. SOD absorbs O^{2-}, converts it to H_2O_2, and then breaks it down into harmless H_2O. Furthermore, quercetin can influence enzyme-free antioxidant defense pathways, which lowers ROS levels [60]. A study conducted by Catalán *et al.* on CCD841 and RKO cell cultures exposed to hermin showed the ability of quercetin and its derivative 3,4-dihydroxyphenylacetic acid to repair cellular damage induced by ROS and delay the onset of CRC [61]. Resveratrol's antioxidant activity is primarily linked to its ability to control antioxidant-related enzymes, lower peroxidation of lipids, and prevent the generation of free radicals [62]. A significant antioxidant enzyme called manganese SOD converts toxic superoxide free radicals into hydrogen peroxide and molecular oxygen. By lowering the expression of this enzyme, resveratrol helps to suppress ROS [62].

12.3.2 Anti-Inflammatory Effects

Chronic inflammation significantly increases the risk of CRC by creating a tumor microenvironment through elevated oxidative stress, increased DNA damage, and enhanced cellular proliferation. Anti-inflammatory medications are essential for cancer prevention and therapy because of the link between chronic inflammation and the development and progression of CRC [63]. Bioactive compounds modulate key signaling pathways involved in inflammation, such as the COX-2, NF-κB, and MAPK pathways [64]. There is a link between oxidative stress and inflammation since inflammatory cells are known to produce a range of ROS at the site of inflammation, leading to oxidative stress [65]. Tomatoes contain lycopene, which has been demonstrated to affect NF-κB activation by reducing the translocation of the NF-κBp65 protein from the cytoplasm to the nucleus and inhibiting the phosphorylation of IκB kinase alpha (IKKα) and IκB alpha (IκBα) [66]. A study indicates that lycopene also suppresses NF-κB and JNK protein expression in SW480 CRC cells, which in turn results in decreased IL-1, IL-6, and TNF-α production as well as suppressed expression of COX-2 and iNOS mRNA, which subsequently suppresses PGE2 and NO production [67]. Similarly, curcumin can also inhibit the transcription factor NF-κB from activating, which is responsible for the production of genes that promote inflammation. Curcumin suppresses the synthesis of pro-inflammatory cytokines like IL-2, IL-6, IL-8, IL-12, IL-13, IL-15, IFN-γ, and TNF-α and enzymes by blocking NF-κB activation, which in turn lessens inflammation in CRC cells and tissues [68].

12.3.3 Anti-Proliferative and Pro-Apoptotic Effects

Inhibition of uncontrolled cell growth, promoting apoptosis, and triggering anti-proliferative responses significantly controls CRC. A preventive mechanism against the development and spread of cancer is the induction of apoptosis in cancer cells [69]. The principal anti-proliferative effects of isoflavone genistein include antioxidants, tyrosine kinase inhibition, cell cycle termination, blockage of estrogen receptors, promoting differentiation, and inducing apoptosis [70]. Genistein induces apoptosis in various malignancies by increasing the expression of *P21* and *BAX*, decreasing the expression of *BCL-2*, and activating caspase enzymes [71]. Mitogen-activated protein kinases (MAPKs) are a class of protein kinases that include JNK, p38 MAPK, and ERK. These kinases have been associated with several cellular processes, such as differentiation, proliferation, and apoptosis [72]. According to reports, genistein can prevent phosphorylation of the tyrosine residue on p38 MAPK, which in turn causes the MAPK pathway to become inactive, hence blocking the activation of p38 MAPK [73]. Likewise, the active form of vitamin D, known as calcitriol, increases the synthesis of pro-apoptotic proteins like BAD, BAK, and BAX, while inhibiting the expression of anti-apoptotic proteins like BAG1, BCL-XL, and BCL-2 [74]. By suppressing the p53, an increased modulator of apoptosis, a crucial proapoptotic regulator, the vitamin D receptor in colonic epithelial cells prevents apoptosis. In addition to lowering inflammation, this activity helps to preserve the mucosal barrier [74].

12.3.4 Epigenetic Modulatory Effects

The expression of genes associated with CRC can be influenced by bioactive compounds that modify non-coding RNA expression, histone patterns, and DNA methylation. DNA methylation occurs when a methyl group becomes attached to the cytosine residues of CpG dinucleotides, which frequently results in the silencing of genes [75]. The tumor suppressor gene p53 is commonly activated in CRC via oncogene activation and DNA damage. It controls several biological reactions, including DNA repair, autophagy, invasive metastasis, senescence, apoptosis, and ferroptosis [76]. The flavonoid kaempferol reduces A4CT2 methylation levels in HT-29 and HCT-116 cells by inhibiting DNA methyltransferases (DNMTs), which in turn promotes gene expression [76]. In HCT-116 cells, kaempferol reduced the expression of genes like *AXIN2* and *Cyclin D1*, which are involved in the β-catenin and Wnt signaling pathways [77]. Resveratrol was shown to have protective effects on SW480 cells by Tili *et al.*. The results showed that while resveratrol treatment decreased the activity of Dicer-1, tumor inhibitors PDCD4 and PTEN, and the TGF-β signal pathway, it enhanced the production of miR-663, a tumor-suppressive microRNA-targeting TGF-β-1 [78]. Furthermore, in the HT-29 cell line, the combination of the two bioactive compounds quercetin and resveratrol enhanced the antioxidant action and decreased the generation of ROS. Moreover, quercetin inhibited the expression of microRNA-27a (miR-27a), induced Sp-inhibitor zinc finger protein ZBTB10, and the mRNAs for Sp1, Sp3, and Sp4 [79]. These findings suggested that the interaction of quercetin with the miR-27a-ZBTB10 axis contributed to the downregulation of Sp. These indicated the potential use of polyphenols as organic anticancer drugs [79].

12.3.5 Angiogenesis and Metastasis Effects

Bioactive compounds exhibit strong inhibitory effects on angiogenesis and metastasis, key processes in CRC development and progression. Angiogenesis, the formation of new blood vessels, is essential for tumor growth and metastasis, providing oxygen and nutrients for cancer cells to grow [80]. Flavonoids quercetin and EGCG have been shown to exert anti-angiogenic activity through the downregulation of vascular endothelial growth factor (VEGF), a major mediator of neovascularization [81]. Quercetin inhibits VEGF expression by modulating the PI3K/Akt/mTOR signaling pathway and suppressing hypoxia-inducible factor-1α (HIF-1α), which plays a central role under hypoxic tumor conditions [81]. Similarly, EGCG decreases endothelial cell growth and migration through VEGF receptor phosphorylation and inhibition of downstream signaling cascades [82]. Regarding metastasis, genistein disrupts epithelial–mesenchymal transition (EMT), an obligatory step in metastatic dissemination, by upregulating E-cadherin and downregulating vimentin and matrix metalloproteinases (MMPs), particularly MMP-2 and MMP-9, that degrade extracellular matrix and promote invasion [83]. Curcumin also plays a key role in anti-metastatic effects by suppressing NF-κB and its downstream targets that are responsible for cell adhesion, motility, and invasion [84]. Similarly, luteolin, a flavone in parsley and celery, has demonstrated the capacity to inhibit EMT by suppressing Notch1 signaling and thereby reversing the mesenchymal phenotype and the decrease in cell invasion [85]. In an orthotopic *in vivo* mouse model, treatment with luteolin inhibited liver metastases and increased survival [86]. These combined activities not only inhibit tumor vascularization but also limit the migration and invasion of CRC cells, thus decreasing metastatic capability and enhancing therapeutic outcomes.

12.4 MOLECULAR APPROACHES IN CRC

Advances in cancer therapy emphasize the importance of understanding genetic, epigenetic, and molecular profiles of tumors in developing effective treatment strategies [87]. In contrast to the old therapeutic approaches, individualized therapy is based on the fact that each tumor is biologically distinct, and learning about these unique differences can dramatically improve the effectiveness of treatment, minimize side effects, and enhance overall outcomes [11]. Genomic and epigenomic profiling of CRC allows for the detection of individual mutations, gene expression profiles, DNA methylation patterns, and chromosomal changes that impact cancer initiation and progression [88, 89]. This knowledge is vital for the selection of targeted therapies and patient response prediction. For instance, mutations in the *KRAS* and *BRAF* genes have been typically seen to correlate with resistance to anti-EGFR monoclonal antibodies, and microsatellite instability (MSI) status is a strong marker for response to immune checkpoint inhibitors [90]. Alterations in the p53 tumor suppressor gene are also significant, as they can affect tumor behavior and resistance to certain chemotherapies [91]. Furthermore, the integration of nutritional interventions with conventional therapeutic strategies is emerging as a complementary approach to enhance treatment response and reduce therapy-associated side effects [11]. Nutritional elements can regulate gene expression and signaling pathways, interact with specific molecular targets, and affect the tumor microenvironment [92]. For instance, diet-derived bioactive compounds like polyphenols, flavonoids, and omega-3 fatty acids have anti-inflammatory, antioxidant, and anticancer activities that can complement traditional therapies [93]. Dietary interventions can support immune function, reduce inflammation, and enhance tumor sensitivity to chemotherapy or immunotherapy [94]. Through the integration of molecular diagnostics and nutrition science, individualized medicine in CRC is an integrative strategy that not only aims more accurately at the disease but also improves the quality of life for the patient both during and after treatment. This emerging approach emphasizes the need for a multidisciplinary approach that crosses genomics, pharmacology, and dietetics against CRC.

12.5 BIOACTIVE COMPOUNDS IN CRC

The incorporation of bioactive compounds in CRC management is gaining increasing attention, as studies highlight their selective activity against specific genetic and molecular aberrations found in various CRC subtypes Curcumin has shown great promise in targeting KRAS-mutant CRC, which is especially resistant to anti-EGFR therapies [95]. Curcumin exerts its effects by modulating key downstream signaling pathways such as MAPK/ERK and PI3K/AKT, thereby reducing cellular proliferation and enhancing apoptosis [95, 96]. It also inhibits NF-κB activity, resulting in reduced expression of pro-inflammatory cytokines and angiogenic factors that promote tumor growth [96]. Resveratrol has also demonstrated remarkable activity in MSI-high CRC, a subtype with defective DNA mismatch repair and elevated mutational burden [97, 98]. Resveratrol augments the anti-tumor immune response by stimulating $CD8^+$ T cells, boosting interferon-gamma (IFN-γ) production, and suppressing pro-tumor inflammatory mediators such as IL-6 and TNF-α, and thus is a viable synergist in immunotherapy regimens [99]. A dietary flavonoid, quercetin, demonstrates efficacy in p53-mutated CRC, a common mutation that disrupts the cell's intrinsic tumor-suppressor functions [100]. Quercetin bypasses p53 dependence by inducing mitochondria-dependent apoptosis directly, modulating pro- and anti-apoptotic proteins (e.g., Bax/Bcl-2), and blocking cell cycle progression via cyclin control [100, 101]. Furthermore, sulforaphane, a sulfur isothiocyanate from cruciferous plants, is known for its epigenetic reprogramming functions such as inhibition of HDACs, modification of DNA methylation, and regulation of non-coding RNAs like microRNAs. These functions restore tumor suppressor gene expression, decrease cancer cell stemness, and impair metastatic capability [102]. Preclinical studies have consistently confirmed the mechanistic functions of these compounds in inhibiting tumor burden, sensitizing tumors to chemotherapy, and preventing metastasis. For example, curcumin-treated animal models of *KRAS*-mutant CRC exhibit decreased tumor intensity and increased survival, whereas xenografts treated with sulforaphane have inhibited tumor growth and epigenetic normalization [103, 104]. Curcumin co-administered with FOLFOX chemotherapy has enhanced survival in metastatic CRC patients, and resveratrol-based nutritional interventions have given immunological benefits in MSI-high CRC groups [105]. Together, these results highlight that certain bioactive compounds, acting on specific tumor characteristics such as gene mutations (*KRAS*, *p53*), epigenetic alterations, or immune profiles, represent a highly promising, low-toxicity, and integrative strategy for management. These compounds not only enhance the efficacy of conventional therapies but also counteract resistance pathways and enhance quality of life for patients, pointing toward precision nutrition in cancer.

12.6 EMERGING CHALLENGES

Over the last few years, bioactive compounds from natural origins have gained significant attention due to their therapeutic promise in the targeted treatment of CRC. These compounds offer targeted anticancer effects with relatively low toxicity, making them promising candidates for integrative cancer therapy. However, despite their promising advantages, the clinical application of these bioactive compounds in CRC faces several key challenges, including limited bioavailability, variable pharmacokinetics, heterogeneous patient responses, and the absence of standardized dosing protocols. A comparative overview of these advantages and emerging challenges is presented in **Figure 12.2**, illustrating the complexities involved in translating bioactive compounds into effective

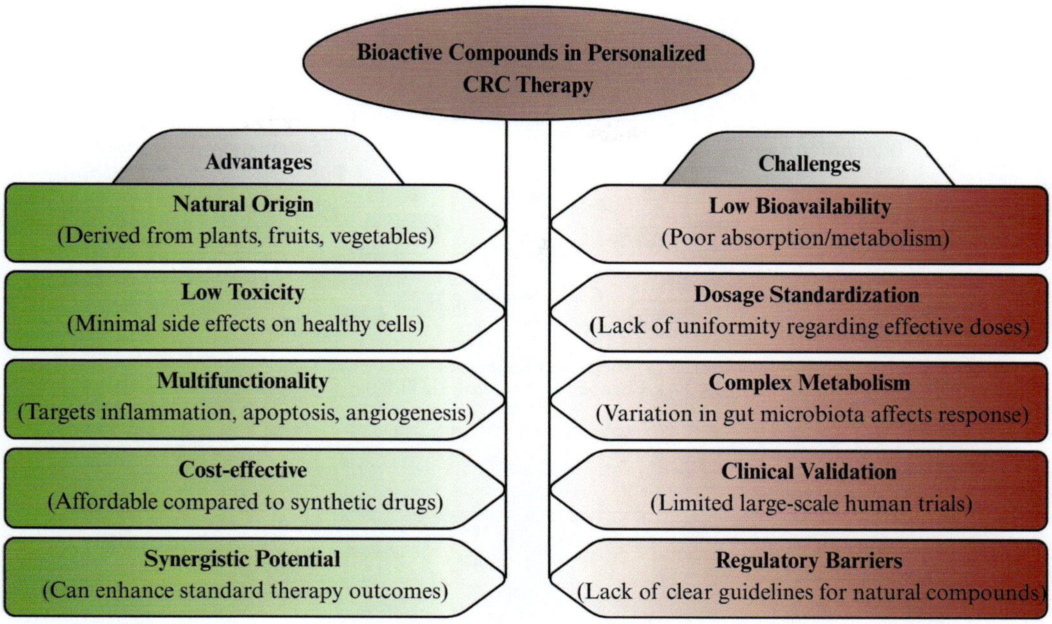

FIGURE 12.2 Comparative overview of the advantages and emerging challenges of bioactive compounds in CRC therapy.

colorectal cancer treatments. The following are the key emerging challenges associated with the clinical use of bioactive compounds in CRC.

12.6.1 Bioavailability and Metabolism

One of the main challenges in using bioactive compounds for CRC is their low bioavailability, primarily because of low gastrointestinal absorption and high metabolic degradation. Reduced bioavailability can result from the poor solubility of bioactive compounds, which may limit their absorption in the gastrointestinal tract [106]. Fast metabolism also affects the body's capacity to produce therapeutic effects by limiting the amount of time and concentration of these compounds in circulation. Inadequate gastric absorption is another important reason for the bioavailability of bioactive compounds [109]. Certain bioactive compounds might have problems associated with the effective passage through the intestinal barrier, which would lower their bioavailability and restrict their ability to reach the targeted areas, thereby affecting the expression of desired therapeutic effects [107]. Compounds such as curcumin and resveratrol have good anticancer activity *in vitro* but tend to be ineffective in the human body due to extensive metabolism and rapid clearance [108, 109]. In addition, gut microbiota has a dual effect: while it has the ability to activate some phytochemicals into bioactive metabolites, it can also deactivate or inactivate others. An example is that ellagic acid, which exists in pomegranates, is transformed into urolithins by gut microbiota, responsible for its anticancer and anti-inflammatory activities **(Figure 12.3)** [110]. However, not all individuals possess the microbial species required for this transformation, leading to variability in therapeutic response.

12.6.2 Dual Role of Bioactive Compounds

Phytochemicals, while being anticancer agents, under some circumstances unexpectedly trigger carcinogenesis. In CRC, flavonoids and polyphenols possess antioxidant activity, inhibit inflammation, and influence signal pathways like the Wnt/β-catenin pathway [111]. Yet, excessive intake

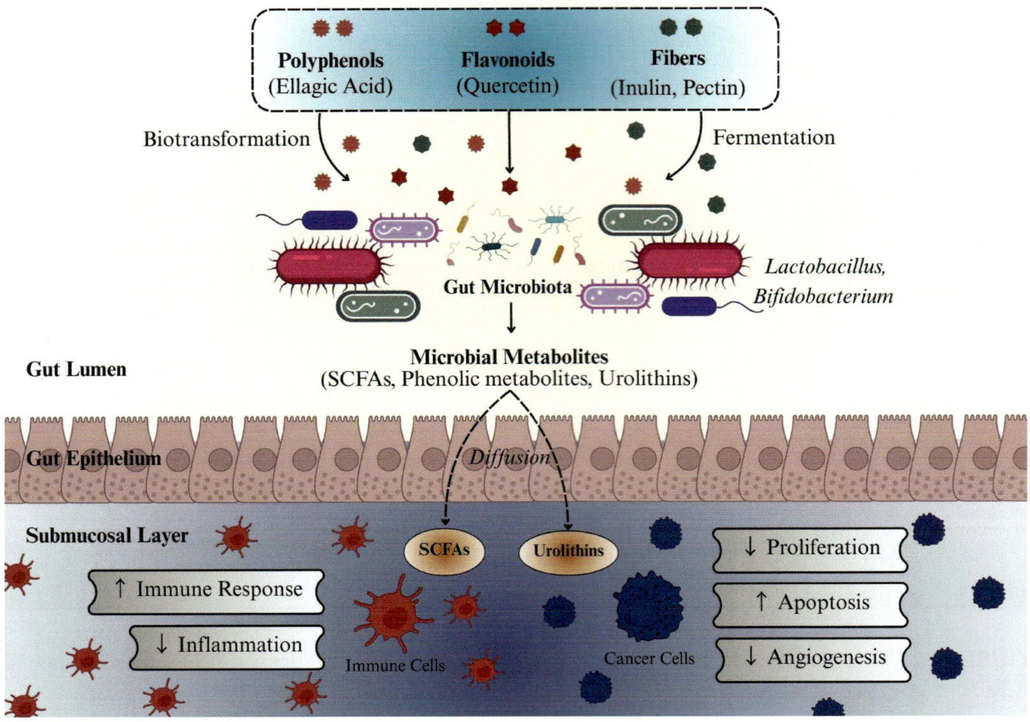

FIGURE 12.3 Interaction between gut microbiota and bioactive compounds, illustrating microbial transformation that enhances anticancer and anti-inflammatory activities.

or chronic exposure to some, such as safrole or high-dose quercetin, can produce ROS or create DNA damage [112]. These dual effects make it difficult to predict outcomes, particularly without precise dosing. Inappropriate use could potentially stimulate tumor initiation or growth, especially in genetically susceptible patients or in individuals with pre-existing inflammatory colonic disease. This emphasizes the need for carefully controlled usage and a detailed understanding of each compound's dose–response relationship.

12.6.3 Standardization and Dosing

The absence of consistent doses for bioactive compounds may lead to variations in the therapeutic benefits. Ensuring the right levels of bioactive compounds and consistency are major barriers in treating CRC. Accurately identifying and quantifying individual bioactive compounds is difficult due to the complex molecular compositions present in natural products [113]. Patients may not obtain regular dosages of bioactive compounds required for therapeutic benefit, which raises issues about therapy efficiency. Treatment response and effectiveness may also vary among patients due to differences in how well they absorb or metabolize bioactive compounds [114]. In CRC therapy, ensuring consistent delivery of bioactive compounds at therapeutic concentrations remains a key challenge. Innovative delivery systems like liposomes, nanoparticles, and micelles are being explored to enhance stability and absorption, but they are not yet established or verified in clinical practice [115].

12.6.4 Genetic Variability

Therapeutic efficacy can be influenced by the genetic and metabolic profile of patients. In particular, polymorphisms in genes encoding drug-metabolizing enzymes, such as CYP450, can significantly affect the metabolism of phytochemicals. Polymorphisms in CYP1A1 or CYP3A4 can alter the metabolism of flavonoids and other phytochemicals, impacting both efficacy and toxicity [116]. Moreover, the microbiome diversity of individuals introduces another layer of variability. Two patients consuming identical dietary bioactive compounds will have a radically different therapeutic response because of differences in their microbial composition [117]. This makes it difficult and emphasizes the need for microbiome profiling in therapeutic planning.

12.6.5 Antinutrient Effects

Many phytochemicals can act as antinutrients, impairing the absorption of essential nutrients critical for CRC patients. The oxalates in *Terminalia ferdinandiana* (Kakadu plum) bind with calcium and magnesium, which may result in deficiencies and gastrointestinal discomfort in prolonged CRC treatment [118]. CRC patients undergoing chemotherapy often face impaired absorption, through the addition of antinutrient phytochemicals that may lead to malnutrition. Furthermore, tannins and phytates found in herbs such as sorghum or legumes may interfere with iron absorption, which leads to anemia, a frequent side effect of chemotherapy [119]. These interactions need to be taken into consideration in diet planning, particularly for multimodal CRC patients. A balance between the advantages of bioactive compounds and their nutrient-interfering capacity is important in CRC dietary interventions.

12.6.6 Pharmacokinetics and Drug-Bioactive Interactions

Understanding how a compound is absorbed, distributed, metabolized, and excreted is essential for predicting how it will act in the body. Several bioactive compounds, such as quercetin and berberine, have poor water solubility, which restricts their systemic distribution [120]. Once absorbed, they can be conjugated quickly in the liver, decreasing their active availability in target tissues like the colon. Furthermore, bioactive compounds can interact with conventional chemotherapeutics, either synergistically or antagonistically. Grapefruit-derived naringin inhibits CYP3A4, potentially increasing the toxicity of drugs metabolized by this enzyme [121]. Similarly, St. John's Wort induces CYP enzymes, potentially reducing the efficacy of co-administered cancer therapies [122]. Consequently, comprehensive preclinical and clinical studies are essential to assess these interactions prior to including bioactive compounds in therapeutic protocols, particularly when multiple drugs are administered concurrently.

12.6.7 Potential Side Effects

Bioactive compounds are usually seen as beneficial; however, prolonged use or excessive dosages may have unfavorable effects. Polyphenols, which are abundant in plant-based diets and herbal extracts frequently utilized in complementary medicine, are examples of substances that can be harmful if taken in excess or for a prolonged period [123]. The possibility of gastrointestinal discomfort is one of the main issues. Overconsumption of polyphenols and herbal extracts can irritate the digestive tract and cause symptoms such as nausea, diarrhea, and an upset stomach [123]. Intentionally using large amounts of dietary supplements containing apigenin may slightly increase the chance of negative side effects like sleepiness, muscular relaxation, and indigestion. Topical products containing apigenin may cause skin irritation in certain individuals [124]. Similarly, lycopene from tomatoes and watermelon is usually considered safe, but it can also cause side effects such as gastrointestinal effects like diarrhea, nausea, and low blood pressure. Overconsumption of lycopene may also result in lycopenemia, characterized by orange skin discoloration [125]. Patients receiving treatment for CRC may find these side effects more challenging because they may already be experiencing digestive problems due to the disease.

12.6.8 Clinical Integration and Regulatory Gaps

Although there has been widespread *in vitro* and animal research demonstrating anticancer properties of natural compounds, there remains a translational gap between laboratory findings and clinical application. One of the reasons is the absence of strong, large-scale, randomized clinical trials to assess these compounds in humans. For instance, while curcumin has shown tumor-suppressing properties in *in vitro* and *in vivo* models, its efficacy in clinical trials involving CRC patients has been confusing, mainly because of low bioavailability and poor systemic retention [126]. Furthermore, regulatory agencies like the FDA, EMA, and MFDS require extensive documentation on safety, efficacy, and quality control [127], which most natural molecules cannot provide because of limited data. This limits their approval for therapeutic use, keeping many potentially beneficial bioactive compounds in the domain of dietary supplements rather than approved therapies.

12.6.9 Complexity of Studying Plant Metabolites

Plant extracts have several hundred metabolites that can interact synergistically or antagonistically with each other, making it challenging to describe the activity of a single compound in CRC treatment. For example, grape seed extract has proanthocyanidins, catechins, and gallic acid with various bioactivities and metabolic fates [128]. Investigating them separately *in vitro* may not represent their collective activity *in vivo*. Besides, differences in plant genetics, methods of harvesting, and extraction techniques result in batch-to-batch variability. This complexity delays reproducibility and regulatory acceptance [129]. Comprehensive metabolomic profiling and systems pharmacology are required to better characterize and standardize these extracts for CRC treatment.

12.6.10 Intellectual Property Issues

The availability and study of naturally occurring bioactive compounds for therapeutic application are severely limited by the problem of patents and intellectual property rights in CRC. Patents that are awarded for certain materials, processes of extraction, or compositions may result in legal conflicts and reduce chances for scientific progress [17]. Patent-holding companies may implement access restrictions on bioactive molecules, which may prevent research initiatives and the development of potentially advantageous medicines. Furthermore, the costs associated with licensing patented chemicals can significantly increase research and development expenditures for pharmaceutical companies and scientists. This limitation could slow down the rate of novel and more effective discoveries for CRC therapies [114]. These regulatory norms may impose many challenges in the commercialization phase. This may result in a significant delay in the development of bioactive compounds or the application of semi-synthetic techniques to enhance the medicinal efficacy of the bioactive compound [17].

12.7 CONCLUSION AND FUTURE DIRECTIONS

The therapeutic application of bioactive compounds like polyphenols, flavonoids, carotenoids, terpenoids, and glucosinolates has revealed promising potential to regulate major signaling pathways like Wnt/β-catenin, NF-κB, Notch, PI3K/Akt, TGF-β, and JAK/STAT, inhibit tumor growth, and improve conventional treatment efficacy. These molecules, derived from fruits, vegetables, nuts, and oils, provide advantages such as natural origin, low toxicity, availability, and affordability. However, issues including efficiency, solubility, bioavailability, ideal dosage, and standardization may continue to be problematic, and they demand additional study and development for the CRC treatment. Studies are being conducted to explain the underlying mechanisms via which bioactive compounds are effective in CRC. To overcome this, molecular biology and genetic advancements will probably provide more information about how bioactive compounds affect signaling pathways associated with the development of CRC. Incorporating nano-formulations and sophisticated delivery systems, including liposomes, nanoparticles, and micelles, to improve bioavailability and targeted release, are other future directions. Additionally, the integration of technologies such as genomics, proteomics, metabolomics, and gut microbiome profiling can provide valuable insights to optimize therapeutic strategies and improve treatment efficacy. Furthermore, it is expected that system biology and bioinformatics would work together to accelerate the identification of new bioactive compounds and their targets. By using computer modeling and large-scale screening, we can predict how bioactive compounds would interact with cancer-associated proteins. This method makes it easier to find possible treatment strategies. Moreover, computational modeling and artificial intelligence are emerging as critical tools to predict patient responses and discover novel compound-target interactions. Designing nutraceutical interventions based on molecular and microbiome profiles represents a novel approach in oncology. Combining insights from nutrition science, molecular biology, and microbiome research may offer transformative strategies for CRC management. A multidisciplinary approach combining translational research, clinical trials, and systems biology will be essential to realize the complete potential of bioactive compounds in CRC management, ultimately bridging the gap between natural compound research and oncology.

STATEMENTS AND DECLARATIONS

Acknowledgment: All authors are thankful to the Chettinad Academy of Research and Education for providing infrastructural support to complete this work.

Ethics Approval: NA.

Conflict of Interest: None. All authors declare that there are no conflicts of competing interests.

Availability of Data: NA

Author's Contribution: The chapter was designed, conceptualized, and supervised by AB. ASP and SnP were involved in drafting the chapter. ASP and SnP were involved in designing the images and tables. SuP and AB critically reviewed the chapter. All authors read, reviewed, and approved the final chapter.

ABBREVIATIONS

CRC: colorectal cancer
DNMT: DNA methyltransferase
EGCG: epigallocatechin gallate
HIF-1α: hypoxia-inducible factor-1α
I3C: indole-3-carbicol
IFN-γ: interferon-gamma
IL: interleukin
MSI: microsatellite instability
MAPK: mitogen-activated protein kinase
MMP2: matrix metalloproteinase-2
PEITC: phenethyl isothiocyanate
ROS: reactive oxygen species
SOD: superoxide dismutase
TGF-β: transforming growth factor β
TNF-α: tumor necrosis factor α
VEGF: vascular endothelial growth factor

REFERENCES

1. Ochoa-Sanchez, A., Sahare, P., Pathak, S., Banerjee, A., Estevez, M., Duttaroy, A. K., Luna-Bárcenas, G., & Paul, S. (2024). Evaluation of the synergistic effects of curcumin-resveratrol co-loaded biogenic silica on colorectal cancer cells. *Frontiers in Pharmacology*, *15*, 1341773. https://doi.org/10.3389/fphar.2024.1341773
2. Bray, F., Laversanne, M., Sung, H., Ferlay, J., Siegel, R. L., Soerjomataram, I., & Jemal, A. (2024). Global cancer statistics 2022: GLOBOCAN estimates of incidence and mortality worldwide for 36 cancers in 185 countries. *CA: A Cancer Journal for Clinicians*, *74*(3), 229–263. https://doi.org/10.3322/caac.21834
3. Akhtar, M. F., Saleem, A., Rasul, A., Faran Ashraf Baig, M. M., Bin-Jumah, M., & Abdel Daim, M. M. (2020). Anticancer natural medicines: An overview of cell signaling and other targets of anticancer phytochemicals. *European Journal of Pharmacology*, *888*, 173488. https://doi.org/10.1016/j.ejphar.2020.173488
4. Rawla, P., Sunkara, T., & Barsouk, A. (2019). Epidemiology of colorectal cancer: incidence, mortality, survival, and risk factors. *Gastroenterology Review*, *14*(2), 89–103. https://doi.org/10.5114/pg.2018.81072
5. Zhang, Y., Wang, Y., Zhang, B., Li, P., & Zhao, Y. (2023). Methods and biomarkers for early detection, prediction, and diagnosis of colorectal cancer. *Biomedicine & Pharmacotherapy*, *163*, 114786. https://doi.org/10.1016/j.biopha.2023.114786
6. Jain, S. M., Nagainallur Ravichandran, S., Murali Kumar, M., Banerjee, A., Sun-Zhang, A., Zhang, H., Pathak, R., Sun, X. F., & Pathak, S. (2024). Understanding the molecular mechanism responsible for developing therapeutic radiation-induced radioresistance of rectal cancer and improving the clinical outcomes of radiotherapy – a review. *Cancer Biology & Therapy*, *25*(1), 2317999. https://doi.org/10.1080/15384047.2024.2317999
7. Sewitch, M. J., & Rajput, Y. (2010). A literature review of complementary and alternative medicine use by colorectal cancer patients. *Complementary Therapies in Clinical Practice*, *16*(1), 52–56. https://doi.org/10.1016/j.ctcp.2009.10.001
8. Anand, U., Dey, A., Chandel, A. K. S., Sanyal, R., Mishra, A., Pandey, D. K., De Falco, V., Upadhyay, A., Kandimalla, R., Chaudhary, A., Dhanjal, J. K., Dewanjee, S., Vallamkondu, J., & Pérez de la Lastra, J. M. (2022). Cancer chemotherapy and beyond: Current status, drug candidates, associated risks and progress in targeted therapeutics. *Genes & Diseases*, *10*(4), 1367–1401. https://doi.org/10.1016/j.gendis.2022.02.007
9. Wang, K., & Tepper, J. E. (2021). Radiation therapy-associated toxicity: Etiology, management, and prevention. *CA: A Cancer Journal for Clinicians*, *71*(5), 437–454.
10. Krzyszczyk, P., Acevedo, A., Davidoff, E. J., Timmins, L. M., Marrero-Berrios, I., Patel, M., White, C., Lowe, C., Sherba, J. J., Hartmanshenn, C., O'Neill, K. M., Balter, M. L., Fritz, Z. R., Androulakis, I. P., Schloss, R. S., & Yarmush, M. L. (2018). The growing role of precision and personalized medicine for cancer treatment. *Technology*, *6*(3–4), 79–100. https://doi.org/10.1142/S2339547818300020
11. Su, J., Yang, L., Sun, Z., & Zhan, X. (2024). Personalized drug therapy: innovative concept guided with proteoformics. *Molecular & Cellular Proteomics: MCP*, *23*(3), 100737. https://doi.org/10.1016/j.mcpro.2024.100737
12. Golshani, G., & Zhang, Y. (2020). Advances in immunotherapy for colorectal cancer: a review. *Therapeutic Advances in Gastroenterology*, *13*, 1756284820917527. https://doi.org/10.1177/1756284820917527
13. Xie, Y. H., Chen, Y. X., & Fang, J. Y. (2020). Comprehensive review of targeted therapy for colorectal cancer. *Signal Transduction and Targeted Therapy*, *5*(1), 22. https://doi.org/10.1038/s41392-020-0116-z
14. Sorrenti, V., Burò, I., Consoli, V., & Vanella, L. (2023). Recent advances in health benefits of bioactive compounds from food wastes and by-products: biochemical aspects. *International Journal of Molecular Sciences*, *24*(3), 2019. https://doi.org/10.3390/ijms24032019
15. Asma, S. T., Acaroz, U., Imre, K., Morar, A., Shah, S. R. A., Hussain, S. Z., Arslan-Acaroz, D., Demirbas, H., Hajrulai-Musliu, Z., Istanbullugil, F. R., Soleimanzadeh, A., Morozov, D., Zhu, K., Herman, V., Ayad, A., Athanassiou, C., & Ince, S. (2022). Natural products/bioactive compounds as a source of anticancer drugs. *Cancers*, *14*(24), 6203. https://doi.org/10.3390/cancers14246203
16. Roy, S., Deka, D., Kondaveeti, S. B., Ayyadurai, P., Siripragada, S., Philip, N., Pathak, S., Duttaroy, A. K., & Banerjee, A. (2025). An overview of potential of natural compounds to regulate epigenetic modifications in colorectal cancer: a recent update. *Epigenetics*, *20*(1), 2491316. https://doi.org/10.1080/15592294.2025.2491316

17. Esmeeta, A., Adhikary, S., Dharshnaa, V., Swarnamughi, P., Ummul Maqsummiya, Z., Banerjee, A., Pathak, S., & Duttaroy, A. K. (2022). Plant-derived bioactive compounds in colon cancer treatment: An updated review. *Biomedicine & Pharmacotherapy, 153*, 113384. https://doi.org/10.1016/j.biopha.2022.113384
18. Yuan, M., Zhang, G., Bai, W., Han, X., Li, C., & Bian, S. (2022). The role of bioactive compounds in natural products extracted from plants in cancer treatment and their mechanisms related to anticancer effects. *Oxidative Medicine and Cellular Longevity, 2022*, 1429869. https://doi.org/10.1155/2022/1429869
19. Mir, M. A., & Banik, B. K. (2025). Sustainable healing: natural compounds facilitating the future cancer treatment. *World Development Sustainability, 6*, 100215. https://doi.org/10.1016/j.wds.2025.100215
20. Zhang, Y., Liu, K., Yan, C., Yin, Y., He, S., Qiu, L., & Li, G. (2022). Natural polyphenols for treatment of colorectal cancer. *Molecules (Basel, Switzerland), 27*(24), 8810. https://doi.org/10.3390/molecules27248810
21. Pandey, K. B., & Rizvi, S. I. (2009). Plant polyphenols as dietary antioxidants in human health and disease. *Oxidative Medicine and Cellular Longevity, 2*(5), 270–278. https://doi.org/10.4161/oxim.2.5.9498
22. Unnikrishnan Meenakshi, D., Narde, G. K., Ahuja, A., Al Balushi, K., Francis, A. P., & Khan, S. A. (2024). Therapeutic applications of nanoformulated resveratrol and quercetin phytochemicals in colorectal cancer-an updated review. *Pharmaceutics, 16*(6), 761. https://doi.org/10.3390/pharmaceutics16060761
23. Kciuk, M., Alam, M., Ali, N., Rashid, S., Głowacka, P., Sundaraj, R., Celik, I., Yahya, E. B., Dubey, A., Zerroug, E., & Kontek, R. (2023). Epigallocatechin-3-gallate therapeutic potential in cancer: mechanism of action and clinical implications. *Molecules, 28*(13), 5246. https://doi.org/10.3390/molecules28135246
24. Mosieniak, G., Adamowicz, M., Alster, O., Jaskowiak, H., Szczepankiewicz, A. A., Wilczynski, G. M., Ciechomska, I. A., & Sikora, E. (2012). Curcumin induces permanent growth arrest of human colon cancer cells: link between senescence and autophagy. *Mechanisms of Ageing and Development, 133*(6), 444–455. https://doi.org/10.1016/j.mad.2012.05.004
25. Kim, K. C., & Lee, C. (2010). Curcumin induces downregulation of E2F4 expression and apoptotic cell death in HCT116 human colon cancer cells; involvement of reactive oxygen species. *The Korean Journal of Physiology & Pharmacology, 14*(6), 391–397. https://doi.org/10.4196/kjpp.2010.14.6.391
26. Hollman, P. C., & Katan, M. B. (1999). Dietary flavonoids: intake, health effects and bioavailability. *Food and Chemical Toxicology, 37*(9–10), 937–942. https://doi.org/10.1016/s0278-6915(99)00079-4
27. Manach, C., Scalbert, A., Morand, C., Rémésy, C., & Jiménez, L. (2004). Polyphenols: food sources and bioavailability. *The American Journal of Clinical Nutrition, 79*(5), 727–747. https://doi.org/10.1093/ajcn/79.5.727
28. Dubey, N., Dubey, N., Bhadoria, U., Shah, K., & Chauhan, N. S. (2023). Targeting colorectal cancer using dietary flavonols. *Cancer Innovation, 3*(1), e99. https://doi.org/10.1002/cai2.99
29. Anand David, A. V., Arulmoli, R., & Parasuraman, S. (2016). Overviews of biological importance of quercetin: a bioactive flavonoid. *Pharmacognosy Reviews, 10*(20), 84–89. https://doi.org/10.4103/0973-7847.194044
30. Zhong, Y., Krisanapun, C., Lee, S. H., Nualsanit, T., Sams, C., Peungvicha, P., & Baek, S. J. (2010). Molecular targets of apigenin in colorectal cancer cells: involvement of p21, NAG-1 and p53. *European Journal of Cancer, 46*(18), 3365–3374. https://doi.org/10.1016/j.ejca.2010.07.007
31. Singh, T., Sharma, D., Sharma, R., Tuli, H. S., Haque, S., Ramniwas, S., Mathkor, D. M., & Yadav, V. (2024). The role of phytonutrient kaempferol in the prevention of gastrointestinal cancers: recent trends and future perspectives. *Cancers, 16*(9), 1711. https://doi.org/10.3390/cancers16091711
32. Lee, H. S., Cho, H. J., Yu, R., Lee, K. W., Chun, H. S., & Park, J. H. (2014). Mechanisms underlying apoptosis-inducing effects of Kaempferol in HT-29 human colon cancer cells. *International Journal of Molecular Sciences, 15*(2), 2722–2737. https://doi.org/10.3390/ijms15022722
33. Cho, H. J., & Park, J. H. (2013). Kaempferol induces cell cycle arrest in HT-29 human colon cancer cells. *Journal of Cancer Prevention, 18*(3), 257–263. https://doi.org/10.15430/jcp.2013.18.3.257
34. Sharma, I., Khare, N., & Rai, A. (2024). Carotenoids: Sources, Bioavailability and Their Role in Human Nutrition. In *Dietary Carotenoids-Sources, Properties, and Role in Human Health*. IntechOpen. https://doi.org/10.5772/intechopen.113012
35. Han, X., Zhao, R., Zhang, G., Jiao, Y., Wang, Y., Wang, D., & Cai, H. (2022). Association of retinol and carotenoids content in diet and serum with risk for colorectal cancer: a meta-analysis. *Frontiers in Nutrition, 9*, 918777. https://doi.org/10.3389/fnut.2022.918777
36. Rao, A. V., & Agarwal, S. (2000). Role of antioxidant lycopene in cancer and heart disease. *Journal of the American College of Nutrition, 19*(5), 563–569. https://doi.org/10.1080/07315724.2000.10718953

37. Alhoshani, N. M., Al-Johani, N. S., Alkeraishan, N., Alarifi, S., & Alkahtani, S. (2022). Effect of lycopene as an adjuvant therapy with 5-florouracil in human colon cancer. *Saudi Journal of Biological Sciences*, *29*(9), 103392. https://doi.org/10.1016/j.sjbs.2022.103392
38. Tang, F. Y., Shih, C. J., Cheng, L. H., Ho, H. J., & Chen, H. J. (2008). Lycopene inhibits growth of human colon cancer cells via suppression of the Akt signaling pathway. *Molecular Nutrition & Food Research*, *52*(6), 646–654. https://doi.org/10.1002/mnfr.200700272
39. Ambati, R. R., Phang, S. M., Ravi, S., & Aswathanarayana, R. G. (2014). Astaxanthin: sources, extraction, stability, biological activities and its commercial applications – a review. *Marine Drugs*, *12*(1), 128–152. https://doi.org/10.3390/md12010128
40. Kim, H. Y., Kim, Y. M., & Hong, S. (2019). Astaxanthin suppresses the metastasis of colon cancer by inhibiting the MYC-mediated downregulation of microRNA-29a-3p and microRNA-200a. *Scientific Reports*, *9*(1), 9457. https://doi.org/10.1038/s41598-019-45924-3
41. Terasaki, M., Maeda, H., Miyashita, K., Tanaka, T., Miyamoto, S., & Mutoh, M. (2017). A marine bio-functional lipid, fucoxanthinol, attenuates human colorectal cancer stem-like cell tumorigenicity and sphere formation. *Journal of Clinical Biochemistry and Nutrition*, *61*(1), 25–32. https://doi.org/10.3164/jcbn.16-112
42. Sharma, S. H., Thulasingam, S., & Nagarajan, S. (2017). Terpenoids as anti-colon cancer agents - A comprehensive review on its mechanistic perspectives. *European Journal of Pharmacology*, *795*, 169–178. https://doi.org/10.1016/j.ejphar.2016.12.008
43. El-Baba, C., Baassiri, A., Kiriako, G., Dia, B., Fadlallah, S., Moodad, S., & Darwiche, N. (2021). Terpenoids' anti-cancer effects: focus on autophagy. *Apoptosis: An International Journal on Programmed Cell Death*, *26*(9–10), 491–511. https://doi.org/10.1007/s10495-021-01684-y
44. Jia, S. S., Xi, G. P., Zhang, M., Chen, Y. B., Lei, B., Dong, X. S., & Yang, Y. M. (2013). Induction of apoptosis by D-limonene is mediated by inactivation of Akt in LS174T human colon cancer cells. *Oncology Reports*, *29*(1), 349–354. https://doi.org/10.3892/or.2012.2093
45. Cho, M., So, I., Chun, J. N., & Jeon, J. H. (2016). The antitumor effects of geraniol: modulation of cancer hallmark pathways (review). *International Journal of Oncology*, *48*(5), 1772–1782. https://doi.org/10.3892/ijo.2016.3427
46. Quiñonero, F., Mesas, C., Peña, M., Cabeza, L., Perazzoli, G., Melguizo, C., …, & Prados, J. (2023). Vegetal-derived bioactive compounds as multidrug resistance modulators in colorectal cancer. *Applied Sciences*, *13*(4), 2667. https://doi.org/10.3390/app13042667
47. Wei, C., Liu, H., Cao, X., Zhang, M., Li, X., Chen, K., & Zhang, B. (2021). Synthesis of flavour-related linalool is regulated by PpbHLH1 and associated with changes in DNA methylation during peach fruit ripening. *Plant Biotechnology Journal*, *19*(10), 2082–2096. https://doi.org/10.1111/pbi.13638
48. Hou, M., Zhang, Y., Huang, Q., Zhan, H., Jia, T., Li, M., … & Zhao, Y. (2022). [Retracted] linalool impress colorectal cancer deterioration by mediating AKT/mTOR and JAK2/STAT3 signaling pathways. *BioMed Research International*, *2022*(1), 4801703. https://doi.org/10.1155/2022/4801703
49. Fahey, J. W., Zalcmann, A. T., & Talalay, P. (2001). The chemical diversity and distribution of glucosinolates and isothiocyanates among plants. *Phytochemistry*, *56*(1), 5–51. https://doi.org/10.1016/s0031-9422(00)00316-2
50. Vuong, L. D., Nguyen, Q. N., & Truong, V. L. (2019). Anti-inflammatory and anti-oxidant effects of combination between sulforaphane and acetaminophen in LPS-stimulated RAW 264.7 macrophage cells. *Immunopharmacology and Immunotoxicology*, *41*(3), 413–419. https://doi.org/10.1080/08923973.2019.1569049
51. Wang, M., Chen, S., Wang, S., Sun, D., Chen, J., Li, Y., …, & Gao, H. Q. (2012). Effects of phytochemicals sulforaphane on uridine diphosphate-glucuronosyltransferase expression as well as cell-cycle arrest and apoptosis in human colon cancer Caco-2 cells. *Chinese Journal of Physiology*, *55*(2), 134–144. https://doi.org/10.4077/CJP.2012.BAA085
52. McAlpine, P. L., Fernández, J., Villar, C. J., & Lombó, F. (2024). Organosulfur compounds in colorectal cancer prevention and progression. *Nutrients*, *16*(6), 802. https://doi.org/10.3390/nu16060802
53. Lee, J. Y., Lim, H. M., Lee, C. M., Park, S. H., & Nam, M. J. (2021). Indole-3-carbinol inhibits the proliferation of colorectal carcinoma LoVo cells through activation of the apoptotic signaling pathway. *Human & Experimental Toxicology*, *40*(12), 2099–2112. https://doi.org/10.1177/09603271211021475
54. Rejhová, A., Opattová, A., Čumová, A., Slíva, D., & Vodička, P. (2018). Natural compounds and combination therapy in colorectal cancer treatment. *European Journal of Medicinal Chemistry*, *144*, 582–594. https://doi.org/10.1016/j.ejmech.2017.12.039

55. Chen, Y., Li, Y., Wang, X. Q., Meng, Y., Zhang, Q., Zhu, J. Y., Chen, J. Q., Cao, W. S., Wang, X. Q., Xie, C. F., Li, X. T., Geng, S. S., Wu, J. S., Zhong, C. Y., & Han, H. Y. (2018). Phenethyl isothiocyanate inhibits colorectal cancer stem cells by suppressing Wnt/β-catenin pathway. *Phytotherapy Research: PTR*, *32*(12), 2447–2455. https://doi.org/10.1002/ptr.6183
56. Liu, Y., & Dey, M. (2017). Dietary phenethyl isothiocyanate protects mice from colitis associated colon cancer. *International Journal of Molecular Sciences*, *18*(9), 1908. https://doi.org/10.3390/ijms18091908
57. Aggarwal, B. B., & Shishodia, S. (2006). Molecular targets of dietary agents for prevention and therapy of cancer. *Biochemical Pharmacology*, *71*(10), 1397–1421. https://doi.org/10.1016/j.bcp.2006.02.009
58. Sorolla, M. A., Hidalgo, I., Sorolla, A., Montal, R., Pallisé, O., Salud, A., & Parisi, E. (2021). Microenvironmental reactive oxygen species in colorectal cancer: involved processes and therapeutic opportunities. *Cancers*, *13*(20), 5037. https://doi.org/10.3390/cancers13205037
59. Xu, D., Hu, M. J., Wang, Y. Q., & Cui, Y. L. (2019). Antioxidant activities of quercetin and its complexes for medicinal application. *Molecules*, *24*(6), 1123. https://doi.org/10.3390/molecules24061123
60. Neamtu, A. A., Maghiar, T. A., Alaya, A., Olah, N. K., Turcus, V., Pelea, D., Totolici, B. D., Neamtu, C., Maghiar, A. M., & Mathe, E. (2022). A comprehensive view on the quercetin impact on colorectal cancer. *Molecules*, *27*(6), 1873. https://doi.org/10.3390/molecules27061873
61. Catalán, M., Ferreira, J., & Carrasco-Pozo, C. (2020). The microbiota-derived metabolite of quercetin, 3,4-dihydroxyphenylacetic acid prevents malignant transformation and mitochondrial dysfunction induced by hemin in colon cancer and normal colon epithelia cell lines. *Molecules*, *25*(18), 4138. https://doi.org/10.3390/molecules25184138
62. Honari, M., Shafabakhsh, R., Reiter, R. J., Mirzaei, H., & Asemi, Z. (2019). Resveratrol is a promising agent for colorectal cancer prevention and treatment: focus on molecular mechanisms. *Cancer Cell International*, *19*, 180. https://doi.org/10.1186/s12935-019-0906-y
63. Nardone, O. M., Zammarchi, I., Santacroce, G., Ghosh, S., & Iacucci, M. (2023). Inflammation-driven colorectal cancer associated with colitis: from pathogenesis to changing therapy. *Cancers*, *15*(8), 2389. https://doi.org/10.3390/cancers15082389
64. Cuevas-Cianca, S. I., Romero-Castillo, C., Gálvez-Romero, J. L., Juárez, Z. N., & Hernández, L. R. (2023). Antioxidant and anti-inflammatory compounds from edible plants with anti-cancer activity and their potential use as drugs. *Molecules*, *28*(3), 1488. https://doi.org/10.3390/molecules28031488
65. Hewlings, S. J., & Kalman, D. S. (2017). Curcumin: a review of its effects on human health. *Foods*, *6*(10), 92. https://doi.org/10.3390/foods6100092
66. Feng, D., Ling, W. H., & Duan, R. D. (2010). Lycopene suppresses LPS-induced NO and IL-6 production by inhibiting the activation of ERK, p38MAPK, and NF-kappaB in macrophages. *Inflammation Research*, *59*(2), 115–121. https://doi.org/10.1007/s00011-009-0077-8
67. Cha, J. H., Kim, W. K., Ha, A. W., Kim, M. H., & Chang, M. J. (2017). Anti-inflammatory effect of lycopene in SW480 human colorectal cancer cells. *Nutrition Research and Practice*, *11*(2), 90–96. https://doi.org/10.4162/nrp.2017.11.2.90
68. Jurenka J. S. (2009). Anti-inflammatory properties of curcumin, a major constituent of *Curcuma longa*: a review of preclinical and clinical research. *Alternative Medicine Review: A Journal of Clinical Therapeutic*, *14*(2), 141–153.
69. D'Angelo, S., Martino, E., Ilisso, C. P., Bagarolo, M. L., Porcelli, M., & Cacciapuoti, G. (2017). Pro-oxidant and pro-apoptotic activity of polyphenol extract from Annurca apple and its underlying mechanisms in human breast cancer cells. *International Journal of Oncology*, *51*(3), 939–948. https://doi.org/10.3892/ijo.2017.4088
70. Shafiee, G., Saidijam, M., Tavilani, H., Ghasemkhani, N., & Khodadadi, I. (2016). Genistein induces apoptosis and inhibits proliferation of HT29 colon cancer cells. *International journal of Molecular and Cellular Medicine*, *5*(3), 178–191.
71. Maru, G. B., Hudlikar, R. R., Kumar, G., Gandhi, K., & Mahimkar, M. B. (2016). Understanding the molecular mechanisms of cancer prevention by dietary phytochemicals: from experimental models to clinical trials. *World Journal of Biological Chemistry*, *7*(1), 88–99. https://doi.org/10.4331/wjbc.v7.i1.88
72. Yue, J., & López, J. M. (2020). Understanding MAPK signaling pathways in apoptosis. *International Journal of Molecular Sciences*, *21*(7), 2346. https://doi.org/10.3390/ijms21072346
73. Kong, A. N., Yu, R., Hebbar, V., Chen, C., Owuor, E., Hu, R., Ee, R., & Mandlekar, S. (2001). Signal transduction events elicited by cancer prevention compounds. *Mutation Research*, *480–481*, 231–241. https://doi.org/10.1016/s0027-5107(01)00182-8

74. Li, Y. C., Chen, Y., & Du, J. (2015). Critical roles of intestinal epithelial vitamin D receptor signaling in controlling gut mucosal inflammation. *The Journal of Steroid Biochemistry and Molecular Biology*, *148*, 179–183. https://doi.org/10.1016/j.jsbmb.2015.01.011
75. Jia, Y., & Guo, M. (2013). Epigenetic changes in colorectal cancer. *Chinese Journal of Cancer*, *32*(1), 21–30. https://doi.org/10.5732/cjc.011.10245
76. Geng, Z., Chen, M., Yu, Q., Guo, S., Chen, T., & Liu, D. (2023). Histone modification of colorectal cancer by natural products. *Pharmaceuticals*, *16*(8), 1095. https://doi.org/10.3390/ph16081095
77. Haroon, M., & Kang, S. C. (2025). Kaempferol promotes apoptosis and inhibits proliferation and migration by suppressing HIF-1α/VEGF and Wnt/β-catenin activation under hypoxic condition in colon cancer. *Applied Biological Chemistry*, *68*(1), 19.
78. Tili, E., Michaille, J. J., Alder, H., Volinia, S., Delmas, D., Latruffe, N., & Croce, C. M. (2010). Resveratrol modulates the levels of microRNAs targeting genes encoding tumor-suppressors and effectors of TGFβ signaling pathway in SW480 cells. *Biochemical Pharmacology*, *80*(12), 2057–2065. https://doi.org/10.1016/j.bcp.2010.07.003
79. Del Follo-Martinez, A., Banerjee, N., Li, X., Safe, S., & Mertens-Talcott, S. (2013). Resveratrol and quercetin in combination have anticancer activity in colon cancer cells and repress oncogenic microRNA-27a. *Nutrition and Cancer*, *65*(3), 494–504. https://doi.org/10.1080/01635581.2012.725194
80. Saman, H., Raza, S. S., Uddin, S., & Rasul, K. (2020). Inducing angiogenesis, a key step in cancer vascularization, and treatment approaches. *Cancers*, *12*(5), 1172. https://doi.org/10.3390/cancers12051172
81. Mirossay, L., Varinská, L., & Mojžiš, J. (2017). Antiangiogenic effect of flavonoids and chalcones: an update. *International Journal of Molecular Sciences*, *19*(1), 27. https://doi.org/10.3390/ijms19010027
82. Shirakami, Y., Shimizu, M., Adachi, S., Sakai, H., Nakagawa, T., Yasuda, Y., Tsurumi, H., Hara, Y., & Moriwaki, H. (2009). (–)-Epigallocatechin gallate suppresses the growth of human hepatocellular carcinoma cells by inhibiting activation of the vascular endothelial growth factor-vascular endothelial growth factor receptor axis. *Cancer Science*, *100*(10), 1957–1962. https://doi.org/10.1111/j.1349-7006.2009.01241.x
83. Pavese, J. M., Farmer, R. L., & Bergan, R. C. (2010). Inhibition of cancer cell invasion and metastasis by genistein. *Cancer Metastasis Reviews*, *29*(3), 465–482. https://doi.org/10.1007/s10555-010-9238-z
84. Davoodvandi, A., Farshadi, M., Zare, N., Akhlagh, S. A., Alipour Nosrani, E., Mahjoubin-Tehran, M., Kangari, P., Sharafi, S. M., Khan, H., Aschner, M., Baniebrahimi, G., & Mirzaei, H. (2021). Antimetastatic effects of curcumin in oral and gastrointestinal cancers. *Frontiers in Pharmacology*, *12*, 668567. https://doi.org/10.3389/fphar.2021.668567
85. Rauf, A., Wilairatana, P., Joshi, P. B., Ahmad, Z., Olatunde, A., Hafeez, N., Hemeg, H. A., & Mubarak, M. S. (2024). Revisiting luteolin: an updated review on its anticancer potential. *Heliyon*, *10*(5), e26701. https://doi.org/10.1016/j.heliyon.2024.e26701
86. Cook, M. T., Liang, Y., Besch-Williford, C., & Hyder, S. M. (2016). Luteolin inhibits lung metastasis, cell migration, and viability of triple-negative breast cancer cells. *Breast Cancer (Dove Medical Press)*, *9*, 9–19. https://doi.org/10.2147/BCTT.S124860
87. Goetz, L. H., & Schork, N. J. (2018). Personalized medicine: motivation, challenges, and progress. *Fertility and Sterility*, *109*(6), 952–963. https://doi.org/10.1016/j.fertnstert.2018.05.006
88. Ruiz-Bañobre, J., & Goel, A. (2021). Genomic and epigenomic biomarkers in colorectal cancer: from diagnosis to therapy. *Advances in Cancer Research*, *151*, 231–304. https://doi.org/10.1016/bs.acr.2021.02.008
89. Jung, G., Hernández-Illán, E., Moreira, L., Balaguer, F., & Goel, A. (2020). Epigenetics of colorectal cancer: biomarker and therapeutic potential. *Nature Reviews. Gastroenterology & Hepatology*, *17*(2), 111–130. https://doi.org/10.1038/s41575-019-0230-y
90. Garcia-Carbonero, N., Martinez-Useros, J., Li, W., Orta, A., Perez, N., Carames, C., Hernandez, T., Moreno, I., Serrano, G., & Garcia-Foncillas, J. (2020). *KRAS* and *BRAF* mutations as prognostic and predictive biomarkers for standard chemotherapy response in metastatic colorectal cancer: a single institutional study. *Cells*, *9*(1), 219. https://doi.org/10.3390/cells9010219
91. Michel, M., Kaps, L., Maderer, A., Galle, P. R., & Moehler, M. (2021). The role of p53 dysfunction in colorectal cancer and its implication for therapy. *Cancers*, *13*(10), 2296. https://doi.org/10.3390/cancers13102296
92. Goenka, A., Khan, F., Verma, B., Sinha, P., Dmello, C. C., Jogalekar, M. P., Gangadaran, P., & Ahn, B. C. (2023). Tumor microenvironment signaling and therapeutics in cancer progression. *Cancer Communications*, *43*(5), 525–561. https://doi.org/10.1002/cac2.12416
93. Hossain, M. S., Wazed, M. A., Asha, S., Amin, M. R., & Shimul, I. M. (2025). Dietary phytochemicals in health and disease: mechanisms, clinical evidence, and applications—a comprehensive review. *Food Science & Nutrition*, *13*(3), e70101. https://doi.org/10.1002/fsn3.70101

94. Golonko, A., Pienkowski, T., Swislocka, R., Orzechowska, S., Marszalek, K., Szczerbinski, L., Swiergiel, A. H., & Lewandowski, W. (2024). Dietary factors and their influence on immunotherapy strategies in oncology: a comprehensive review. *Cell Death & Disease*, *15*(4), 254. https://doi.org/10.1038/s41419-024-06641-6
95. Ameer, S. F., Mohamed, M. Y., Elzubair, Q. A., Sharif, E. A. M., & Ibrahim, W. N. (2024). Curcumin as a novel therapeutic candidate for cancer: can this natural compound revolutionize cancer treatment?. *Frontiers in Oncology*, *14*, 1438040. https://doi.org/10.3389/fonc.2024.1438040
96. Tong, W., Wang, Q., Sun, D., & Suo, J. (2016). Curcumin suppresses colon cancer cell invasion via AMPK-induced inhibition of NF-κB, uPA activator and MMP9. *Oncology Letters*, *12*(5), 4139–4146. https://doi.org/10.3892/ol.2016.5148
97. Battaglin, F., Naseem, M., Lenz, H. J., & Salem, M. E. (2018). Microsatellite instability in colorectal cancer: overview of its clinical significance and novel perspectives. *Clinical Advances in Hematology & Oncology: H&O*, *16*(11), 735–745.
98. Gianchecchi, E., & Fierabracci, A. (2020). Insights on the effects of resveratrol and some of its derivatives in cancer and autoimmunity: a molecule with a dual activity. *Antioxidants (Basel, Switzerland)*, *9*(2), 91. https://doi.org/10.3390/antiox9020091
99. Zhang, Q., Huang, H., Zheng, F., Liu, H., Qiu, F., Chen, Y., Liang, C. L., & Dai, Z. (2020). Resveratrol exerts antitumor effects by downregulating $CD8^+CD122^+$ Tregs in murine hepatocellular carcinoma. *Oncoimmunology*, *9*(1), 1829346. https://doi.org/10.1080/2162402X.2020.1829346
100. Siddiqui, S. S., Rahman, S., Rupasinghe, H. P. V., & Vazhappilly, C. G. (2020). Dietary flavonoids in p53-mediated immune dysfunctions linking to cancer prevention. *Biomedicines*, *8*(8), 286. https://doi.org/10.3390/biomedicines8080286
101. Bhatiya, M., Pathak, S., Jothimani, G., Duttaroy, A. K., & Banerjee, A. (2023). A comprehensive study on the anti-cancer effects of quercetin and its epigenetic modifications in arresting progression of colon cancer cell proliferation. *Archivum Immunologiae et Therapiae Experimentalis*, *71*(1), 6. https://doi.org/10.1007/s00005-023-00669-w
102. Tortorella, S. M., Royce, S. G., Licciardi, P. V., & Karagiannis, T. C. (2015). Dietary sulforaphane in cancer chemoprevention: the role of epigenetic regulation and HDAC inhibition. *Antioxidants & Redox Signaling*, *22*(16), 1382–1424. https://doi.org/10.1089/ars.2014.6097
103. Deng, W., Xiong, X., Lu, M., Huang, S., Luo, Y., Wang, Y., & Ying, Y. (2024). Curcumin suppresses colorectal tumorigenesis through restoring the gut microbiota and metabolites. *BMC Cancer*, *24*(1), 1141. https://doi.org/10.1186/s12885-024-12898-z
104. Martin, S. L., Kala, R., & Tollefsbol, T. O. (2018). Mechanisms for the inhibition of colon cancer cells by sulforaphane through epigenetic modulation of microRNA-21 and human telomerase reverse transcriptase (hTERT) down-regulation. *Current Cancer Drug Targets*, *18*(1), 97–106. https://doi.org/10.2174/1568009617666170206104032
105. Howells, L. M., Iwuji, C. O. O., Irving, G. R. B., Barber, S., Walter, H., Sidat, Z., Griffin-Teall, N., Singh, R., Foreman, N., Patel, S. R., Morgan, B., Steward, W. P., Gescher, A., Thomas, A. L., & Brown, K. (2019). Curcumin combined with FOLFOX chemotherapy is safe and tolerable in patients with metastatic colorectal cancer in a randomized phase iIa trial. *The Journal of Nutrition*, *149*(7), 1133–1139. https://doi.org/10.1093/jn/nxz029
106. Rein, M. J., Renouf, M., Cruz-Hernandez, C., Actis-Goretta, L., Thakkar, S. K., & da Silva Pinto, M. (2013). Bioavailability of bioactive food compounds: a challenging journey to bioefficacy. *British Journal of Clinical Pharmacology*, *75*(3), 588–602. https://doi.org/10.1111/j.1365-2125.2012.04425.x
107. Lippolis, T., Cofano, M., Caponio, G. R., De Nunzio, V., & Notarnicola, M. (2023). Bioaccessibility and bioavailability of diet polyphenols and their modulation of gut microbiota. *International Journal of Molecular Sciences*, *24*(4), 3813. https://doi.org/10.3390/ijms24043813
108. Sohn, S. I., Priya, A., Balasubramaniam, B., Muthuramalingam, P., Sivasankar, C., Selvaraj, A., Valliammai, A., Jothi, R., & Pandian, S. (2021). Biomedical applications and bioavailability of curcumin—an updated overview. *Pharmaceutics*, *13*(12), 2102. https://doi.org/10.3390/pharmaceutics13122102
109. Aqil, F., Munagala, R., Jeyabalan, J., & Vadhanam, M. V. (2013). Bioavailability of phytochemicals and its enhancement by drug delivery systems. *Cancer Letters*, *334*(1), 133–141. https://doi.org/10.1016/j.canlet.2013.02.032
110. Kujawska, M., & Jodynis-Liebert, J. (2020). Potential of the ellagic acid-derived gut microbiota metabolite – urolithin A in gastrointestinal protection. *World Journal of Gastroenterology*, *26*(23), 3170–3181. https://doi.org/10.3748/wjg.v26.i23.3170

111. Pandey, P., Khan, F., Seifeldin, S. A., Alshaghdali, K., Siddiqui, S., Abdelwadoud, M. E., Vyas, M., Saeed, M., Mazumder, A., & Saeed, A. (2023). Targeting Wnt/β-catenin pathway by flavonoids: implication for cancer therapeutics. *Nutrients*, *15*(9), 2088. https://doi.org/10.3390/nu15092088
112. Galati, G., & O'Brien, P. J. (2004). Potential toxicity of flavonoids and other dietary phenolics: significance for their chemopreventive and anticancer properties. *Free Radical Biology & Medicine*, *37*(3), 287–303. https://doi.org/10.1016/j.freeradbiomed.2004.04.034
113. Barba-Ostria, C., Carrera-Pacheco, S. E., Gonzalez-Pastor, R., Heredia-Moya, J., Mayorga-Ramos, A., Rodríguez-Pólit, C., Zúñiga-Miranda, J., Arias-Almeida, B., & Guamán, L. P. (2022). Evaluation of biological activity of natural compounds: current trends and methods. *Molecules*, *27*(14), 4490. https://doi.org/10.3390/molecules27144490
114. Pai, S., Hebbar, A., & Selvaraj, S. (2022). A critical look at challenges and future scopes of bioactive compounds and their incorporations in the food, energy, and pharmaceutical sector. *Environmental Science and Pollution Research International*, *29*(24), 35518–35541. https://doi.org/10.1007/s11356-022-19423-4
115. Patra, J. K., Das, G., Fraceto, L. F., Campos, E. V. R., Rodriguez-Torres, M. D. P., Acosta-Torres, L. S., Diaz-Torres, L. A., Grillo, R., Swamy, M. K., Sharma, S., Habtemariam, S., & Shin, H. S. (2018). Nano based drug delivery systems: recent developments and future prospects. *Journal of Nanobiotechnology*, *16*(1), 71. https://doi.org/10.1186/s12951-018-0392-8
116. Zhang, Y., Wang, Z., Wang, Y., Jin, W., Zhang, Z., Jin, L., Qian, J., & Zheng, L. (2024). CYP3A4 and CYP3A5: the crucial roles in clinical drug metabolism and the significant implications of genetic polymorphisms. *PeerJ*, *12*, e18636. https://doi.org/10.7717/peerj.18636
117. Johnson K. V. (2020). Gut microbiome composition and diversity are related to human personality traits. *Human Microbiome Journal*, *15*, 100069. https://doi.org/10.1016/j.humic.2019.100069
118. Akter, S., Netzel, M., Tinggi, U., Fletcher, M., Osborne, S., & Sultanbawa, Y. (2020). Interactions between phytochemicals and minerals in *Terminalia ferdinandiana* and implications for mineral bioavailability. *Frontiers in Nutrition*, *7*, 598219. https://doi.org/10.3389/fnut.2020.598219
119. Delimont, N. M., Haub, M. D., & Lindshield, B. L. (2017). The impact of tannin consumption on iron bioavailability and status: a narrative review. *Current Developments in Nutrition*, *1*(2), 1–12. https://doi.org/10.3945/cdn.116.000042
120. Ai, X., Yu, P., Peng, L., Luo, L., Liu, J., Li, S., Lai, X., Luan, F., & Meng, X. (2021). Berberine: a review of its pharmacokinetics properties and therapeutic potentials in diverse vascular diseases. *Frontiers in Pharmacology*, *12*, 762654. https://doi.org/10.3389/fphar.2021.762654
121. Kiani, J., & Imam, S. Z. (2007). Medicinal importance of grapefruit juice and its interaction with various drugs. *Nutrition Journal*, *6*, 33. https://doi.org/10.1186/1475-2891-6-33
122. Borrelli, F., & Izzo, A. A. (2009). Herb-drug interactions with St John's wort (*Hypericum perforatum*): an update on clinical observations. *The AAPS Journal*, *11*(4), 710–727. https://doi.org/10.1208/s12248-009-9146-8
123. Duda-Chodak, A., & Tarko, T. (2023). Possible side effects of polyphenols and their interactions with medicines. *Molecules*, *28*(6), 2536. https://doi.org/10.3390/molecules28062536
124. Daneshvar, S., Zamanian, M. Y., Ivraghi, M. S., Golmohammadi, M., Modanloo, M., Kamiab, Z., Pourhosseini, S. M. E., Heidari, M., & Bazmandegan, G. (2023). A comprehensive view on the apigenin impact on colorectal cancer: focusing on cellular and molecular mechanisms. *Food Science & Nutrition*, *11*(11), 6789–6801. https://doi.org/10.1002/fsn3.3645
125. Khan, U. M., Sevindik, M., Zarrabi, A., Nami, M., Ozdemir, B., Kaplan, D. N., Selamoglu, Z., Hasan, M., Kumar, M., Alshehri, M. M., & Sharifi-Rad, J. (2021). Lycopene: food sources, biological activities, and human health benefits. *Oxidative Medicine and Cellular Longevity*, *2021*, 2713511.
126. Lambring, C., Varga, K., Livingston, K., Lorusso, N., Dudhia, A., & Basha, R. (2022). Therapeutic applications of curcumin and derivatives in colorectal cancer. *Onco Therapeutics*, *9*(1), 51–62. https://doi.org/10.1615/OncoTherap.2022044575
127. Kang, S. L., Woo, J. H., Kim, N. H., Kwon, J. Y., & Kim, S. M. (2023). Necessity of strengthening the current clinical regulatory for companion diagnostics: an institutional comparison of the FDA, EMA, and MFDS. *Molecular Therapy. Methods & Clinical Development*, *30*, 447–458. https://doi.org/10.1016/j.omtm.2023.08.008
128. Rodríguez-Pérez, C., García-Villanova, B., Guerra-Hernández, E., & Verardo, V. (2019). Grape seeds proanthocyanidins: an overview of in vivo bioactivity in animal models. *Nutrients*, *11*(10), 2435. https://doi.org/10.3390/nu11102435
129. Li, S., Han, Q., Qiao, C., Song, J., Lung Cheng, C., & Xu, H. (2008). Chemical markers for the quality control of herbal medicines: an overview. *Chinese Medicine*, *3*, 7. https://doi.org/10.1186/1749-8546-3-7

13 Evidence-Based Blood Transfusion Practices

R. Raj Bharath
SRM Medical College Hospital and Research Centre,
SRM Institute of Science and Technology,
Kattankulathur, Tamil Nadu, India

13.1 INTRODUCTION

Patients undergoing treatment for oncological diseases require blood transfusion support during or following surgery and after chemotherapy. Blood center provides a variety of blood components such as packed red cells, platelets, and fresh frozen plasma for different clinical indications in malignancy. The frequent transfusion of blood components results in production of red cell antibodies and other transfusion-associated adverse events. The transfusion-associated adverse events may be mild such as febrile or allergic and also severe such as hemolytic transfusion reaction. Blood transfusion always carried an inherent risk, and informed written consent should be obtained from the patient explaining the benefits and risk of transfusion. There is also limited literature regarding blood transfusion practices and well-defined transfusion guidelines to be followed in oncological disorders compared to other transfusion dependent diseases.

Anemia in oncological patients can either be directly due to poor nutritional uptake and cancer cells invading bone marrow or indirectly due to inflammation and red cell autoantibodies developing in the patient [1]. Chemotherapy-induced anemia and thrombocytopenia are also featured in cancer patients, leading to frequent red blood cell (RBC) and platelet transfusion. Anemia in patients with oncological or hematological malignancies has a prevalence of between 26% and 53% and is reported to be as high as 75% in patients with solid tumors who are receiving chemotherapy. The evidence suggests that anemia in cancer patients is associated with increased morbidity and mortality as well as poorer functional status and healthcare-related quality of life [2].

Patient blood management (PBM) is an evidence-based, multidisciplinary approach to caring for patients who might need a blood transfusion. It was implemented to limit the transfusion of allogeneic blood with the aim of improving the patient's clinical morbidity and mortality [3]. When considering a patient for a blood component transfusion, a multifaceted "Patient Centric" approach is necessary. The World Health Organization (WHO) underscores that the promotion of patient safety, patient education, autonomy and empowerment, informed consent, and shared decision-making are integral to PBM. PBM fundamentally shifts from a focus on blood as a product to be replaced if anemia or bleeding occurs, to a focus on improving with the patient in the center, protecting and preserving the patient's own unique and precious blood. The objectives of PBM are to increase the red cell mass by erythropoietin-stimulating agents, minimizing surgical blood loss using advanced techniques, and following restrictive transfusion threshold. PBM encompasses strategies aimed at minimizing practices that contribute to iatrogenic anemia, establishing preoperative anemia management pathways, and utilizing electronic decision-making tools for transfusion orders [4].

DOI: 10.1201/9781003644309-13

13.1.1 RBC Transfusion Practices

RBC transfusion is given to correct the hemoglobin level, thereby increasing the oxygen carrying capacity of the blood to deliver oxygen to the tissues. Red cells are also given during surgical procedures in resecting tumors when significant blood loss is imminent [5]. Blood can be collected by either autologous (using one's own blood by collecting and storing before surgery) or allogenic (blood derived from voluntary blood donors) method. While autologous blood is preferable because of its safety, patients with malignancy often have a low hemoglobin level and are not suitable for autologous donation. So allogenic transfusion is given, but they carry inherent risks such as post-operative infections and other transfusion reactions. A meta-analysis of various studies from 5635 patients with liver malignancy reported that patients who received allogeneic RBCs perioperatively had a higher risk of mortality and cancer recurrence than those non-transfused during the five years after surgery for hepatocellular carcinoma. The meta-analysis revealed odds ratio for all-cause death during the five years after surgery was 1.60 for those who were transfused compared with those who were not transfused with allogenic blood [6]. The mechanisms reported for the underlying adverse effects of blood transfusion are believed to be suppression of host immune system. Another systematic review done in 20,795 colorectal cancer patients who had undergone surgery has reported high mortality in transfused patients [7]. The mean length of hospital stay was significantly longer in transfused compared with non-transfused patients (17.8 ± 4.8 vs. 13.9 ± 4.7 days). Blood transfusion should be required only when there is a clear clinical indication and other options are ruled out. PBM can be initiated in oncology patients by implementing a restrictive transfusion threshold (Hb < 7 gm/dL) in stable patients with anemia [8]. Numerous investigations have indicated that reduced Hb levels in cancer patients have a minimal effect on mortality or morbidity-related outcomes. In individuals with hematological disorders, Hb levels falling below 7 g/dL did not correlate with notable adverse outcomes. Restrictive transfusion strategies decreased the likelihood of at least one RBC transfusion by 41% across a diverse array of clinical settings (orthopedic, cardiac, or vascular surgery; critical care, hematological malignancies) involving 21,433 patients from 48 clinical trials. Implementing the lower threshold consistently in hospitals would significantly decrease the demand for blood [9]. The transfusion of RBCs using a restrictive strategy of 7.0 g/dL–8.0 g/dL, in contrast to a liberal hemoglobin threshold of 9.0 g/dL–10.0 g/dL, does not negatively impact clinical outcomes. Implementation of a restrictive blood transfusion protocol can be an important blood-saving and cost-saving strategy.

13.2 SINGLE UNIT RBC TRANSFUSIONS

The transfusion of a single unit of RBCs has been demonstrated to be safe when applied with a restrictive transfusion trigger, such as pre-transfusion hemoglobin levels or symptoms of anemia, according to several randomized controlled trials (RCTs). A dose of 4 ml red cells per kg increases hemoglobin concentration by approximately 1 g/dL, which is equivalent to the increase seen with one unit of red cells in a 70 kg patient. Transfusion of RBCs is not an appropriate treatment for iron deficiency anemia, except in cases of acute bleeding or when symptoms of acute physiological stress arise due to inadequate oxygen delivery, which may be alleviated by administering a single unit of RBCs. Subsequently, additional transfusions may be deferred or substituted with alternative approaches to managing anemia. The administration of a single unit should be followed by a clinical or laboratory evaluation of the patient to determine whether the transfusion therapy is sufficient or if additional units are required [10]. Transfusion of multiple RBC units is associated with an increased risk of pulmonary edema or transfusion-associated circulatory overload (TACO) in elderly patients and also with patients with heart or kidney failure. Studies have found increased use of single-unit transfusions, combined with lower transfusion thresholds, contributed to a 35% reduction in RBC transfusions in patients with a primary diagnosis of malignancy. The mean RBC units transfused per inpatient and outpatient episode decreased from 0.067 to 0.038 unit ($p < 0.001$) [11]. The study advocated ordering RBCs one unit at a time, following a conservative (restrictive) transfusion hemoglobin threshold, and increased use of intravenous iron to manage anemia can result in a significant decrease in transfusion exposure to all patients.

13.3 ERYTHROPOIESIS-STIMULATING AGENTS

Anemia frequently occurs in individuals diagnosed with solid or hematological malignancies. The factors contributing to anemia associated with malignancy can be diverse, encompassing the toxicity of cancer treatments, elevated inflammatory states, ongoing bleeding, and nutritional deficiencies. The presence of anemia and its associated symptoms, such as fatigue, considerably affect the quality of life for individuals experiencing cancer or receiving treatment for it. Increased levels of inflammatory cytokines produced by cancer cells, along with the toxic effects of chemotherapy or radiotherapy, could contribute to disruptions in iron homeostasis and hindered erythropoietic activity. Therapeutic strategies for addressing chemotherapy-induced anemia encompass RBC transfusions and erythropoiesis-stimulating agents (ESAs). Erythropoiesis-stimulating agents (ESAs) play a significant role in minimizing the need for transfusions associated with chemotherapy-induced anemias. The recommendations issued by the American Society of Clinical Oncology (ASCO) and the American Society of Hematology (ASH) advocate for the use of ESAs in the management of chemotherapy-induced anemia when hemoglobin levels fall below 10 g/dL, particularly in cases where the cancer treatment is not aimed at a cure [12]. It is essential to exclude iron deficiency in cancer patients (ferritin > 100 µg/L and transferrin saturation > 20%) prior to initiating treatment with ESA. Additionally, the supplementation of ESA therapy with intravenous iron is advised. In the absence of a response within six to eight weeks (indicated by a change in Hb of less than 1 g/dL–2 g/dL or no decrease in transfusion frequency), it is advisable to reassess iron stores. The available erythropoiesis-stimulating agents, including epoetin, darbepoetin, and biosimilars of epoetin alfa, appear to demonstrate comparable effectiveness and safety profiles [13]. ESA therapy provides benefits that develop over weeks to months; thus, RBC transfusion should be considered for patients requiring immediate symptom relief.

The application of ESA in patients who fulfill the specified criteria results in a reduction of RBC transfusions by approximately 35%. ESAs could serve as a potential option for patients who are at risk of volume overload or have a history of immune-mediated transfusion reactions resulting from the formation of alloantibodies in their blood. Individuals for whom compatible blood cannot be located or who decline transfusion due to personal or religious convictions (such as Jehovah's Witnesses) should be evaluated for treatment with ESA if appropriate. It is essential for clinicians to thoroughly reassess the application of ESA in patients who are at an elevated risk of thromboembolism [14]. ESAs should also be used with caution in certain tumor entities such as metastatic breast cancer receiving chemotherapy, and thrombotic vascular events were reported in 2.8% of erythropoietin group vs. 1.4% ($p = 0.038$) in standard of care group, respectively [15].

13.4 INTRAVENOUS (IV) IRON

Preoperative anemia in patients is linked to higher rates of morbidity and mortality, as well as an increased likelihood of postoperative complications and extended hospital stays. During surgical procedures and subsequent hospital stays, patients often experience blood loss, leading to varying degrees of anemia upon discharge. Traditionally, the focus of iron therapy has been on oral iron. The presence of symptoms like nausea, diarrhea, or constipation as a consequence of cancer therapy frequently indicates that only a small percentage of cancer patients are able to tolerate oral iron. The advancement of novel intravenous iron–carbohydrate formulations enables the safe administration of a substantial dose (1000 mg) within a 15-minute timeframe. The application of intravenous iron has seen a significant rise across various domains of clinical practice, such as surgery, women's health, cardiology, and hematology. Intravenous iron has the ability to circumvent the iron sequestration effect mediated by hepcidin during inflammation in cancer. A comprehensive review was conducted utilizing data from 23 RCTs that assessed intravenous iron therapy in patients with cancer and anemia, along with their respective outcomes [16]. Trials examining intravenous iron in patients with colorectal cancer-associated anemia revealed that hemoglobin levels were notably elevated in the IV iron group at the time of surgery. Additionally, a larger percentage of individuals in the IV iron group achieved hemoglobin normalization on the day of surgery when compared to those receiving oral iron. Nonetheless, there were no observed differences in the complication rates (including infections) or the duration of postoperative hospital stays. An RCT involving women with anemia and gynecological cancer who underwent platinum-based adjuvant chemotherapy demonstrated a reduced need for RBC transfusions in the intravenous iron group compared to the oral iron group (22.7% vs. 63.6%, respectively, $p < 0.01$) during the subsequent chemotherapy cycle. A total of ten RCTs assessed the impact of intravenous iron supplementation alongside erythropoiesis-stimulating agents in various patient populations suffering from breast, colorectal, lung, and gynecological cancers, specifically focusing on anemia associated with cancer and/or chemotherapy. The results demonstrated that the use of IV iron was associated with a significant increase in Hb levels, marked by an elevation of ≥20 g/L from baseline and/or a decreased requirement for RBC transfusion (20%) in comparison to the administration of oral iron and ESAs alone. The aim for patients with cancer who are facing anemia is to improve their quality of life and to effectively complete adjuvant therapies. Four trials demonstrated a beneficial impact on quality of life, while eight trials reported no significant differences in quality-of-life outcomes. Jayne Lim and colleagues concluded that intravenous iron can enhance hemoglobin levels and can be safely administered to patients throughout their treatment journey, from primary surgery to the palliative phase [16].

13.5 COMPUTERIZED PHYSICIAN ORDER ENTRY (CPOE) SYSTEM

The crucial aspect of executing a PBM program in a hospital involves effectively sharing evidence-based transfusion information with physicians, ensuring they are informed during each transfusion decision-making process. Decision support systems (DSSs) have been applied across multiple areas in medicine, including diagnosis, disease management, and the dosing and prescribing of medications. The utilization of electronic tools is essential for effectively engaging clinicians in the decision-making process regarding the appropriateness of transfusions for their patients. Decision-making regarding blood transfusion can be supported by having patient-centric assessments or recommendations as warnings or alerts using electronic health records. They are defined as "any software designed to directly aid in clinical decision making in which characteristics of individual patients are matched to a computerized knowledge base and presented to clinicians for consideration" [17]. For example, if an RBC transfusion was done for a patient with an Hb level of >9.5 g/dL, an email is sent to the ordering physician asking them to justify why the transfusion was administered. When there is linkage of laboratory data within the electronic health records, the laboratory results can be used to drive clinical decision support (CDS) warnings. This CDS has significantly improved quality of care and patient outcomes. This was improvised by using computerized physician order entry (CPOE) system to automatically generate alerts when an ordered transfusion was not substantiated by the laboratory evidence. Studies have reported that appropriate use of warnings can reduce RBC and platelet transfusions. These warning alerts in the system were based on existing laboratory data or guidelines prescribing blood transfusion. The alert could be overridden if the physician felt that the patient required blood transfusion and clinically indicated. Similarly, alert systems are followed for preoperative anemia management. When a low Hb value is detected, an email report is sent to the patient's surgeon indicating that the patient is anemic, and the reason should be investigated before the date of surgery. These alerts have been very successful in helping to decrease the number of blood components transfused to a patient. A CPOE system with CDS is a useful tool in maintaining reductions in RBC utilization achieved through compliance with application of evidence-based transfusion guidelines. The same alerts can also be implemented for plasma and platelet transfusion. If prophylactic transfusion was given for a stable patient with more than 10,000/μl, an alert is sent to the concerned clinician. However, the alert does not trigger if there is platelet dysfunction, underlying coagulation abnormalities or massive bleeding indication. A systematic review on DSS regarding blood transfusion practices concluded that there is good evidence that implementation of a DSS improves RBC usage and also resulted in cost savings [18].

13.6 PROPHYLACTIC VS. THERAPEUTIC PLATELET TRANSFUSION

Oncohematologic diseases induce thrombocytopenia and hemorrhagic manifestations as a result of bone marrow failure caused by the disease itself and also if radiotherapy or chemotherapy is used for the treatment of malignancy [19]. Platelet transfusion is given in the prevention and treatment of bleeding in cancer patients with treatment-related thrombocytopenia. The ASCO Panel recommends a threshold of less than 10,000/μl for prophylactic platelet transfusion in patients receiving therapy for hematologic malignancies. Transfusion at higher levels may be advisable in patients with signs of hemorrhage, high fever, hyperleukocytosis, sudden drop of platelet count, and coagulation abnormalities. The Panel recommends a threshold of 40,000/μl–50,000/μl for performing major invasive procedures in the absence of associated coagulation abnormalities. Platelets for transfusion can be prepared by blood component separation of platelet concentrates from whole blood using the buffy coat or platelet-rich plasma (PRP) method. These platelets produced by PRP method result in a final volume of 50 ml–70 ml of platelets which contains a minimum of $3.5–4.5 \times 10^{10}$ platelets, while buffy coat method yields a platelet count of minimum of 6×10^{10} platelets per unit. However, the more efficient way of collecting high yield of platelets from a single donor is through plateletpheresis method. In plateletpheresis, blood is withdrawn from a donor or patient in an anticoagulant solution and separated into blood components by using apheresis equipment. The platelet component is retained, and the remaining constituents are returned to the individual through the apheresis equipment. The volume collected is more than 200 ml with a minimum platelet count of 3×10^{11} per unit. So transfusing one unit of single donor platelets will give a significant increment of platelet count to the patient and also reduce multiple donor exposures. This is because platelets collected from whole blood will require four to five units to have the same increment as seen with single donor platelets. The PLADO trial was conducted on 1272 patients undergoing hematopoietic stem cell transplantation or chemotherapy for hematologic cancers or solid tumors who received prophylactic platelet transfusions at different platelet doses [20]. They concluded that when prophylactic transfusions are given after a trigger threshold of 10,000 platelets or lower is reached, the platelet dose has no significant effect on the incidence of bleeding possibly because few platelets are needed to maintain hemostasis.

Eltrombopag and romiplostim are thrombopoietic stimulating agents (TSAs) which have been studied in patients with malignancy to mitigate thrombocytopenia although they are not currently approved for such use. The frequency of platelet transfusions could be safely lowered by following a more restrictive transfusion strategy that takes account of the risk of bleeding, as recommended by the guidelines [21].

13.7 MANAGEMENT OF PLATELET REFRACTORINESS

Hematopoietic stem cell transplantation and the more aggressive use of chemotherapy in the treatment of malignancies have led to a sudden increase in platelet transfusions. Platelet refractoriness is defined as a repeated suboptimal response to platelet transfusions with lower-than-expected post-transfusion count increments. Refractoriness can be caused by immune and nonimmune factors, with nonimmune factors responsible for a majority of cases. Nonimmunologic factors are involved in about 80% of cases with underlying sepsis, fever, splenomegaly, bone marrow and peripheral blood progenitor cell transplantation, and disseminated intravascular coagulation. Immune-mediated factors play a role in 10%–25% of patients with platelet refractoriness which includes

Corrected Count Increment (CCI)

$$\text{CCI} = \frac{\text{Post-transfusion plt count} - \text{Pre-transfusion plt count (/L)} \times \text{BSA (m}^2\text{)}}{\text{platelets transfused } (10^{11})^*}$$

Percentage Platelet Recovery (PPR)

$$\text{PPR} = \frac{\text{Post-transfusion plt count} - \text{Pre-transfusion plt count (/L)} \times \text{TBV} \times 100\%}{\text{platelets transfused } (10^{11})^*}$$

*If exact platelet count is unavailable use 3×10^{11}
plt – platelet; BSA – body surface area; TBV – total blood volume

FIGURE 13.1 Calculation of corrected count increment (CCI) and the percent platelet response (PPR) in patients receiving platelet transfusion.

antibodies against human leukocyte antigen (HLA) class I, human platelet antigens (HPAs), and ABO red cell antibodies. Refractoriness to platelet transfusions due to immunological factors is the result of previous sensitization history (pregnancies and frequent transfusions) which triggered the production of corresponding antibodies [21]. Platelet refractoriness is associated with a number of adverse outcomes, including longer hospital stays, increased risk of bleeding, and decreased survival. Platelet counts should be repeated 10–60 minutes following platelet transfusion when refractoriness is suspected [22]. A diagnosis of refractoriness to platelet transfusion should only be made when at least two consecutive transfusions of ABO-compatible units have resulted in poor increments. The corrected count increment (CCI) and the percent platelet response (PPR) are frequently used formulas (**Figure 13.1**) for monitoring the post-transfusion increment based on the size of the patient and the dosage administered. Alloimmunization due to transfusion of platelet component is usually due to antibody against HLA antigens and rarely to platelet-specific antigens. Patients with alloimmune refractory thrombocytopenia are best managed with platelet transfusions from histocompatible donors matched for HLA-A and HLA-B antigens or by platelet crossmatching (**Figure 13.2**). Anti-HLA antibodies are described as Panel Reactive Antibodies (PRA). The PRA–HLA test is considered to be highly sensitive and specific for the identification of HLA class I alloantibodies. PRA detection using methods based on enzyme-linked immunosorbent assay (ELISA) and fluorescence-based flow cytometry or single antigen bead (SAB) technologies has high sensitivity and specificity. The presence of alloimmunization to HPAs should be confirmed with more specific tests such as the Monoclonal Antibody Immobilization of the Platelets Antigens Assay (MAIPA). Platelet crossmatching technique detects antibodies against HLA class I and platelet-specific antigens.

13.8 SPECIALIZED RBCs

Leukoreduced RBCs are red cell components that have undergone processes to eliminate white blood cells through various techniques. Leukoreduced RBCs mitigate the risk of febrile non-hemolytic transfusion reactions (FNHTR), reduce HLA alloimmunization in patients receiving multiple transfusions, and prevent the transmission of leukotropic viruses like cytomegalovirus (CMV).

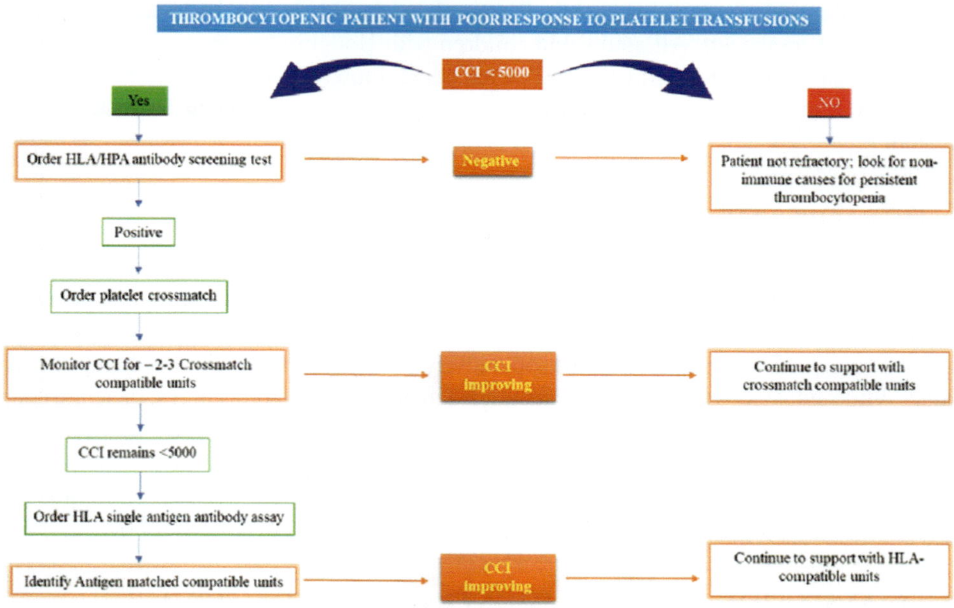

FIGURE 13.2 Management of patient with platelet refractoriness.

The occurrence of HLA alloimmunization after transfusions can differ based on the patient's diagnosis and treatment. HLA antibodies are identifiable in 25%–30% of patients with leukemia who have received transfusions, and their presence can reach up to 80% in patients with aplastic anemia. To minimize HLA alloimmunization, it is essential to decrease the leukocyte content to below 5×10^6, a goal that can be accomplished through the use of leukocyte-reduction filters.

Prestorage leukofiltration serves as an effective approach for leukoreduction, typically conducted shortly after or within five days of whole blood collection. This process utilizes either inline filter blood bags or supplementary filters connected to the tubing via a sterile connecting device. The primary benefits of prestorage leukoreduction include the elimination of leukocytes prior to their disintegration and the subsequent release of cytokines into the plasma. The presence of these cytokines in the blood unit, when released into the bloodstream of the patient, can lead to immune modulation and transfusion reactions in the recipient. The occurrence of alloantibody-mediated refractoriness to platelet transfusion can be reduced in patients with leukemia and those undergoing induction chemotherapy when both platelet and RBC units are subjected to leukoreduction prior to transfusion. In developed nations, the majority of blood components are currently subjected to leukoreduction during the processes of blood collection and component preparation.

Irradiated RBCs are given to prevent transfusion-associated graft-versus-host disease (TA-GVHD) in patients who are immunocompromised or with immature immune system [23]. Transfusion-associated graft-versus-host disease (TA-GVHD) is a rare, usually fatal, complication of transfusion of blood components containing lymphocytes. Irradiated red cells are given to recipients of marrow or peripheral blood stem cell transplantation and patients with hematologic malignancies or solid tumors in oncology. Irradiation leads to the inactivation of T lymphocytes in the blood unit and can be done either using gamma or X-rays using an irradiator. All patients undergoing autologous or allogenic bone marrow transplant or peripheral blood stem cell transplant should receive irradiated cellular blood components from time of initiation of conditioning chemo/radiotherapy. Irradiated components should be continued in allogenic bone marrow transplant until all of the following criteria are met – six months have elapsed since the transplant date, the lymphocyte count is $>1.0 \times 10^9$/L, and the patient is free of active chronic GVHD and off all immunosuppression.

All patients undergoing autologous stem cell transplant should receive irradiated red cells until three months post-transplant. All adults and children with Hodgkin lymphoma at any stage of the disease should have irradiated red cells and platelets indefinitely. For all at-risk patients of developing TaGVHD, all red cell, platelet, and granulocyte concentrates should be irradiated before transfusion.

13.9 INTRAOPERATIVE CELL SALVAGE

Adverse effects of allogenic blood transfusion could be reduced or avoided by using intraoperative autologous blood cell salvage. Autologous transfusion is the procedure of collecting the patient's own blood and transfusing it later during the surgery. This autologous blood can be made available either by preoperative autologous collection or by intraoperatively using hemodilution method and cell salvage technique. While autologous transfusion is encouraged in other surgical procedures, there are concerns with regard to oncological patients as this will result in patient cancerous cells being transfused back to the bloodstream of the patient. A meta-analysis on IOCS in cancer surgery concluded that this is associated with a reduced risk ratio for cancer recurrence and metastasis. They also reported the safest option is to use intraoperative cell salvage in combination with leukofiltration of red cells [24].

13.10 TRANSFUSION-RELATED IMMUNOMODULATION (TRIM)

Transfusion-related immunomodulation (TRIM) represents a specific immune-mediated reaction that can occur subsequent to a blood transfusion. The mechanisms involved in TRIM encompass residual leukocytes, apoptotic cells, immunosuppressive cytokines, the transfer of metabolically active growth factor–loaded microparticles and extracellular vesicles, as well as the presence of free hemoglobin or extracellular vesicle-bound hemoglobin found in donor blood components [25]. Transfusions of RBCs could adversely affect the outcomes for cancer patients, with TRIM potentially playing a crucial role in this process. The impact of TRIM leading to adverse effects is significant in individuals with gastrointestinal, head and neck, and urological cancers, while its influence is expected to be less evidently seen in breast, gynecological, and prostate tumors [25].

13.11 HOSPITAL TRANSFUSION POLICY AND ROLE OF AUDITS

It is essential for all hospitals to establish a transfusion policy that aligns with the standards set forth by national blood policy, regulations, and guidelines for transfusion practices. The objective of the policy is to guarantee adherence to the rational, effective, and safe utilization of blood and its components. The policy is developed by the hospital transfusion committee, and for it to be effectively implemented, all staff members must grasp the significance of quality and the potential repercussions of failing the quality system for patients [26].

Audits in transfusion medicine must encompass every aspect of the processes and workflows conducted within the blood center and during transfusion therapy. The aim of performing audits is to enhance patient care and outcomes through systematic reviews, monitoring compliance with transfusion guidelines, identifying key areas for improvement, and fostering a culture of consistently delivering quality service to patients. Audits can be conducted in either a prospective or retrospective manner for the evaluation of data. Concurrent audits may be conducted, which include, for instance, collecting information on a transfusion administered to a patient and providing feedback within the duration of the patient's hospital stay. Audits play a crucial role in a PBM strategy and can take place in both the blood center and the hospital wards and operating rooms where transfusions are performed. An audit entails a thorough examination of both a process and its outcomes to verify that they align with established performance expectations. Audits conducted concerning transfusion encompass the hospital's transfusion metrics (the number of units transfused per hospital bed annually), the crossmatch/transfusion ratio, and the transfusion index. A straightforward evaluation that can be conducted involves the consistent observation of the crossmatch:transfusion (C:T) ratio for either an individual or entire services. Ratios that greatly exceed 2:1 indicate a hospital's tendency to overestimate the quantity of RBC units they anticipate transfusing to a patient. The audit feedback must be structured as an audit report and reviewed within the hospital transfusion committee to facilitate the implementation of recommendations. This may involve staff education or training, the utilization of computer software for blood requisitioning, and suggestions for electronic patient identification systems to reduce clerical errors within the hospital. A comprehensive hospital transfusion policy, an efficient PBM program, and thorough audits to encompass all transfusion processes are crucial. The hospital transfusion committee serves as a vital tool for enhancing blood transfusion practices.

13.12 IMPLEMENTATION OF PBM

The effective execution of the PBM program necessitates critical components, including adequately trained personnel, the development of new standard operating procedures, and suitable systems to track outcomes resulting from the changes introduced as part of the PBM [1]. The primary participants consist of the PBM coordinator, alongside other stakeholders such as physicians, surgeons, nurses, members of the transfusion committee, quality personnel, and administrative officers. The involvement of the laboratory and information technology department is vital for its success. PBM requires a message that encompasses the "Triple E," i.e. using evidence, economics, and ethics to motivate stakeholders to implement PBM [27]. The costs of implementing a PBM program are modest, predicated on education, strong clinical leadership, and redirecting existing resources. Not implementing PBM as a global standard of care means hampering a sound medical model that offers multiple health benefits, reduces and avoids disease burden, and benefits the individual patient. It is essential to establish mechanisms that facilitate the evaluation of changes and the monitoring of the effectiveness of the PBM program's implementation. A scorecard system can be implemented to track compliance with blood transfusion guidelines, utilizing benchmarking to pinpoint clinicians and departmental units that consistently deviate significantly from the average blood usage for particular procedures. A comprehensive project management plan for PBM should encompass the identification of champion coordinators, key clinical areas or patient groups, and ongoing education on best practices for blood transfusion for all hospital staff.

There is still a common misperception regarding the PBM. There is a clear difference between the concept of optimum blood use and PBM. Optimum blood use is a blood component–centered approach, with a focus on limiting transfusion when clinically indicated and given at the minimal effective dose, while PBM is broad, patient-centered approach to manage blood failure [2]. Transfusion of blood products is still an essential therapeutic intervention. Since there are few alternatives to blood transfusion, deliberate handling and distribution of blood products is essential. PBM also helps to avoid costs related to cancelation or delay in care secondary to seasonal- or pandemic-related blood shortages by reducing the demand for blood, thus mitigating imbalances between supply and demand.

13.13 FUTURE PERSPECTIVES

The future perspectives of transfusion of blood components should be a decision-making process that is shared between clinicians and their patients. Clinicians must explain evidence-based options for treatment, inclusive of their benefits and risks, and patients must be allowed to express their goals and preferences. The optimal threshold for hemoglobin might vary among various patient populations and with various medical and surgical interventions. The availability of electronic health data have expanded the role of PBM, allowing for transfusion-related high-quality data collection, data mining, and big data analytics that can promote informed PBM healthcare decisions [28]. Hospital clinical information system and laboratory information system with well-defined data acquisition can collect a massive amount of relevant data. Efforts are underway to incorporate machine learning into the clinical decision-making for transfusion, using data sets and stochastic dynamic programming to predict need and optimize ordering. Mobile and web-based application such as blood component app and iTransfuse app promotes safe and appropriate use of blood components to anyone with access to a smartphone. Artificial intelligence will not replace informed clinical decisions but will support transfusion medicine to be more cost-effective and personalized.

13.14 CONCLUSION

Early identification of anemia is critical in malignancy and evaluation for suboptimal iron stores, including increased use of IV iron to ensure patients are iron replete. The role of management of functional iron deficiency in patients can be achieved through the implementation of restrictive transfusion thresholds and a focus on single-unit transfusions. Personalized transfusion support of cancer patients can be achieved through CDS system using patient-centric data and prescribed transfusion guidelines. Evidence-based transfusion demonstrates effectiveness by decreasing the number of blood transfusions, which results in lower hospital costs and enhanced patient outcomes.

REFERENCES

1. Friedman MT (2020) Patient blood management in hematology and oncology.
2. World Health Organization. World Health Organization; Geneva, Switzerland: 2021. The urgent need to implement patient blood management: Policy brief. https://iris.who.int/bitstream/handle/10665/346655/9789240035744-eng.pdf?sequence=1
3. Franchini M, Marano G, Veropalumbo E, et al (2019) Patient Blood Management: A Revolutionary Approach to Transfusion Medicine. Blood Transfusion 17:191–195.
4. World Health Organization (2024). Guidance on implementing patient blood management to improve global blood health status. World Health Organization. https://iris.who.int/handle/10665/380784
5. Iqbal N, Haider K, Sundaram V, et al (2017) Red Blood Cell Transfusion and Outcome in Cancer. Transfusion and Apheresis Science 56:287–290. https://doi.org/10.1016/j.transci.2017.05.014
6. Liu L, Wang Z, Jiang S, et al (2013) Perioperative Allogenenic Blood Transfusion Is Associated with Worse Clinical Outcomes for Hepatocellular Carcinoma: A Meta-Analysis. PLoS One 8:e64261. https://doi.org/10.1371/journal.pone.0064261
7. Acheson AG, Brookes MJ, Spahn DR (2012) Effects of Allogeneic Red Blood Cell Transfusions on Clinical Outcomes in Patients Undergoing Colorectal Cancer Surgery. Annals of Surgery 256:235–244. https://doi.org/10.1097/SLA.0b013e31825b35d5
8. Schaap CM, Klanderman RB, Peters A-L, et al (2025) Ultra-Restrictive Transfusion Thresholds in Critically Ill Adults: Are We Ready for the Next Step? Transfusion Medicine Reviews 39:150893. https://doi.org/10.1016/j.tmrv.2025.150893
9. Carson JL, Stanworth SJ, Dennis JA, et al (2021) Transfusion Thresholds for Guiding Red Blood Cell Transfusion. Cochrane Database of Systematic Reviews 2022. https://doi.org/10.1002/14651858.CD002042.pub5
10. Norgaard AB, McQuilten Z. Single unit transfusion. In: International society of blood transfusion. https://doi.org/10.1182/blood-2021-148270
11. Gross I, Trentino KM, Andreescu A, et al (2016) Impact of a Patient Blood Management Program and an Outpatient Anemia Management Protocol on Red Cell Transfusions in Oncology Inpatients and Outpatients. Oncologist 21:327–332. https://doi.org/10.1634/theoncologist.2015-0406
12. Schiffer CA, Bohlke K, Anderson KC (2018) Platelet Transfusion for Patients with Cancer: American Society of Clinical Oncology Clinical Practice Guideline Update Summary. Journal of Oncology Practice 14:129–133. https://doi.org/10.1200/JOP.2017.028902
13. Fujisaka Y, Sugiyama T, Saito H, et al (2011) Randomised, Phase III Trial of Epoetin-B to Treat Chemotherapy-Induced Anaemia According to the EU Regulation. British Journal of Cancer 105:1267–1272. https://doi.org/10.1038/bjc.2011.395

14. Heregger R, Greil R (2023) Erythropoiesis-stimulating agents—benefits and harms in the treatment of anemia in cancer patients. Magazine of European Medical Oncology 16:259–262. https://doi.org/10.1007/s12254-023-00902-4
15. Leyland-Jones B, Bondarenko I, Nemsadze G, et al (2016) A Randomized, Open-Label, Multicenter, Phase III Study of Epoetin Alfa versus Best Standard of Care in Anemic Patients with Metastatic Breast Cancer Receiving Standard Chemotherapy. Journal of Clinical Oncology 34:1197–1207. https://doi.org/10.1200/JCO.2015.63.5649
16. Lim J, Auerbach M, MacLean B, et al (2023) Intravenous Iron Therapy to Treat Anemia in Oncology: A Mapping Review of Randomized Controlled Trials. Current Oncology 30:7836–7851. https://doi.org/10.3390/curroncol30090569
17. Atia J, Evison F, Gallier S, et al (2022) Effectiveness of Clinical Decision Support in Controlling Inappropriate Red Blood Cell and Platelet Transfusions, Speciality Specific Responses and Behavioural Change. BMC Medical Informatics and Decision Making 22:342. https://doi.org/10.1186/s12911-022-02045-8
18. Hibbs SP, Nielsen ND, Brunskill S, et al (2015) The Impact of Electronic Decision Support on Transfusion Practice: A Systematic Review. Transfusion Medicine Reviews 29:14–23. https://doi.org/10.1016/j.tmrv.2014.10.002
19. Ferreira AA, Zulli R, Soares S, et al (2011) Identification of Platelet Refractoriness in Oncohematologic Patients. Clinics 66:35–40. https://doi.org/10.1590/S1807-59322011000100007
20. Slichter SJ, Kaufman RM, Assmann SF, et al (2010) Dose of Prophylactic Platelet Transfusions and Prevention of Hemorrhage. New England Journal of Medicine 362:600–613. https://doi.org/10.1056/NEJMoa0904084
21. Wandt H, Schäfer-Eckart K, Greinacher A (2014) Platelet Transfusion in Hematology, Oncology and Surgery. Dtsch Arztebl Int. https://doi.org/10.3238/arztebl.2014.0809
22. Youk H-J, Hwang S-H, Oh H-B, Ko D-H (2022) Evaluation and Management of Platelet Transfusion Refractoriness. Blood Research 57:S6–S10. https://doi.org/10.5045/br.2022.2021229
23. Foukaneli T, Kerr P, Bolton-Maggs PHB, et al (2020) Guidelines on the Use of Irradiated Blood Components. British Journal of Haematology 191:704–724. https://doi.org/10.1111/bjh.17015
24. Esper SA, Waters JH (2011) Intra-Operative Cell Salvage: A Fresh Look at the Indications and Contraindications. Blood Transfusion 9:139–147.
25. Goubran H, Sheridan D, Radosevic J, et al (2017) Transfusion-Related Immunomodulation and Cancer. Transfusion and Apheresis Science 56:336–340. https://doi.org/10.1016/j.transci.2017.05.019
26. Saran RK (Ed.). (2003) Transfusion medicine: technical manual. Directorate General of Health Services, Ministry of Health and Family Welfare, Government of India.
27. Hofmann A, Shander A, Blumberg N, et al (2022) Patient Blood Management: Improving Outcomes for Millions While Saving Billions. What Is Holding It Up? Anesthesia & Analgesia 135:511–523. https://doi.org/10.1213/ANE.0000000000006138
28. Gammon RR, Almozain N, Jindal A, et al (2024) Patient Blood Management, Past, Present and Future. Annals of Blood 9:7–7. https://doi.org/10.21037/aob-22-45

Index

Note: **Bold** and *italic* page numbers refer to **tables** and figures, respectively.

A

Abiraterone, 5
Absorption distribution metabolism excretion (ADME), 22
Acquired immune responses, 97, *102*
Actinobacteria, 33, 36
Adenoma detection rate (ADR), 120
ADMET actions (absorption, distribution, metabolism, and excretion), 50
Adoptive cell therapy (ACT), 136–137
  CAR-NK cell therapy, 137
  chimeric antigen receptor T cell (CAR-T cell) therapy, 136
  TIL therapy, 137
AI designs, 49–73
AImmunoscore, 120
AI-powered precision medicine, GI tract cancers, 55, *55*
AI tools-based drugs, 14–15
  BMS-986205, AI for targeted therapy, 15, **15**
  DSP-1181, AI-designed cancer drug, 14, **15**
  ibrutinib, AI-driven drug repurposing, 14–15, **15**
ALK protein, 11, 12
Alkylating agents, 126
Alloprevotella, 86
Anemia, 235, 237
ANN models, 118
Anthracyclines, 126
Anticancer agents, natural origin, 21–22
Antimetabolites, 126
Antimicrobial peptides (AMPs), 104
Arif, T., 180
Artificial intelligence (AI), 5–8, *7,* 16, 64, 106, 121
  in chemotherapy, 7
  in immunotherapy, 8
  in radiotherapy, 7–8
Artificial intelligence-integrated precision oncology, 115–121
Aspergillus flavus, 96
Aspergillus parasiticus, 96
Astaxanthin, 216
Audits, 242–243
Axitinib, 12–13, **14**

B

Bacillus coagulans, 43
Bacteria, 94–95
  resistance and infectious agents, 94–95
Bacteroides pseudolongum, 39
Baekeland, Leo, 194
BCR-ABL tyrosine kinase protein, 8, 9
BenevolentAI, 14
Beta diversity, 68, 69
Beta-glucuronidase enzymes, 51
B. fragilis, 83
B. fragilis toxin (BFT), 83
Bft gene, 83
Bifidobacterium bifidum, 38, 39
Bifidobacterium lactis, 38
Bifidobacterium longum, 37, 38, 155
Bifidobacterium pseudolongum, 39
Binding affinity, 13
Bioactive compounds, 24–25, 215
  carotenoids, 216
  in colorectal cancer therapy, 214–227
  CRC therapy and sources, 215–217
  emerging challenges, CRC therapy, 222–226, *223*
    antinutrient effects, 225
    bioavailability and metabolism, 223, *224*
    clinical integration and regulatory gaps, 226
    dual role, bioactive compounds, 223–224
    genetic variability, 224–225
    intellectual property issues, 226
    pharmacokinetics and drug-bioactive interactions, 225
    potential side effects, 225
    standardization and dosing, 224
    studying plant metabolites, complexity, 226
  flavonoids, 216
  glucosinolates, 217
  mechanism of action, 217–221, *219*
    angiogenesis and metastasis effects, 221
    anti-inflammatory effects, 220
    antioxidant effects, 219
    anti-proliferative and pro-apoptotic effects, 220
    epigenetic modulatory effects, 220–221
  polyphenols, 215–216
  as potential anticancer agents, 24–25
  terpenoids, 217
Bioinformatic techniques, **59**
Biomarker discovery
  AI-impact on, 116–117, **118**
  prediction approaches, 117, *117*
Black phosphorus quantum dots (BPQDs), 43
Blood based immunological biomarkers, *130*
Blood–brain barrier (BBB), 166, 182
Blood transfusion practices, evidence-based, 235–244
Bluestone, Jeffrey, 138
BMS-986205, AI for targeted therapy, 15, **15**
Brain cancer, 199–200
Brain tumor, 165
Bray–Curti's dissimilarity, 68
BRCA mutations, 10, 11
Breast cancer (BC)
  conventional cancer treatment therapies in, 126–127
  immuno-oncology approach, 125–139
  immunotherapy, 132–136
    liquid biopsy, 127–131
    significance, 127
  precision medicine in, 125–139
  probiotics in, 152–154
  traditional screening methods, 127

Bruton's tyrosine kinase (BTK), 15
Bufuralol, 19
Burns, C.A., 80

C

cagA oncoprotein, 83
C. albicans, 96
Calcium homeostasis, 167
Camptothecin derivatives (irinotecanand topotecan), 21
Campylobacter jejuni, 84
Cancer research
  microbiome, drugs, and cancer progression, interaction, 52–53
  microbiome and artificial intelligence, 53–54
  paradigms and challenges, 52
Candida glabrata, 96
Candida tropicalis, 96
Carbon nanomaterials (CNMs), 206, 207
Carcinogenesis, mechanisms, 198, *198*
Cardia GC, 32
CAR-NK cell therapy, 137
Catalán, M., 219
Cellular metabolism, glioma cells, 168, *169*
Chaib, M., 37
Chemoimmunotherapy, 138
Chemoresistance, 126
Chemotherapy, 7, 20, 126
Chimeric antigen receptor T cell (CAR-T cell) therapy, 136
Chlamydia pneumoniae, 95
Choi, Kihwan, 118
Chronic inflammation, 80
Chronic lymphocytic leukemia (CLL), 14
Chronic myeloid leukemia (CML), 8
Climate change, 105
Clinical decision-making, transfusion, 244
Clinical translation, 157–158
Clostridium butyricum, 44
Clostridium difficile, 60
Clostridium septicum, 83
c-Met/HGFR (hepatocyte growth factor receptor), 11
Colorectal cancer (CRC), 32, 63
  artificial intelligence-integrated precision oncology, 115–121
  bioactive compounds in, 214–227
  diagnostic and therapeutic modalities, *116*
  gut microbial metabolites and, 85, *86*
  microbial prognostic markers, *87*
  microbiome-based biomarkers, diagnosis, 86–87
  molecular approaches in, 221–222
  mycobiome and virome, dysbiosis, 85
  novel screening tool, 79–88
  pathogenesis, bacteria in, 80–81
    Streptococcus bovis/gallolyticus, 80–81
  probiotics in, 154–155
  prognosis, neural networks, 118–119, **119**
  sulphidogenic bacteria, 81–84
Combination chemotherapy, 20
Combination therapies, 138–139
Complement activation, 99
Comprehensive genomic profiling (CGP), 10
Computational biology, 16
  software, 11
Computational drug discovery (CDD), 5
Computational modeling, 15
Computational tools-based drugs, 11–14
  axitinib, 12–13, **14**
  crizotinib, 11–12, **14**
  gefitinib, 13–14, **14**
Computerized physician order entry (CPOE) system, 238–239
Conjugated linoleic acid (CLA), 151
Conventional methods, 2
Convolutional NNs (CNNs), 116, 119
CQSAR (Chem Quant Struct Act Rel), 13
CRC-precision oncology, AI tools, 120, *120*
Crizotinib, 5, 11–12, **14**
CTLA-4 inhibitors, 134
Curcumin, 222
Curtobacterium proimmune, 42
Cyclophosphamide, 25
Cytolethal distending toxin (CDT), 84

D

Decision support systems (DSSs), 237
Deep learning (DL), 56, 57, 115, 116
Deoxycholic acid (DCA), 85
Disease conscription
  microbial dysbiosis and disease states, 58
  microbial implications, disease development, 58
  microbial signatures, 58
  personalized medicine, 59
Disease-modifying antirheumatic drug (DMARD), 25
Disease prognosis, 52–53
DL-based NNs, 121
D-limonene, 217
Drug likeness, 22
Drug–microbe–host processes, 57, *57*
Drug–microbiomics nexus, 61–62, *62*
  collaborative platform integration, 61
  diverse datasets, repository, 61
  personalized treatment development, 61–62
Drug sensitivity prediction model, 6
DSP-1181, AI-designed cancer drug, 14, **15**
Dynamic host–pathogen interactions, *104*
Dysbiosis, 79, 80, 203
  defined, 58
  mycobiome and virome, 85

E

Early onset colorectal cancer (EOCRC), 79
Ebola virus epidemic, 61
E. coli, 43
EGCG, 221
Ehrlich, Paul, 100
Entamoeba histolytica, 96
Enterococcus faecalis, 83–84
Enterotoxigenic *B. fragilis* (ETBF), 83
Enzalutamide, 7
Epigenetic reprogramming functions, 222
Epigenomic biomarker discovery, AI-impact on, 116–117
Epigenomics, 2
Epithelial–mesenchymal transition (EMT), 221
Epstein–Barr virus (EBV), 95
Eribulin mesylate, 21
Erythropoiesis-stimulating agents (ESAs), 237

Esophageal cancer, 64
Evidence-based blood transfusion practices, 235–244
Exemestane, 205
Exopolysaccharides (EPSs), 150

F

Fecal microbiota transplantation (FMT), 53, 60, 64, 65, 67
Firmicutes, 33, 36
Flavonoids, 21
Fucoxanthin, 216
Fucoxanthinol, 216
Fungal microbiome atlas, 96
Fungi, 95–96
Fusarium proliferatum, 96
Fusarium verticillioides, 96
Fusobacterium nucleatum, 38, 53, 58, 82, 86

G

Gastric cancer (GC), 32, 64
Gastrointestinal (GI) tract cancers, 31
  comorbidities, 71–72, *72*
    cardiovascular disease (CVD), 71
    chronic inflammatory and autoimmune diseases, 71
    depression and anxiety, 72
    malnutrition, 72
    metabolic disorders, 71
    pharmacomicrobiomics, 72–73
    pulmonary diseases, 71
    renal dysfunction, 71
  diagnosing and treating, challenges, 65
    accurate diagnosis, 66
    clinical disease monitoring, 66
    early diagnosis, 66
    personalized treatment selection, 66
    treatment resistance, overcoming, 67
  global burden, 33, 62, *63*
  incidence and mortality rates, 62, **63**
  microbiome contribution, paramount, 62–67
  new research avenues, 67
  overview, 31–33
  pharmacomicrobiomics, statistical analysis, 67–69
    correlational and regression analysis, 68
    descriptive and inferential statistics, 68
    microbiome profiling and analysis, 68
    ML/AI algorithms, 68
    survival analysis, 68
  pharmacomicrobiomics and AI designs, 49–73
  preventive medicine, managing, 69–70, *70*
    chemoprevention, 69
    lifestyle modifications, 70
    screening programs, 70
    vaccinations, 69
  treatment response and resistance, microbiome, 65, **66**
  worldwide, prevalence, 62
Gefitinib, 5, 13–14, **14**
Gemella, 86
"Generally Recognized As Safe" (GRAS) microorganisms, 157
Genetic algorithms, 13
Genetic mutations, 1
Genomics, 2, 15
Geraniol, 217
Gliomas, 165–183
  mitochondria and radiotherapy resistance, 171–172
  mitochondria and temozolomide resistance, 171
  mitochondrial apoptosis, avoidance, 170
  mitochondrial dynamics and mitophagy, tumor adaptation, 173–174
  mitochondrial functions in, 176, **177–178**
  neuro-tumor microenvironment, 175–176, *176*
  precision neuro-oncology, 166
  reactive oxygen species and antioxidant defense, 171
  redox imbalance and oxidative stress, 172–173
  TCA cycle rewiring and glutamine dependence, 169
  therapeutic approaches and innovations, mitochondria, 176–179
  Warburg effect and extensions, 169
Glioma stem-like cells (GSCs), 173, 174
  and mitochondrial plasticity, 174–175
Glutaminase, 169
Glutamine, 169
Glutathione S-transferase (GSTP), 19
Goserelin, 205
G-protein-coupled receptors (GPRs), 149
Group D Streptococci, 80
Gut disease axis, 52–53
Gut flora, 53
Gut microbes, 51
  probiotics, impact, 33–34
Gut microbial metabolites, 85, *86*
Gut microbiome, 49, 53, 65, 73, 79–88, *81*
  techniques to characterize, 87–88, *88*
Gut microbiota, 54, 65, 148

H

Halichondrin B, 21
Helicobacter pylori, 37, 95
Hepatitis viruses, 95
Hepatocellular carcinoma (HCC), 32
HER2-CAR-T cells, 136
HER2 gene *(ERBB2),* 9, 10
Heterocyclic compounds, anticancer drugs, **23**
Heterocyclic compounds, nitrogen atom, 22–23
Heterocyclic compounds, oxygen atom, 23–24
Heterocyclic sulfonamides, 23
Heydari, Z., 38
High-density neutrophils (HDN), 128
Histone deacetylases (HDACs), 149
Horizontal gene transfer (HGT), 103
Hospital transfusion policy, 242–243
Host–microbiota–tumor interactions, 152
Hou, M., 217
Huang, Ming Jun, 120
Human gut microbiota, 33
Human immune system, 97–103
  adaptive or specific immunity, 100–101
    tailored and specific responses, 100–101
  body against infection, defending, 97–103
  immune evasion mechanisms, pathogens and cancer, 101–103
  inborn immune system, early defense, 98–100
Huo, R.X., 86
2-hydroxyglutarate, 170
Hypoxia-inducible factors (HIFs), 23

I

Ibrutinib, AI-driven drug repurposing, 14–15, **15**
Imatinib (Gleevec), 8–9, **11**, 26
Immune checkpoint inhibitors, 132–136, **135**
  CTLA-4 inhibitors, 134
  LAG-3, 134
  PD-1/PDL-1 inhibitors, 132–133, *133*
  TIGIT, 134–136
Immune gene signatures, 131
Immune modulation, checkpoint inhibitors, 206
Immune score, 131
Immunohistochemistry (IHC), 9
Immunotherapy, 8, 132–136
  challenges, 137–138
  circulating immune cells, 127–129
  cytokine profiles, 129–130
  immune cells, circulating, 127–129
  immune checkpoint inhibitors, 132–136, **135**
  immune score/immune gene signatures, 131
  liquid biopsy, 127–131
  MDSCs, 128
  monocyte–lymphocyte ratio (MLR), 129
  monocytes, 129
  neutrophil–lymphocyte ratio (NLR), 129
  neutrophils, 128–129
  significance, 127
Indole-3-carbinol (I3C), 217
Infectious diseases, 92–108
  worldwide impact, 104–105
Infectious pathogens, 93
Information statistics, 67–70
Ingenol mebutate, 21
Innate immune responses (IIR), 97, *100*
Insilico Medicine, 15
Intraoperative cell salvage, 242
Intravenous (IV) iron, 237–238
Invasive fungal infections (IFIs), 96
Irinotecan, 51, 65
Ixabepilone, 21

J

Jia, S. S., 217

K

Kaempferol, 216, 220
Kaposi sarcoma herpesvirus (KSHV), 95
Karpel-Massler, G., 170
Kuugbee, E. D., 38

L

Lacticaseibacillus paracasei, 38, 42, 154
Lactobacillus acidophilus, 37–39
Lactobacillus acidophilus 10307, 150
Lactobacillus casei, 37, 151
Lactobacillus delbrueckii, 148
Lactobacillus gasseri, 37
Lactobacillus kefiranofaciens, 151
Lactobacillus reuteri, 37, 152
Lactobacillus rhamnosus, 37, 38, 151
Lactobacillus rhamnosus GG (LGG), 148, 155
LAG-3, 134
Late-onset colorectal cancer (LOCRC), 79
Li, Y., 86
Ligand-based drug discovery, 5
Ligilactobacillus salivarius, 38
Lilley, 31
Limosilactobacillus fermentum, 41, 42
Linalool, 217
Lipinski's rule of five, 22
Liu, Y., 217
Low density neutrophils (LDN), 128–129
L. pantheris, 38
L. plantarum, 37, 38
Lung cancer, probiotics in, 154
Lycopene, 216, 225

M

Machine learning (ML), 2, 53, 56, 69, 106, 115, 116
Macrophage Marker Genes (MMGs), 131
Malasseziomycetes, 87
Memory cells, 101
Metabolic reprogramming, 168–169
Metabolomics, 15, 59–60
Metagenomic sequencing, 61
Metformin, 205
Methicillin-resistant *S. aureus* (MRSA), 103
Methotrexate, 25
Microbes, 33, 50
Microbiome-based biomarkers, 66
  discovery, **59**
Microbiome-based disease markers, 64
Microbiome-guided oncology, 158–159
Microbiomes, 49–50
  GI carcinogenesis, 33, **34**
  in human physiology and metabolism, 49–50
Microbiota biobank, 148
Microplastics (MPs), oncology, 194–207, *195*
  affect on body organs, lungs, 199
  brain, 199–200
  breast cancer (BC), 200–201
  carcinogenesis, mechanisms, 198, *198*
  cervix and ovaries, 200
  gastrointestinal tract, 203–204
  human exposure, 197–198
  kidney-testis microfluidic platform (KTP), 201
  penile cancer, 201
  pharmacological approaches, 204–205
    anticancer drugs, existing, 204–205
    hormonal therapies, 205
    repurposed drugs, 205
  potential therapeutic interventions, 204, *204*
  skin, 202
  types and sources, 195–197, *196*
Microtubules, 24
Microtubule-targeting agents, 24
Mitochondria-based neuro-oncology, 180–182
Mitochondrial biology, neural tissues, 166–168
  energy generation and metabolic adjustments, 167
  fission, fusion, and trafficking, 167
  mitochondrial dynamics, 167
  neurogenesis and neural maturation, mitochondrial contribution, 167
  neurological disorders, implications, 167–168

Mitochondrial biomarkers, precision oncology, 179–180, **181**
Mitochondrial dysfunction, gliomas, 165–183
progression, 168
Mitochondria-mediated resistance, 170–171
mitochondrial DNA (mtDNA) and genomic instability, 171
reactive oxygen species and antioxidant defense, 171
Mitochondria-targeted therapy approaches, *179*
Mitogen-activated protein kinases (MAPKs), 220
Molecular docking, 5, 11, 13
Molecular dynamics (MD) simulations, 12, 13
Molecular profiling, 1
Momo, C. H. K., 38
Mono-ethylhexyl phthalate (MEHP), 200
Mozaffari Namin, B., 37
M. tuberculosis, 102
Multidrug-resistant (MDR) strains, 19, 94
Mutant IDH inhibitors, 166
Myeloid-derived suppressor cells (MDSCs), 206

N

Nanoplastics (NPs), 197, 202
Narunsky-Haziza, L., 96
Natural language processing (NLP), 56
Natural products, 27
Neisseria elongata, 155
Neoadjuvant chemotherapy (NACT), 129
Neural Stem Cell (NSCs), 167
Neuro-tumor microenvironment, 175–176, *176*
Next-generation probiotics, 158
Next-generation sequencing (NGS), 88, 107
techniques, 2
Nigella sativa, 42
Nisin, 150
Nitrogen-containing heterocycles, 22–23
Non-cardia GC, 32
NONMEM, 5
Non-steroidal anti-inflammatory drugs (NSAIDs), 69
Novel technologies, 206

O

Olaparib (Lynparza), 10–11, **11**
Omacetaxine mepesuccinate, 21
Omics-based technologies, 2–4, *3*
epigenomics, 2
genomics, 2
lipidomics, 3
metabolomics, 3
proteomics, 3
single-cell and imaging approaches, 4
transcriptomics, 3
Omics-based tools drugs, 8–11
imatinib (Gleevec), 8–9, **11**
olaparib (Lynparza), 10–11, **11**
trastuzumab (Herceptin), 9–10, **11**
Omics technologies, 16
Oncogenic viruses, 95
Oncology, 92–108
and infectious diseases, intersection, 92–108
Oncometabolism, 168–169
Oncometabolites, 170
Oncotherapeutic drug discovery, 8–15
Oncotherapeutics
artificial intelligence, role, 5–8, *7*
computational tools, role, 4–5, *6*
ligand-based drug discovery, 5
molecular docking, 5
multi-omics, role, 4
QSAR modeling, 5
structure-based drug discovery, 5
Oral cancers, probiotics in, 155–156
Oral dysbiosis, 155–156; *see also* Dysbiosis
Oral squamous cell carcinoma (OSCC), 155
Oxidative phosphorylation (OXPHOS), 166, 167, 172, 182
Oxygen-based heterocycle, 23–24

P

Paclitaxel, 204
Pahumunto, 38
Pancreatic cancer, probiotics in, 155
Pancreatic ductal adenocarcinoma (PDAC), 32
Pancreatic neuroendocrine tumors (PanNET), 32
PARP (poly ADP-ribose polymerase), 10
inhibitors, 7
Parvimonas, 86
Parvimonas micra, 84
Pathogen associated molecular patterns (PAMPs), 98
Pathogens, nature, 93–97, **94**
bacteria, 94–95
emergence and re-emergence, 96
protozoa and fungi, 95–96
viruses, 95
zoonotic diseases, 96–97
Pathogens and humans
antimicrobial resistance, 103
evolutionary conflict, 103–104
fighting resistance, 104
novel approaches, drug development, 104
human behavior's contribution, resistance, 103
pathogens' genetic adaptability, 103
Pathological angiogenesis, 20
Patient blood management (PBM), 235, 242–243
implementation, 243
Pattern-recognition molecules or receptors (PRMs/PRRs), 98
Pediococcus pentosaceus, 38
Pembrolizumab, 133
Peptostreptococcus anaerobius, 84, 86
Perou, 125
Persistent organic pollutants (POPs), 198
Personalized cancer therapy
harnessing probiotics for, 147–159
microbiome-guided oncology, 158–159
next-generation strategy, 31–44
probiotics, applications, *32*
Personalized medicine, 20, 25, 31, 105–107, *107*, 108, 148
infectious disease and cancer management, 105–107
Personalized oncology, 15, 31
Personalized probiotic strategies, 148, 152–156, **153**
in cancer immunotherapy, 156, *157*
Pharmacogenomics, 107

Pharmacomicrobiomics, 49–73
AI role, personalized therapy, 56–57
concept and aspects, disease, 50–51, **51**
disease analysis and microbiomics, 59–60
disease conscription, 57–59
drug–microbiomics nexus, 61–62, *62*
elements, 57–62
gaps and new insights, disease analysis, 59–60
incorporating with AI, treatment approaches, 64–65
progression trends, health disasters, 60–61
Phenethyl isothiocyanate (PEITC), 217
Plasmodium falciparum, 101
Plasmodium species, 96
Plastic pollution, 194–207
Platelet refractoriness, management, 239–240, *240, 241*
P. micra, 86
Polystyrene microplastics (PS-MPs), 199
Precision medicine, 121, 139
AI and GI tract cancers, 54–56
drug research and repurposing, 55–56
early evaluation and diagnosis, 54
predictive modeling, treatment response, 54–55
prognostications, 54
in breast cancer, 125–139
Precision neuro-oncology, 166, 179
Preoperative anemia, 237
Preventive medicine, 67–70
Principal coordinate analysis (PCoA), 68
Probiotic-based nanomedicine, 31–44
Probiotic microbes, 36
Probiotic nano-formulations (PNF), 33, **35–36**, 39–41, *40*, 44
advantages, 40–41, *41*
application against GI cancers, 41–44
in combating colon cancer, 43
effective medication, gastric cancer, 41–43
induction, apoptosis, *42*
medication for treating pancreatic cancer, 44
need for, 39–40
in personalized cancer therapy, *40*
Probiotics, 31
anti-oncogenic components, production, 149–151
as apoptosis inducer, 151
in breast cancer, 152–154
in colorectal cancer, 154–155
in combating pancreatic cancer, 37
defined, 147
against esophageal cancer, 36–37
gut microbiome, altering, 148–149
immunomodulatory effects, 151
impact on gut microbes, 33–34
in lung cancer, 154
mechanism of action, anticancer agent, 148–151, *149*
in oral cancers, 155–156
in pancreatic cancer, 155
for personalized cancer therapy, 147–159
significance, GI cancers, *32*, 34–39, **35–36**
in suppressing colorectal cancer, 38
in thwarting liver cancer, 38–39
in treating gastric cancer, 37
Prophylactic *vs.* therapeutic platelet transfusion, 239
Proteobacteria, 33
Proteomics, 15, 107, 108
techniques, 9
Protozoa, 95–96

Q

QSAR modeling, 12, 13
Quantitative structure–activity relationship modeling (QSAR) modeling, 5
Quercetin, 216, 221

R

Radiation therapy, 214
Radiotherapy, 7–8, 126
Reactive oxygen species (ROS), 151, 165, 172, 198, 199, 202, 214
Real-time sequencing technologies, 61
Red blood cell (RBC), 235
specialized, 240–242
transfusion practices, 236
Region proposal networks (RPN), 119
Resveratrol, 215, 219, 221
Rodrigues, F. A., 24
Romidepsin, 21

S

Saccharomycetes, 87
Salmonella spp., 84
Salmonella typhi, 95
S. aureus, 102
Semi-synthetic epipodophyllotoxins (etoposide, teniposide, and etoposide phosphate), 21
S. gallolyticus, 86
Sheng, S., 38
Shigella, 101
Short-chain fatty acids (SCFAs), 80, 149, 150
Single unit RBC transfusions, 236–237
16S ribosomal RNA gene, 50, 87
Small heterocyclic compounds, 19–27
Small-molecule triazole, heterocyclic component, 25
Smith, 180
Sorafenib, 204–205
Spatial transcriptomics (ST), 4
Specialized RBCs, 240–242
Specific heterocyclic compounds, anticancer drug, 25–26, **26**
Stillwell, 31
Stomach cancer, *see* Gastric cancer
Streptococcus bovis, 80–81, 95
Streptococcus gallolyticus, 80–81, 95
Streptococcus mitis, 155
Streptococcus thermophilus, 148
Structure–activity relationship (SAR), 20
Structure-based drug design, 13
Structure-based drug discovery, 5
Structure-based pharmacophore (SBP) mapping, 5
Sulforaphane, 217
Sulphidogenic bacteria, 81–84
B. fragilis, 83
Campylobacter jejuni, 84
Clostridium septicum, 83
Enterococcus faecalis, 83–84
F. nucleatum, 82
Helicobacter pylori, 82–83
Parvimonas micra, 84
Peptostreptococcus anaerobius, 84
Salmonella spp., 84

Superoxide dismutase (SOD), 219
Sympatric machine learning algorithm, 7
Synergistic approaches, 207

T

Tan, 131
Targeted probiotics, 64
Targeting MP-activated pathways, 205–206
Taxanes (paclitaxel, docetaxel, and cabazitaxel), 21, 126
Teanpaisan, 38
Temozolomide (TMZ), 170
Terminalia ferdinandiana, 225
Three-dimensional (3D) convolutional neural network (3D CNN), 8
TIGIT, 134–136
Tili, E., 221
Tiragolumab, 134
Toprak, N.U., 83
Trabectedin (ET-743), 21
Transcriptomics, 15
Transfusion-related immunomodulation (TRIM), 242
Trastuzumab (Herceptin), 9–10, **11**
Triazolothiadiazines, 22
Triazolothiadiazoles, 22
Triple-negative breast cancers (TNBCs), 125
Tumor adipose features (TAF), 117
Tumor angiogenesis, 23
Tumor-associated macrophages (TAMs), 148
Tumor atlases, 4
Tumor cell biological traits, 107
Tumor heterogeneity, 126
Tumorigenesis, 1
Tumor-infiltrating lymphocytes (TILs), 131–132
Tumor–neuron communication, 176
Tyrosine kinase inhibitor (TKI), 23, 26

V

Vascular endothelial growth factor receptors (EGFRs) (VEGFRs), 12, 13, 19, 22, 23, 26
Vemurafenib, 205
Vinblastine, 24
Vincristine, 24
Viruses, 95
  multifaceted microbial invaders, 95
Voriconazole, 25

W

Warburg effect, 166, 169
Warfarin, 50
Wen, 131
Whole exome sequencing (WES), 4
Whole genome sequencing (WGS), 4

Y

Yu, J., 82

Z

ZEN-3694, 7
Zhang, J., 38
Zoonotic diseases, 96–97
  human–animal transmission, pathogens, 96–97
Zumkeller, N., 82

For Product Safety Concerns and Information please contact our
EU representative GPSR@taylorandfrancis.com Taylor & Francis
Verlag GmbH, Kaufingerstraße 24, 80331 München, Germany